Current Clinical Psychiatry

Series Editor:

Jerrold F. Rosenbaum
Department of Psychiatry
Massachusetts General Hospital
Boston, MA, USA

Current Clinical Psychiatry offers concise, practical resources for clinical psychiatrists and other practitioners interested in mental health. Covering the full range of psychiatric disorders commonly presented in the clinical setting, the Current Clinical Psychiatry series encompasses such topics as cognitive behavioral therapy, anxiety disorders, psychotherapy, ratings and assessment scales, mental health in special populations, psychiatric uses of nonpsychiatric drugs, and others. Series editor Jerrold F. Rosenbaum, MD, is Chief of Psychiatry, Massachusetts General Hospital, and Stanley Cobb Professor of Psychiatry, Harvard Medical School.

More information about this series at http://www.springer.com/series/7634

Abigail L. Donovan • Suzanne A. Bird
Editors

Substance Use and the Acute Psychiatric Patient

Emergency Management

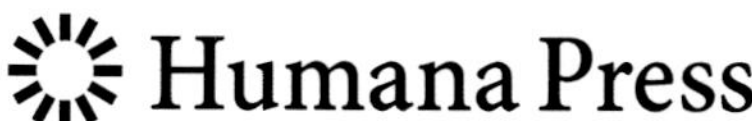

Editors
Abigail L. Donovan
Massachusetts General Hospital
Boston, MA
USA

Suzanne A. Bird
Massachusetts General Hospital
Boston, MA
USA

ISSN 2626-241X ISSN 2626-2398 (electronic)
Current Clinical Psychiatry
ISBN 978-3-319-23960-6 ISBN 978-3-319-23961-3 (eBook)
https://doi.org/10.1007/978-3-319-23961-3

This Humana imprint is published by the registered company Springer Nature Switzerland AG
The registered company address is: Gewerbestrasse 11, 6330 Cham, Switzerland

We would like to dedicate this book to our patients and their families: may you be treated with expertise and compassion at every encounter.

Preface

Through more than 50 years of combined emergency psychiatric practice, we have seen endless permutations of psychiatric and medical crisis, illness, and suffering. The common thread throughout much of this work has been the impact of substance use. There are few factors as overreaching, prevalent, and stigma-ridden as substance use in the lives of our patients. The vast majority of the patients we see every day in the emergency department (ED) have illnesses and lives that have been complicated, in one way or another, by substance use. We have lived and worked through the cocaine epidemic, the methamphetamine epidemic, and, now, the opioid epidemic (all while alcohol has remained the unnamed epidemic). The substance changes, but our patients' need for our care, our understanding, and our expertise never does.

Despite the prevalence of substance use disorders (SUDs) in EDs, when we started planning for this book, we realized that there was almost no literature on the assessment and management of SUDs in EDs. Our goal was to change that, to provide the frontline practitioners, the emergency medicine physicians, ED and consult-liaison psychiatrists, social workers, nurse practitioners, physician assistants, and trainees of all professions with information, guidance, and, hopefully, wisdom. We sought to provide practical, accessible, clinically relevant information for the medical and psychiatric care of these complex patients. Where the literature was lacking, we relied on clinical experience. Where our own clinical experience was lacking, we relied on the expertise of colleagues, near and far. This book is the result of all of our combined efforts, to improve the emergency care of patients with substance use and comorbid disorders.

Boston, MA, USA

Abigail L. Donovan
Suzanne A. Bird

Acknowledgments

We would like to thank every author for their contributions to this book. We appreciate your time, expertise, and dedication to this important project. We would also like to thank our Chair, Jerrold Rosenbaum, MD, for the opportunity to produce this book and for his commitment to the Acute Psychiatric Service.

Contents

Contributors

Allison S. Baker, MD Perinatal Psychiatry, MGH Center for Women's Mental Health, Boston, MA, USA

Massachusetts General Hospital, Department of Psychiatry, Boston, MA, USA

Theodore I. Benzer, MD, PhD Harvard Medical School, Massachusetts General Hospital, Emergency Department, Boston, MA, USA

Suzanne A. Bird, MD Acute Psychiatry Service, Massachusetts General Hospital, Department of Psychiatry, Boston, MA, USA

Daryl Blaney Jr., MD Boston University Medical Center, Department of Psychiatry, Boston, MA, USA

Hannah E. Brown, MD Wellness and Recovery After Psychosis Program, Boston Medical Center, Boston, MA, USA

Boston University School of Medicine, Boston, MA, USA

Michelle Chaney, MD, MScPH Resident in Child and Adolescent Psychiatry, Massachusetts General Hospital and McLean Hospital, Boston, MA, USA

Massachusetts General Hospital, Department of Psychiatry, Boston, MA, USA

Abigail L. Donovan, MD Massachusetts General Hospital, Department of Psychiatry, Boston, MA, USA

First Episode and Early Psychosis Program, Massachusetts General Hospital, Department of Psychiatry, Boston, MA, USA

Harvard Medical School, Boston, MA, USA

Acute Psychiatry Service, Massachusetts General Hospital, Boston, MA, USA

Anna Fitzgerald

Lior Givon, PhD, MD Psychiatric Emergency Services, Cambridge Hospital, Cambridge Health Alliance, Department of Psychiatry, Cambridge, MA, USA

Amanda S. Green, MD Central Texas Veterans Health Care System, Temple, TX, USA

Charlotte S. Hogan, MD Perinatal Psychiatry, MGH Center for Women's Mental Health, Boston, MA, USA

Massachusetts General Hospital, Department of Psychiatry, Boston, MA, USA

Annise K. Jackson, MD Boston University Medical Center, Department of Psychiatry, Boston, MA, USA

Peter Jackson, MD University of Vermont Medical Center, Burlington, VT, USA

Massachusetts General Hospital, Department of Psychiatry, Waltham, MA, USA

Daniel P. Johnson, PhD Department of Psychiatry, Massachusetts General Hospital, Boston, MA, USA

Yoshio Kaneko, MD First Episode and Early Psychosis Program, Massachusetts General Hospital, Department of Psychiatry, Boston, MA, USA

Harvard Medical School, Boston, MA, USA

Transitional Age Youth Clinic, Massachusetts General Hospital, Boston, MA, USA

Newton-Wellesley Hospital, Newton, MA, USA

Karsten Kueppenbender, MD Pavilion Center, McLean Hospital, Belmont, MA, USA

Melisa W. Lai-Becker, MD Whidden Hospital Emergency Department, Division of Medical Toxicology, Whidden Hosptial Campus of Cambridge Health Alliance, Department of Emergency Medicine, Everett, MA, USA

Michael Murphy, MD, PhD McLean Hospital, Belmont, MA, USA

Mladen Nisavic, MD Massachusetts General Hospital, Department of Psychiatry, Boston, MA, USA

Harvard Medical School, Boston, MA, USA

Joanna Piechniczek-Buczek, MD Boston Medical Center/Boston University School of Medicine, Department of Psychiatry, Boston, MA, USA

Laura M. Prager, MD Harvard Medical School, Boston, MA, USA

Child Psychiatry Emergency Consult Service, Massachusetts General Hospital, Boston, MA, USA

Vinod Rao, MD, PhD Department of Psychiatry, Massachusetts General Hospital, Harvard Medical School, Boston, MA, USA

S. Alex Sidelnik, MD NYU School of Medicine, NYU Langone Health, Department of Psychiatry, New York, NY, USA

Ozan Toy, MD Boston University Medical Center, Department of Psychiatry, Boston, MA, USA

E. Nalan Ward, MD Department of Psychiatry, Massachusetts General Hospital, Harvard Medical School, Boston, MA, USA

Scott G. Weiner, MD, MPH Department of Emergency Medicine, Brigham and Women's Hospital, Boston, MA, USA

Curtis Wittmann, MD Massachusetts General Hospital, Department of Psychiatry, Boston, MA, USA

Harvard Medical School, Boston, MA, USA

Acute Psychiatry Service, Massachusetts General Hospital, Boston, MA, USA

Part I
Management of Acute Substance Use Disorders

Chapter 1
Opioid Use Disorders and Related Emergencies

Vinod Rao and E. Nalan Ward

The Opioid Epidemic

For centuries, people have used compounds derived from the opium plant for their medicinal or psychoactive properties. In the last century, synthetic derivatives, such as methadone, hydromorphone, and fentanyl, have been manufactured for analgesia. Starting in the 1980s, opioid pain medications played an increasing role in the medical management of cancer and chronic pain. This change in pain management practice was, in part, due to clinical experts advocating for pain to become a "vital sign," to be assessed and addressed like any other vital sign. Pharmaceutical companies also played a role in this change with aggressive marketing strategies encouraging the use of "safe" and effective opioid agents. In 2001, the Joint Commission on Accreditation of Healthcare Organizations (JCAHO), now known as the Joint Commission, developed new pain management standards for organizations to adapt [1], emphasizing the importance of adequate pain management. A decade later, it was estimated that the United States consumed 80% of the global opioid supply. As prescriptions for opioid pain medications soared, there was a parallel increase in overdose death rates and in the number of individuals admitted for the treatment of opioid use disorders (OUDs) [2] (see Fig. 1.1). Furthermore, starting in 2008, drug overdose, mostly caused by opioids, became the leading cause of death among Americans, surpassing death rates caused by motor vehicle accidents [3].

V. Rao · E. N. Ward (✉)
Department of Psychiatry, Massachusetts General Hospital, Harvard Medical School, Boston, MA, USA
e-mail: enward@mgh.harvard.edu

A. L. Donovan, S. A. Bird (eds.), *Substance Use and the Acute Psychiatric Patient*, Current Clinical Psychiatry, https://doi.org/10.1007/978-3-319-23961-3_1

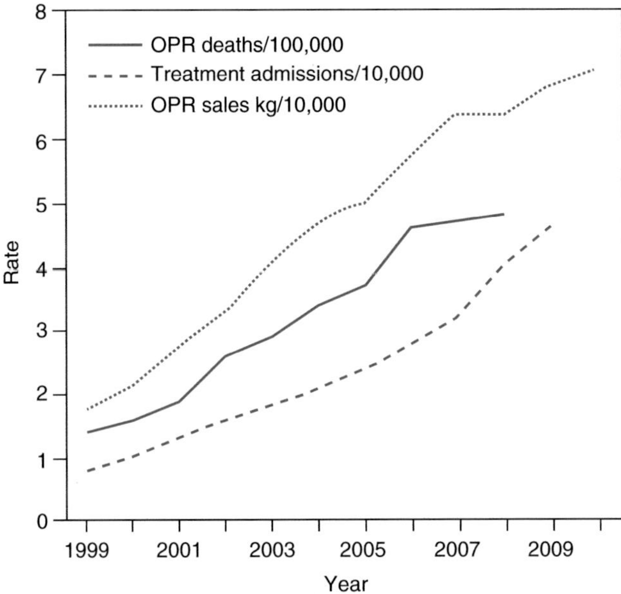

Fig. 1.1 Rates of opioid pain reliever (OPR) overdose deaths, OPR treatment admissions, and kilograms of OPR sold, United States, 1999–2010. (Source: *http://www.cdc.gov/mmwr*)

Epidemiology

In 2016, the opioid epidemic killed, on average, 115 individuals a day nationwide. The entire US healthcare system, including EDs, has been overwhelmed [4] due to increasing numbers of people needing treatment for problems related to opioid misuse or overdose [5].

According to the 2016 National Survey on Drug Use and Health, 11.8 million Americans reported misusing prescription pain medications and/or illicit opioids in the past year. The survey estimated that over 2.1 million individuals struggled with an opioid use disorder, specifically 1.8 million involving prescription pain medications and 626,000 involving heroin [6]. The nation grappled with rapidly increasing overdose death rates during the preceding years, as an illicitly manufactured form of the opioid fentanyl became available in 2013. This extremely potent illicit drug was often mixed with, or sold as, heroin. Many opioid users reported that they were unaware of fentanyl's presence in the drugs they had consumed [7]. Similarly, illicitly manufactured fentanyl was sold as counterfeit prescription opioid pills, compounding the frequency of accidental exposures. In more recent years, illicit forms of fentanyl have been responsible for even more significant increases in overdose death rates, and fentanyl was the leading cause of opioid-related deaths in 2016 [8] (see Fig. 1.2). This surge in fentanyl-related overdoses was caused by illicitly manufactured fentanyl analogs, such as acetylfentanyl, furanylfentanyl, and carfentanil, and not by diverted prescription fentanyl (see Fig. 1.3) [9, 10].

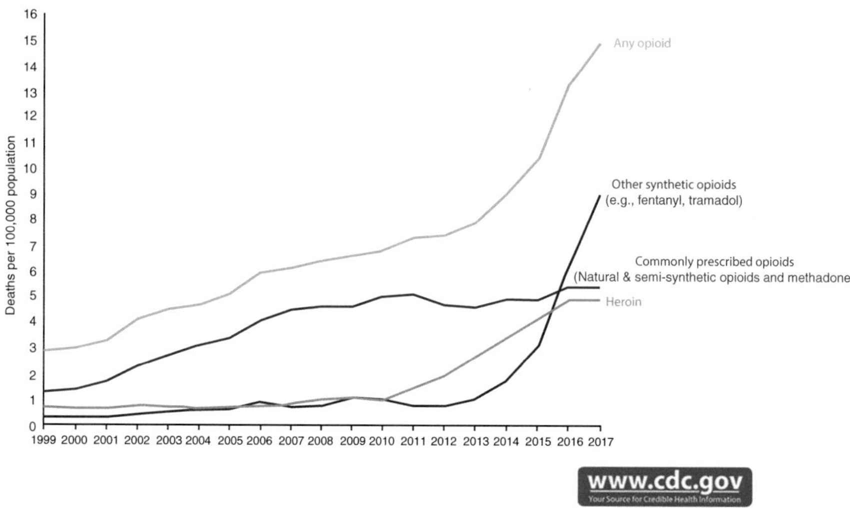

Fig. 1.2 Overdose deaths involving opioids, United States, 2000–2017. (Source: CDC/NCHS [65])

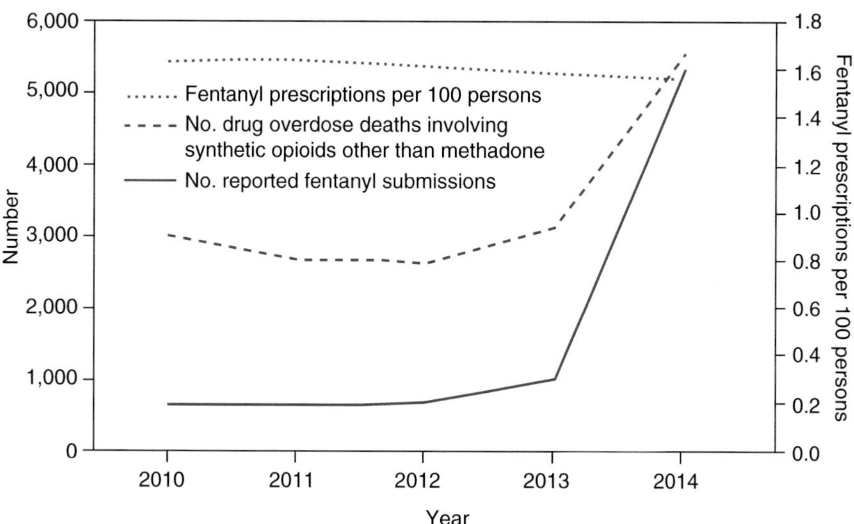

Fig. 1.3 Trends in number of drug overdose deaths involving synthetic opioids other than methadone, number of reported fentanyl submissions (drug products obtained by law enforcement that tested positive for fentanyl), and rate of fentanyl prescriptions, United States, 2010–2014. (Source: CDC/MMWR)

Not surprisingly, the nation's hospitals and EDs have been greatly impacted by an increase in visits related to opioids. For example, between 2005 and 2014, there was a 99.4% increase in opioid-related ED visits [11]. Eighty percent of individuals with an OUD have another comorbid substance use disorder (SUD); therefore, increasing numbers of patients have been presenting to EDs with more than one substance being actively used [12]. The number of ED visits related to particularly concerning combinations, such as non-medical use of opioids and benzodiazepines, more than tripled from 2004 to 2011 [13]. In addition, almost one in five ED visits involving opioid pain medications also involved alcohol [14]. While cocaine-related overdose death rates increased by 57% overall from 2010 to 2015, this increase was entirely driven by cocaine overdoses involving accidental exposure to opioids [15].

Similarly, from 2005 to 2014, the national rate for opioid-related general hospital admissions increased by 64.1% [11] (see Fig. 1.4). One retrospective study showed that 53% of ED visits related to opioid overdoses resulted in hospitalization [16]. These inpatient admissions were due to opioid use, misuse, dependence, and poisoning and opioid-related infections, such as endocarditis, osteomyelitis, septic arthritis, or epidural abscess. Therefore, opioid-related healthcare utilization affects not only the ED but also the inpatient medical hospital.

Another important factor complicating ED presentations of patients with OUDs is comorbid psychiatric illness, which can include depression, PTSD, antisocial personality disorder, as well as other substance use disorders. For instance, among treatment-seeking individuals with OUDs, the prevalence of mood disorders is estimated to be 20–25% [17, 18]. Prescription opioid misuse is significantly associated with suicidal ideation, suicide planning, and suicide attempts, compared to those who do not misuse opioids [19]. Individuals with heroin use disorder have a higher likelihood of dying of suicide than the general population [20].

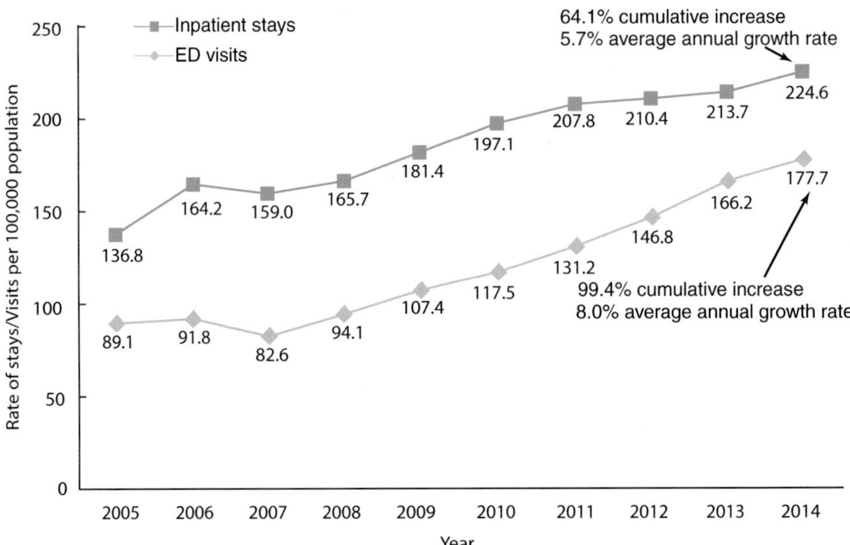

Fig. 1.4 National rates of opioid-related inpatient stays and emergency department visits, 2005–2014. (Source: Agency for Healthcare Research and Quality)

Pharmacology

Opioid effects in the central nervous system (CNS) are mediated through several receptors, most commonly μ-opioid receptors, but also including κ-, δ-, and σ-opioid receptors. The analgesic effects of opioids are mediated by their actions on descending pain-modulating circuits, as well as through effects on the spinal cord. However, μ-opioid receptors in the midbrain reward circuitry modify dopamine responses and are thought to mediate the reinforcing and euphorigenic effects of opioids. Following opioid use, individuals commonly describe a "rush" and/or a feeling of relief from physical or psychic pain, which may include a feeling of euphoria. The duration of action, potency of opioids, and route of use all play a role in the timing and duration of an individual's experience of euphoria. Oral ingestion of an opioid analgesic may cause a delayed sense of euphoria, compared to the more immediate and intense effect of the same amount if crushed and snorted or injected. Repeated use of opioids inevitably results in physical dependence, defined as tolerance and emergence of withdrawal symptoms if stopped abruptly. Individuals who develop tolerance to the effects of opioids need to use increasing amounts to achieve a sense of euphoria and often change the route of use to achieve more rapid onset of action. As tolerance develops, individuals start to experience withdrawal when they stop taking opioids, which then, in turn, reinforces more use. Patients with OUDs who are dependent on opioids with a shorter duration of action, such as heroin, use more frequently to stave off withdrawal symptoms (see Table 1.1). By contrast, in part due to their delayed peak time and long duration of effect, opioids such as methadone and buprenorphine are ideal medications for the treatment of OUDs. Once-a-day dosing ensures steady levels of medication, without causing euphoria after dosing or withdrawal between doses. In addition to euphoria, opioids have a variety of physiological effects, including analgesia, sedation, pupillary constriction, itching, suppression of cough, decreased gastric motility, and respiratory depression.

Table 1.1 Types of opioids, duration of effect, and time to withdrawal

Type of opioid	Duration of effect (hours)[a]	Beginning of withdrawal (hours)[a]	Peak withdrawal (hours)[a]
Methadone	8–12	36–72	96–144
Buprenorphine	24–72	24–48	72–120
Hydrocodone	4–8	8–12	36–72
Codeine	4–8	8–12	36–72
Morphine	4–5	8–12	36–72
Hydromorphone	4–5	4–5	36–72
Heroin	4[b]	8–12[b]	36–72[b]
Oxycodone	3–6	8–12	36–72
Fentanyl	1[b]	3–5[b]	8–12[b]

[a]When taken orally, unless otherwise noted
[b]When used intravenously

Emergency Department Presentations

Reasons for opioid-related ED visits vary greatly. Some patients present with clinical emergencies caused by opioid misuse (defined as taking opioids for non-medical purposes, i.e., taking more than prescribed or for unintended purposes, such as to get high, or taking an opioid medication prescribed to another person), such as intoxication, injuries, or trauma. Other individuals with OUDs may seek help due to medical and psychiatric comorbidities, such as soft tissue infections, endocarditis, HIV, hepatitis C, acute liver toxicity due to consuming opioid combinations containing acetaminophen, acute renal failure due to rhabdomyolysis, overdose or withdrawal, depression, and acute suicidality. Some individuals present seeking treatment specifically for OUDs, such as admission for inpatient detoxification or referral to medication-assisted outpatient treatment.

Overdose

The amount and type of opioid that causes intoxication varies from person to person, depending on their level of tolerance. Milder cases of intoxication may present with apathy, psychomotor retardation, and impairment in cognitive abilities and judgment. More severe opioid intoxication is characterized by miosis, respiratory depression, and stupor. Individuals can develop apnea and pulmonary edema, which can then progress to anoxia, coma, and death. Depending on the environment and the circumstances, patients may also develop hypothermia, rhabdomyolysis, and compartment syndrome from being immobile for an extended time. While heroin overdoses can occur within 20–30 minutes after use, illicitly manufactured fentanyl-related overdoses have been reported to be much more rapid [22, 23]. Opioid intoxication is not associated with seizures, except in children or with use of certain synthetic opioids, such as tramadol, meperidine, and propoxyphene (no longer available in United States).

Withdrawal

Physical dependence on opioids is a reliable consequence of consistent use. How rapidly physical dependence develops varies in individuals, although studies suggest dependence can develop in less than 1 week of daily opioid use for opioid-naïve people or faster in people who have previously been physically dependent [22].

Abstaining from opioid use can induce a withdrawal syndrome within hours to days from the last dose. The specific time of initiation of withdrawal symptoms depends on the half-life of the opioid (see Table 1.1), but usually symptoms peak in 24–48 hours and decrease in 3–5 days. However, iatrogenic withdrawal can occur more quickly in patients receiving an opioid antagonist, such as naloxone or naltrexone. Opioid partial agonists, such as buprenorphine, can also precipitate withdrawal symptoms, if given to someone physically dependent on opioids who is not yet in withdrawal.

Physical symptoms of withdrawal, while not medically dangerous, are extremely uncomfortable and include flu-like symptoms, such as abdominal cramps, nausea, vomiting, diarrhea, motor restlessness, chills, myalgias, and arthralgias. Psychological symptoms can include insomnia, dysphoria, anxiety, and irritability, as well as intense drug cravings, all of which can manifest as complaints or demands for opioids by withdrawing patients in the ED.

Medical Assessment

The evaluation of every ED patient starts with gathering pertinent medical history. The medical history of an individual with OUD can reveal conditions such as abscesses, cellulitis, hepatitis B or C, HIV, endocarditis, thrombophlebitis, liver disease, anoxic brain injury, and trauma. Intranasal fentanyl use has been linked to diffuse alveolar hemorrhage [21].

All patients will also require a review of systems and thorough physical exam. Patients with OUDs are at increased risk of numerous medical illnesses, and they often do not receive regular medical care. The physical exam of an individual with OUD may reveal physical signs of opioid use and/or medical complications, such as cellulitis, abscesses, or endocarditis (see Table 1.2), as well as signs and symptoms of opioid intoxication or withdrawal (see Table 1.3).

Table 1.2 Medical complications and physical exam findings of OUD

Medical complications	Physical exam findings
Infection, acute liver failure, hepatitis C, HIV, rhabdomyolysis, acute renal failure, compartment syndrome	Needle puncture marks (track marks), extremity edema, fever, tachycardia, jaundice, rash, heart murmur, muscle swelling

Table 1.3 Physical and mental status exam findings in overdose and withdrawal

	Physical signs and symptoms	Psychiatric signs and symptoms
Overdose	Miosis, decreased respiration rate, apnea, loud snoring, signs of pulmonary edema on auscultation, hypothermia, cold, clammy skin, cyanosis	Depressed mood, drowsiness, "nodding," stupor
Withdrawal	*Early phase* Diaphoresis, rhinorrhea, lacrimation, yawning *Later phase* Piloerection, dilated pupils, abdominal cramps, nausea, vomiting, diarrhea, tachycardia, fever, tachypnea	Anxiety, irritability, uncooperativeness, restlessness, demanding behavior, agitation, impulsivity, cravings, insomnia, poor insight and judgment, suicidal ideation

Laboratory Findings

Patients with OUDs will also typically benefit from targeted laboratory investigations. Based on clinical concern, a complete blood count (CBC) may help identify the presence of infection, and liver function tests may help identify the presence of hepatitis. In particular, early detection and treatment initiation for intravenously transmitted infections, such as hepatitis B or C and HIV, have tremendous health benefits for patients with OUDs. Although it is not a routine ED practice, patients with OUDs, especially those who inject drugs, should be strongly considered for hepatitis and HIV testing.

Female patients who are in child-bearing age should be tested for pregnancy. A positive pregnancy test result can change the course of management in the ED setting, as discussed further in Chap. 13.

The value of urine toxicology screening is minimal in cases of opioid use or overdose for several reasons. Many commonly used substances, including opioids, are not reliably detected on standard ED toxicology screens. A standard 5 panel urine toxicology screen will typically fail to detect synthetic opioids (i.e., opioids not derived from the opioid plant) – including oxycodone, methadone, buprenorphine, and fentanyl. Therefore, negative screening results do not necessarily rule out opioid use. Naloxone should not be withheld in clinically suggestive situations pending confirmatory toxicology results. Reliable detection of synthetic opioids requires the use of gas chromatography/mass spectrometry (GC/MS). With the recent propagation of fentanyl, some hospitals have also begun using rapid fentanyl detection tests. Checking serum acetaminophen levels can be valuable to detect the presence of toxicity, especially for patients reporting misuse of prescription opioids which often contain acetaminophen. Lastly, although of limited medical value, urine toxicology screening for opioids may be required for admission to some OUD treatment programs.

Psychiatric Evaluation

Given the high rates of comorbidity between OUDs and other psychiatric disorders, such as depression, anxiety, and PTSD, it is important to screen patients with OUDs for the presence of other active psychiatric illnesses, as part of a standard review of systems. Patients who report ongoing psychiatric symptoms will benefit from a more thorough assessment of their psychiatric and substance use histories. The ideal clinician to conduct that assessment (an EM physician, a LICSW, or a psychiatrist) and the depth of that assessment are dependent upon the individual clinical presentation and the resources available. A comprehensive mental health and addiction assessment, including specific assessment of safety, can help determine the most appropriate disposition, including the need for additional substance use and/or psychiatric treatment.

Psychiatric History

Opioid misuse, withdrawal, and intoxication can mimic signs and symptoms of depression and anxiety disorders. OUDs are also highly comorbid with psychiatric illnesses, including depression, bipolar disorder, anxiety, and PTSD. The history of psychiatric symptoms should include past and present depressed or manic mood, anxiety, trauma, suicidal ideation and attempts, intentional overdoses, violence, psychiatric treatment with or without medications, and inpatient psychiatric or dual-diagnosis admissions. History of an independent comorbid psychiatric disorder and psychiatric symptoms induced by substance use, intoxication, or withdrawal should be further distinguished to the extent possible. For accurate diagnosis, the relationship of these symptoms to periods of opioid misuse or abstinence needs to be clarified. Specifically, a comorbid mood or anxiety disorder should only be suspected if the psychiatric symptoms occur during periods of extended sobriety; mood or anxiety symptoms that occur only during periods of intoxication or withdrawal are more likely to be substance induced. Special attention should be paid to those people who present with opioid overdoses, as some overdoses may actually be intentional suicide attempts. A careful safety assessment of any patient who presents after a nonfatal overdose is critical.

Substance Use History

A careful substance use history can be helpful in elucidating the severity and persistence of potential substance use disorders. The history of opioid use should include information about age of first use, route of use, frequency and type of opioids used, cravings or urges to use, symptoms of tolerance and withdrawal, and timing of last use. In addition to obtaining information about medical and psychiatric consequences of opioid use, patients should also be asked about drug-seeking behavior, obtaining prescription opioid medications from multiple prescribers, and social issues such as unstable housing, associated legal problems, involvement of children and family services, and loss of employment. As previously mentioned, polysubstance use is common among patients with OUDs, and, therefore, history of other substance uses, such as alcohol, benzodiazepines, and cocaine, should be obtained. A history of substance use treatment, such as medication treatment with buprenorphine-naloxone (bup-nx) or methadone and/or admissions to inpatient detoxification units or residential programs, is also important to inform assessment and treatment planning.

Due to variable states of intoxication or withdrawal, patients may be unable to provide a linear or accurate history during their ED stay. Therefore, collateral information from family members, healthcare providers, electronic medical records, and online prescription monitoring programs can provide important additional history.

Table 1.4 Adapted from DSM-5 opioid use disorder criteria

1. Taking the opioid in larger amounts and for longer than intended
2. Wanting to cut down or quit but not being able to do it
3. Spending a lot of time obtaining the opioid
4. Craving or a strong desire to use the opioid
5. Repeatedly unable to carry out major obligations at work, school, or home due to opioid use
6. Continued use despite persistent or recurring social or interpersonal problems caused or made worse by opioid use
7. Stopping or reducing important social, occupational, or recreational activities due to opioid use
8. Recurrent use in physically hazardous situations
9. Consistent use despite persistent or recurrent physical or psychological difficulties
10. Tolerance
11. Withdrawal
Severity: Mild, 2–3 positive; moderate, 4–5 positive; severe, 6 or more positive

It can be challenging to screen ED patients for OUDs, even when they present with opioid-related medical complications. On the one hand, clinicians need to attend to the presenting medical problem; on the other hand, there is a need to appropriately recognize signs and symptoms of an opioid use disorder in the acute care setting to provide appropriate patient care and education and to determine appropriate treatment referrals.

Understanding the Diagnostic and Statistical Manual of Mental Disorders (DSM)-5 criteria for OUDs [23] can provide guidance in diagnosing individuals who present to EDs with suggestive presentations (Table 1.4). Out of 11 possible criteria, at least 2 must be met within a 12-month period for an OUD to be diagnosed. While any patient regularly taking opioid medications as prescribed may develop tolerance and risk of withdrawal, the DSM-5 specifies that "the criteria are not considered to be met for those taking opioids solely under appropriate medical supervision" [23].

Accurately diagnosing a patient with OUD in the ED setting can lead to a lifesaving treatment intervention.

Treatment

Management of Overdose

An opioid overdose can be a life-threatening emergency due to respiratory suppression and risk of respiratory arrest. Naloxone, a short-acting, competitive opioid μ-receptor antagonist, reverses the signs and symptoms of overdose. The medication can be administered intravenously, intramuscularly, subcutaneously, intranasally, or endotracheally, depending on the clinical presentation and setting. For suspected opioid overdose in the ED, while the patient is being managed supportively, naloxone can be administered intravenously or intramuscularly. There is considerable variability in the recommended dose of naloxone, with 0.4–2 mg as the initial dose range, repeated every 2–3 minutes as needed. Naloxone's duration of action is about 20–90 minutes [24, 25]. Adverse events such as hypoxia and hypoventilation require treatment with supplemental oxygen and assisted ventilation.

In recent years, in response to the surge in opioid-related overdose deaths, intranasal naloxone has been widely used outside of the hospital setting by first responders and bystanders. This form of naloxone has been shown to be as safe and effective as the intravenous (IV) form [26]. When administered intranasally, the standard dose is one spray (4 mg) into one nostril, which can be repeated as needed every 2–3 minutes. Although the bioavailability of intranasal naloxone is lower than the IV form, intranasal administration bypasses the time needed to obtain intravenous access and may produce a clinical response in the same total time as IV administration.

After naloxone is administered, many patients will require observation, as long-acting opioids, such as methadone, may cause recurrent respiratory depression after naloxone wears off [27]. It has been reported that patients with heroin overdoses can be revived successfully outside of hospital settings with naloxone. In contrast, overdose cases involving prescription opioids, polysubstance use, and long-acting opioids tend to require ED visits, longer observation periods, more repeated administrations of naloxone, or inpatient admission and intubation [28]. Due to its potency, patients with fentanyl-related overdoses may require multiple administrations of naloxone [29], but if no improvement is observed after a total of 10 mg of naloxone has been administered, the diagnosis of opioid overdose should be questioned.

Evidence-based guidelines are lacking for the determination of when an individual can be safely discharged from the ED after naloxone administration post-overdose. In one study, the authors concluded that by using a prediction rule (normal ambulation, normal vital signs, and Glasgow Coma Scale of 15), 40% of individuals, who were mostly users of heroin, could be safely discharged 1 hour after their last naloxone dose [30]. A more conservative review on this topic concluded that individuals presenting with heroin overdose who are observed to be in stable condition can be discharged 2 hours after the last naloxone dose [31].

Most of these studies, however, were conducted before illicit fentanyl and other more potent synthetic analogs became prevalent; therefore, the current relevance of these studies to the management of patients who may be using a combination of heroin and fentanyl, or fentanyl alone, is less clear. More recently, it has been reported that illicitly manufactured fentanyl-related overdoses require higher and repeated doses of naloxone or naloxone infusions and a longer duration of observation [32, 33]. Further research is needed to understand and accurately determine when a patient can be discharged safely after being revived by naloxone in the ED setting. As the chemical content of illicit drugs changes over time, communities, cities, or regions may be affected by location-specific illicit drug products. EDs would benefit from working closely with state public health agencies for further collaboration to determine their specific geographical risks.

The clinical presentation of an individual recovering from an opioid overdose can be complicated by multifaceted psychological sequelae and physical symptoms. Individuals with OUDs who survive an overdose with the help of emergency medical attention, either in the field or in the ED, may resume consciousness with mixed feelings, such as hopelessness or a sense of desperation and anger. Furthermore, after the reversal of an opioid overdose, individuals with OUDs will eventually develop signs and symptoms of opioid withdrawal. If withdrawal symptoms are unaddressed, patients will become increasingly focused on obtaining opioids to reduce the intense discomfort of withdrawal. Despite the recent scare and potential risk of another overdose, it is common for overdose patients to sign out against medical advice (AMA) from the ED in order to use opioids and prevent or relieve withdrawal symptoms. This situation can be difficult for clinicians to accept, but it is important to recognize and acknowledge the physical and psychological discomfort regularly experienced by opioid-dependent patients and to approach them with empathy and understanding. Individuals who survive an opioid overdose should be assessed for suicidality and questioned about whether the overdose was intentional. Individuals may be more forthcoming about their true intentions if they are assured that they will receive appropriate care to treat withdrawal symptoms.

Management of Withdrawal

Gaps in research and clinical guidance exist regarding the optimal management of opioid withdrawal in the emergency setting, but, in response to the recent opioid epidemic, there has been a growing desire to develop evidence-based treatments for OUDs in the ED. Currently, there is no clear consensus, but several options for treatment of withdrawal do exist. In addition to treating symptoms of withdrawal, it is critical to effectively manage cravings to prevent patients from leaving AMA and then being at risk of relapse and overdose. When patients can remain in the ED and engage in their own assessment and care, there is a better opportunity for a thoughtful assessment of treatment needs and discharge planning to meet those needs.

It is important to recognize that opioid withdrawal is an extremely uncomfortable experience for patients. The Clinical Opiate Withdrawal Scale (COWS) is a structured rating instrument for the systematic evaluation and monitoring of opioid withdrawal (see Table 1.5) [34]. The COWS assesses 11 signs and symptoms of withdrawal and has been validated in outpatient and inpatient settings [35]. Its use in busy ED settings can be limited by the demand for regular nursing assessments and documentation, but clinical information from COWS can provide a standardized approach to assessing and managing withdrawal symptoms.

Table 1.5 Clinical Opiate Withdrawal Scale (COWS) [34]

For each item, circle the number that best describes the patient's signs or symptoms. Rate on just the apparent relationship to opiate withdrawal. For example, if heart rate is increased because the patient was jogging just prior to assessment, the increased pulse rate would not add to the score	
Patient's name:	Date and time:
Resting pulse rate: ______beats/minute *Measured after the patient is sitting or lying for 1 minute* 0 pulse rate 80 or below 1 pulse rate 81–100 2 pulse rate 101–120 4 pulse rate greater than 120	**GI upset:** *Over the last half hour* 0 no GI symptoms 1 stomach cramps 2 nausea or loose stool 3 vomiting or diarrhea 4 multiple episodes of diarrhea or vomiting
Sweating: *Over the past half hour not accounted for by room temperature or patient activity* 0 no report of chills or flushing 1 subjective report of chills or flushing 2 flushed face or observable moistness on face 3 beads of sweat on brow or face 4 sweat streaming off face	**Tremor** *Observation of outstretched hands* 0 no tremor 1 tremor can be felt, but not observed 2 slight tremor observable 4 gross tremor or muscle twitching
Restlessness: *Observation during assessment* 0 able to sit still 1 reports difficulty sitting still, but is able to do so 3 frequent shifting or extraneous movements of legs/arms 5 unable to sit still for more than a few seconds	**Yawning:** *Observation during assessment* 0 no yawning 1 yawning once or twice during assessment 2 yawning three or more times during assessment 4 yawning several times/minute
Pupil size 0 pupils pinned or normal size for room light 1 pupils possibly larger than normal for room light 2 pupils moderately dilated 5 pupils so dilated that only the rim of the iris is visible	**Anxiety or irritability** 0 none 1 patient reports increasing irritability or anxiousness 2 patient obviously irritable or anxious 4 patient so irritable or anxious that participation in the assessment is difficult
Bone or joint aches: *If the patient was having pain previously, only the additional component attributed to opiate withdrawal is scored* 0 not present 1 mild diffuse discomfort 2 patient reports severe diffuse aching of joints/muscles 4 patient is rubbing joints or muscles and is unable to sit still because of discomfort	**Gooseflesh skin** 0 skin is smooth 3 piloerection of skin can be felt or hairs standing up on arms 5 prominent piloerection

(continued)

Table 1.5 (continued)

For each item, circle the number that best describes the patient's signs or symptoms. Rate on just the apparent relationship to opiate withdrawal. For example, if heart rate is increased because the patient was jogging just prior to assessment, the increased pulse rate would not add to the score	
Patient's name:	Date and time:
Runny nose or tearing: *Not accounted for by cold symptoms or allergies* 0 not present 1 nasal stuffiness or unusually moist eyes 2 nose running or tearing 4 nose constantly running or tears streaming down cheeks	**Total score** ______ *The total score is the sum of all 11 items* **Score:** 5–12 = *mild* 13–24 = *moderate* 25–36 = *moderately severe* More than 36 = *severe withdrawal*

Adapted from Wesson and Ling [34]

Buprenorphine and methadone are FDA-approved medications for the treatment of opioid use disorders. They are equally effective in relieving physical signs and symptoms of withdrawal and cravings [36, 37], and they can be used safely and effectively in ED settings for the management of withdrawal.

Buprenorphine is a partial agonist at the opioid μ-receptor with a favorable side effect profile, compared to full opioid agonists, such as methadone or heroin. It has high affinity for the opioid receptor and a slow dissociation rate. If buprenorphine is given to a patient who has recently used opioids, i.e., when μ-receptors are occupied with full agonist opioids, buprenorphine will displace the full agonist opioids and precipitate acute withdrawal. Therefore, patients should be experiencing withdrawal symptoms, a signal that the μ-receptors are not fully occupied, before buprenorphine is initiated to avoid precipitated withdrawal. Buprenorphine slowly dissociates from the opioid receptor and is an ideal medication to stabilize patients with a once-a-day dosing regimen. The initial dose is 4 mg, for a COWS score >8. Relief in withdrawal symptoms should be observed within an hour. An additional dose of 4 mg can be given after reassessing signs and symptoms of withdrawal 1–2 hours after the initial dose [38]. The total dose can be up to 8–12 mg during the first 24 hours of the ED stay. Buprenorphine use for the management of withdrawal symptoms in the ED has been shown to be associated with fewer return visits to the ED in the next 30 days, compared to those who received other medications for symptom relief [39].

Methadone, a full opioid agonist, has historically been the preferred medication for treatment of opioid withdrawal, especially in inpatient medical settings, with initial doses in the range of 20–30 mg a day. Methadone may be preferable for patients with OUDs and trauma or for those who may need an inpatient medical admission and surgery, where moderate to severe acute pain is anticipated. The benefit of methadone over buprenorphine is that the methadone dose can be increased as needed for pain relief purposes and short-acting opioid analgesics can be more easily added, if indicated. One regulatory challenge is that patients can only

Table 1.6 Non-opioid agents used in opioid withdrawal

Symptom	Drug	Common dose range
Autonomic instability	Clonidine Lofexidine	0.1–0.2 mg 0.18–0.54 mg
Anxiety	Hydroxyzine Lorazepam	25–100 mg 1–2 mg
Diarrhea	Loperamide	4 mg, followed by 2 mg
Abdominal cramps	Dicyclomine	10–20 mg
Nausea/vomiting	Ondansetron Promethazine	4–8 mg 25 mg
Muscle aches	Ibuprofen Acetaminophen Naproxen	400–600 mg 650 mg–1000 mg 500 mg
Muscle cramps	Baclofen	5–10 mg

be started on methadone in the ED or medical hospital as part of a taper for withdrawal management; therefore, patients cannot be discharged from the ED or hospital on standing methadone, unless they are already a part of a licensed outpatient methadone clinic.

Non-opioid agents for relief of withdrawal symptoms can be used alone or in conjunction with opioid agonists (see Table 1.6). Clonidine is a centrally acting alpha-agonist, which is not FDA approved for the treatment of opioid withdrawal, but it is commonly used for symptomatic management of withdrawal symptoms. It can be given as 0.1–0.2 mg every 6–8 hours. Patients should be monitored for hypotension. Clonidine reduces symptoms of autonomic instability associated with opioid withdrawal but does not provide relief for cravings or for acute pain. Compared to treatment with opioid agonists, management of opioid withdrawal symptoms with clonidine is associated with higher rates of relapse and treatment drop-out after completing detoxification [40, 41].

Recently, lofexidine, a central alpha-2 adrenergic agonist, has been FDA approved for mitigating symptoms of opioid withdrawal by reducing sympathetic tone. The recommended dose is up to 0.54 mg four times daily. Compared to clonidine, it is associated with less severe side effects, including hypotension and sedation [42].

Treatment Initiation and Referral to Treatment

It is a well-known phenomenon that patients with severe OUDs cycle in and out of detox facilities and EDs, due to high relapse rates. In recent years, growing numbers of studies have shown that medically supervised opioid withdrawal management (detoxification) alone is an inferior treatment, compared to ongoing medication treatment of OUDs with opioid agonists [43–45]. Patients who undergo medically supervised withdrawal, and especially those briefly treated for opioid OD or withdrawal in the ED setting, unfortunately typically return to using. Moreover, those who experience a non-fatal opioid OD are at higher risk of a fatal overdose in the following 12 months [44–46]. Therefore, there is an urgent need to expand emergency treatment services beyond symptomatic OUD care with the critical goal of engaging patients in evidence-based treatments. Both providers and patients need to be educated that withdrawal management alone is not an effective long-term treatment for OUDs [47]. Buprenorphine-naloxone, methadone, and injectable naltrexone are FDA-approved medications to treat OUDs. In addition to reducing cravings, illicit opioid use, and withdrawal symptoms, patients who are in long-term treatment with bup-nx or methadone have lower rates of ED use and fewer hospitalizations [48, 49]. Most importantly, treatment with these medications substantially reduces all-cause and overdose mortality in people with OUDs, compared to those who do not receive medication treatment. A visit to the ED by an individual with OUD should be seen as an opportunity to engage the patient in treatment [50], potentially treatment that begins within the ED encounter itself.

There is increasing evidence that buprenorphine-naloxone is an ideal medication to engage patients in treatment in the ED setting. The effectiveness of initiating OUD treatment in the ED has been studied in a randomized clinical trial. In this study, D'onorfio et al. showed that initiating bup-nx in the ED setting and linking the patients to outpatient bup-nx treatment were feasible and superior, compared to screening, brief intervention in the ED, and referral to community-based outpatient treatment services. The group receiving bup-nx medication treatment as part of their ED care had higher rates of engagement in SUD treatment, less self-reported illicit drug use, and decreased use of inpatient SUD services in the following 30 days [51]. The difference was sustained at 2 months, and medication initiation was found to be cost effective, compared to those who received screening, brief intervention, and referral [52, 53]. Interestingly, the interventions did not differ in terms of subsequent number of ED visits.

Ideal candidates for bup-nx initiation are those with a history of OUD, exhibiting signs and symptoms of withdrawal in the ED setting, meeting diagnostic criteria for OUD, and who are willing and able to keep outpatient follow-up appointments. The online prescription monitoring program should be accessed to determine what other controlled substances may have been prescribed before initiating bup-nx. Once the patient is deemed appropriate, bup-nx can be initiated during withdrawal (as explained earlier), and the patient can be discharged home with a 1–2 days' supply of medication and a follow-up appointment for ongoing treatment. However, prescribing bup-nx in the ED has been a challenge due to licensing requirements. In an outpatient setting, bup-nx can only be prescribed by clinicians who obtain a DEA X license waiver, per the Drug Addiction Treatment Act of 2000. Obtaining the waiver requires an 8-hour training for physicians. NPs and PAs are required to have an additional 16 hours of training. ED providers are increasingly obtaining their DEA X licenses, but their numbers remain small overall. The Providers Clinical Support System (www.pcssNOW.org) provides online waiver training and mentoring opportunities without cost. Alternatively, under Title 21, Code of Federal Regulations, Part 1306.07(b), emergency rooms can dispense buprenorphine by a physician who does not have an X waiver for management of opioid withdrawal while arrangements are made for referral to treatment. This exception, also known as the "72-hour rule," allows prescribers to administer buprenorphine for up to 3 days, as long as the patient returns to ED to receive the medication.

EDs with X-waivered practitioners can prescribe bup-nx to appropriate candidates and discharge the patients with home induction instructions and a prescription for 1–2 days' supply of bup-nx to bridge them until an outpatient follow-up appointment for ongoing treatment [54]. A sample home induction is included in Box 1.1. One of the barriers to successful initiation of bup-nx in the ED setting is to identify timely access to an outpatient buprenorphine provider for ongoing treatment. Some hospitals are creating post-discharge "bridge clinics" to serve that purpose [55]. These clinics provide transitional OUD treatment and connect patients to long-term outpatient care. For hospitals without such services, the EDs will benefit from partnering with bup-nx providers in their communities for rapid referral.

Box 1.1 Massachusetts General Hospital Emergency Department Sample Home Induction

Day 1

- Wait until you experience at least three withdrawal symptoms (aches, chills, sweating, tremors, irritability, goose pimples, restlessness, yawning, stomach cramps, nausea, diarrhea).
- Take 4 mg of buprenorphine-naloxone (one-half of an 8 mg sublingual film strip) by placing it under your tongue and letting it dissolve for 15 minutes.
- If you still feel withdrawal after 1 hour, take another 4 mg (one-half film strip).
- Six to twelve hours later, if you have withdrawal, take another 4 mg (one-half film strip).
- Do not take more than 12 mg on the first day.

Day 2

- Please go to the bridge clinic for follow-up on day 2.
- Before your appointment, please take another dose of buprenorphine.
- If you took 4 mg on day 1 and felt fine in the morning, take 4 mg as your day 2 morning dose.
- If you took 8 mg on day 1 and felt fine in the morning, take 8 mg as your day 2 morning dose.
- If you took 4 mg on day 1 and felt withdrawal symptoms in the morning, take 8 mg as your day 2 morning dose.
- If you took 12 mg on day 1 and felt fine in the morning, take 12 mg as your day 2 morning dose.
- If you took 8 mg on day 1 and felt withdrawal symptoms in the morning, take 12 mg as your day 2 morning dose.

In contrast to bup-nx, outpatient methadone treatment of OUDs is restricted to licensed opioid treatment programs (OTPs) by federal law. Patient preference, prior success with methadone treatment, and history of poor response to bup-nx are some of the reasons to choose treatment with methadone. To provide patients with timely treatment initiation, EDs should partner with OTPs in the communities.

Opioid agonist initiation in the ED setting may not be suitable for all patients. Those with comorbid SUDs, such as alcohol or sedative-hypnotics, may require medically supervised withdrawal management and may benefit from inpatient admission for medically supervised withdrawal. Moreover, individuals with OUDs who present with acute psychiatric instability or safety concerns, such as suicidality, severe mood symptoms, or psychosis, may require inpatient psychiatric admission. Patients with less severe, but still significant, comorbid psychiatric symptoms, who express willingness to engage in structured, supportive treatment, will benefit from a referral to an intensive outpatient program or partial hospitalization level of care for further stabilization. Those patients with chronic pain conditions and OUDs will benefit from a consultation by a pain and addiction specialist to determine bup-nx eligibility.

Injectable naltrexone is not a viable treatment option for those who come in to ED after an OD or in acute opioid withdrawal. Individuals need to be free of opioids 5–7 days before they can start naltrexone treatment to avoid precipitated withdrawal and therefore may benefit from a supervised withdrawal in an inpatient setting where they can start naltrexone under medical monitoring.

Individuals with OUDs present with many psychosocial needs and challenges. As mentioned earlier, brief intervention alone has not been found to be effective in the ED setting. EDs are employing recovery coaches or peer supports who can help patients to navigate the system to improve patient engagement and address some of patients' needs.

Special Population: Pregnant Women with OUDs

The recommended treatment for pregnant patients with OUDs is opioid agonist treatment. Withdrawal (detoxification) is associated with high relapse rates and poor outcomes for the mother and the fetus, and, therefore, is not advised [56]. Pregnant women should be counseled about treatment options, and every effort should be made to connect these patients with outpatient medication treatment, as well as psychosocial care. Please see Chap. 13 for further discussion.

Overdose Risk Assessment, Prevention Education, and Naloxone Prescribing

In response to the opioid overdose crisis in the United States, there has been a growing public health focus on implementing overdose prevention practices and promoting interventions aimed at reducing morbidity and mortality from opioid overdoses

[57–59]. Increasing access to naloxone has been one of the hallmarks of the federal response in the fight against the opioid overdose death epidemic. The "standing order" program is a model that has been adopted by many states to increase access to the life-saving antidote naloxone [60]. This model allows patients, family members, and bystanders to have access to naloxone without requiring a prescription. The ED offers a unique opportunity to identify those who may benefit from OD prevention interventions including naloxone, beginning with accurate identification of those patients who are at increased risk of overdose. Characteristics of individuals who are brought to EDs for non-fatal opioid overdoses have been described in various studies [16, 61–63]. Although there is a lack of consensus, patients who carry a diagnosis of OUDs, those with history of opioid overdose and opioid and polysubstance misuse, and those who are prescribed >100 mg per day oral equivalent of morphine are considered at risk of future opioid overdose [64]. These patients should be educated about their risk of overdose, and they should be discharged with naloxone, as well as with teaching on how to use it. If there are family or friends present in the ED, they should also be taught to administer naloxone.

Conclusion

The ED visit can be an opportunity to engage patients and enhance their willingness to accept treatment for OUDs. It is thus imperative for ED clinicians to diagnose OUDs, treat opioid overdoses and withdrawal in ED patients, and be well informed about effective treatments for OUDs following an ED presentation. ED clinicians can potentially initiate treatment from the ED and/or offer appropriate referrals, connecting patients to critical aftercare. This type of intervention requires ED medical staff to be X waiver trained, to develop protocols to identify patients with OUDs and to determine prescribing policies. Ideally, ED clinicians can initiate bup-nx in the ED, provide patients with a bridge prescription, and refer them to outpatient practices where ongoing medication treatment can be provided. To overcome the existing barriers, the US Department of Health and Human Services granted $1 billion to fight the opioid epidemic in 2018. Hospitals and EDs can apply for State Targeted Response Technical Assistance (www.getSTR-TA.org) to implement ED-based OUD treatment services. Providers can also take advantage of the Providers Clinical Support System (www.pcssNOW.org) for training and mentoring opportunities without cost.

References

1. Phillips DM. JCAHO pain management standards are unveiled. JAMA [Internet]. 2000;284(4):428–9. Available from: http://jama.ama-assn.org/content/284/4/428.short.
2. Paulozzi LJ, Jones C, Mack K, Rudd R. Vital signs: overdoses of prescription opioid pain relievers. CDC Morb Mortal Wkly Rep [Internet]. 2011;60(43):1487–92. Available from: http://www.ncbi.nlm.nih.gov/pubmed/22048730.

3. Administration UD of JDE. 2015 national drug threat assessment summary. 2015; Available from: https://www.mendeley.com/research-papers/2015-national-drug-threat-assessment-summary-2/?utm_source=desktop&utm_medium=1.17.13&utm_campaign=open_catalog&userDocumentId=%7Bd6ac7119-2eb0-4128-abe5-5efa229c89dd%7D.
4. Rudd RA, Seth P, David F, Scholl L. Increases in drug and opioid-involved overdose deaths — United States, 2010–2015. Morb Mortal Wkly Rep. 2016;65:1445.
5. Hasegawa K, Espinola JA, Brown DFM, Camargo CA. Trends in U.S. Emergency department visits for opioid overdose, 1993–2010. Pain Med. 2014;15:1765.
6. Substance Abuse and Mental Health Services Administration. Key substance use and mental health indicators in the United States: results from the 2016 National Survey on Drug Use and Health. 2017.
7. Macmadu A, Carroll JJ, Hadland SE, Green TC, Marshall BDL. Prevalence and correlates of fentanyl-contaminated heroin exposure among young adults who use prescription opioids non-medically. Addict Behav. 2017;68:35–8.
8. Hedegaard H, Warner M, Minino AM. Drug overdose deaths in the United States, 1999–2015. NCHS Data Brief, no. 273. 2017.
9. Gladden RM, Martinez P, Seth P. Fentanyl law enforcement submissions and increases in synthetic opioid–involved overdose deaths — 27 states, 2013–2014. MMWR Morb Mortal Wkly Rep [Internet]. 2016;65(33):837–43. Available from: http://www.cdc.gov/mmwr/volumes/65/wr/mm6533a2.htm.
10. O'Donnell JK, Halpin J, Mattson CL, Goldberger BA, Gladden RM. Deaths involving fentanyl, fentanyl analogs, and U-47700 — 10 states, July–December 2016. MMWR Morb Mortal Wkly Rep [Internet]. 2017;66(43):1197–202. Available from: http://www.cdc.gov/mmwr/volumes/66/wr/mm6643e1.htm.
11. Weiss AJ, Elixhauser A, Barrett ML, Steiner CA, Bailey MK, O'Malley L. Opioid-related inpatient stays and emergency department visits by state, 2009–2014. HCUP Stat Br #219 [Internet]. 2016;December:1–21. Available from: http://www.hcup-us.ahrq.gov/reports/statbriefs/sb219-Opioid-Hospital-Stays-ED-Visits-by-State.pdf.
12. Wu L-T, Zhu H, Swartz MS. Treatment utilization among persons with opioid use disorder in the United States. Drug Alcohol Depend [Internet]. 2016;169:117–27. Available from: http://linkinghub.elsevier.com/retrieve/pii/S0376871616309504.
13. Jones C, McAninch J. Emergency department visits and overdose deaths from combined use of opioids and benzodiazepines. Am J Prev Med [Internet]. 2015;49(4):493–501. Available from: http://www.sciencedirect.com/science/article/pii/S0749379715001634.
14. Jones CM, Paulozzi LJ, Mack KA. Alcohol involvement in opioid pain reliever and benzodiazepine drug abuse-related emergency department visits and drug-related deaths – United States, 2010. Morb Mortal Wkly Rep [Internet]. 2014;63(40):881–5. Available from: http://eutils.ncbi.nlm.nih.gov/entrez/eutils/elink.fcgi?dbfrom=pubmed&id=25299603&retmode=ref&cmd=prlinks%5Cnpapers3://publication/uuid/272038A5-2298-49E0-886A-83E2C07621C0.
15. McCall Jones C, Baldwin GT, Compton WM. Recent increases in cocaine-related overdose deaths and the role of opioids. Am J Public Health. 2017;107(3):430–2.
16. Hasegawa K, Brown DFM, Tsugawa Y, Camargo CA. Epidemiology of emergency department visits for opioid overdose: a population-based study. Mayo Clin Proc. 2014;89(4):462–71.
17. Savant JD, Barry DT, Cutter CJ, Joy MT, Dinh A, Schottenfeld RS, et al. Prevalence of mood and substance use disorders among patients seeking primary care office-based buprenorphine/naloxone treatment. Drug Alcohol Depend. 2013;127:243.
18. Manhapra A, Quinones L, Rosenheck R. Characteristics of veterans receiving buprenorphine vs. methadone for opioid use disorder nationally in the Veterans Health Administration. Drug Alcohol Depend. 2016;160:82.
19. Ashrafioun L, Bishop TM, Conner KR, Pigeon WR. Frequency of prescription opioid misuse and suicidal ideation, planning, and attempts. J Psychiatr Res. 2017;92:1.
20. Pan CH, Jhong JR, Tsai SY, Lin SK, Chen CC, Kuo CJ. Excessive suicide mortality and risk factors for suicide among patients with heroin dependence. Drug Alcohol Depend. 2014;145:224.

21. Ruzycki S, Yarema M, Dunham M, Sadrzadeh H, Tremblay A. Intranasal fentanyl intoxication leading to diffuse alveolar hemorrhage. J Med Toxicol. 2016;12(2):185–8.
22. Jaffe J, Martin W. Narcotic analgesics and antagonists. In: The pharmacological basis of therapeutics. 5th ed. New York: Macmillian Publishing Company, Inc; 1975. p. 245–324.
23. American Psychiatric Association. Diagnostic and statistical manual of mental disorders fifth edition. Arlington: American Psychiatric Association; 2013.
24. Rzasa Lynn R, Galinkin JL. Naloxone dosage for opioid reversal: current evidence and clinical implications. Ther Adv Drug Saf. 2018;9(1):63–88.
25. Hospira. Naloxone Hydrochloride. Packag Inser.
26. Robinson A, Wermeling DP. Intranasal naloxone administration for treatment of opioid overdose. Am J Health Syst Pharm. 2014;71(24):2129–35.
27. Boyer EW. Management of opioid analgesic overdose. N Engl J Med. 2012;367:146.
28. Willman MW, Liss DB, Schwarz ES, Mullins ME. Do heroin overdose patients require observation after receiving naloxone? Clin Toxicol (Phila). 2017;55(2):81–7.
29. Bode AD, Singh M, Andrews J, Kapur GB, Baez AA. Fentanyl laced heroin and its contribution to a spike in heroin overdose in Miami-Dade County. Am J Emerg Med. 2017;35:1364.
30. Christenson J, Etherington J, Grafstein E, Innes G, Pennington S, Wanger K, et al. Early discharge of patients with presumed opioid overdose: development of a clinical prediction rule. Acad Emerg Med. 2000;7(10):1110–8.
31. Dixon P. Managing acute heroin overdose. Emerg Nurse [Internet]. 2007;15(2):30–5. Available from: http://www.ncbi.nlm.nih.gov/pubmed/17542332.
32. Sutter ME, Gerona RR, Davis MT, Roche BM, Colby DK, Chenoweth JA, et al. Fatal fentanyl: one pill can kill. Acad Emerg Med. 2017;24(1):106–13.
33. Somerville NJ, O'Donnell J, Gladden RM, et al. Characteristics of fentanyl overdose. Massachusetts, 2014–2016. MMWR Morb Mortal Wkly Report. 2017;66(14):382–6.
34. Wesson DR, Ling W. The clinical opiate withdrawal scale (COWS). J Psychoactive Drugs. 2003;35(2):253–9.
35. Tompkins DA, Bigelow GE, Harrison JA, Johnson RE, Fudala PJ, Strain EC. Concurrent validation of the Clinical Opiate Withdrawal Scale (COWS) and single-item indices against the Clinical Institute Narcotic Assessment (CINA) opioid withdrawal instrument. Drug Alcohol Depend. 2009;105(1–2):154–9.
36. Meader N. A comparison of methadone, buprenorphine and alpha2 adrenergic agonists for opioid detoxification: a mixed treatment comparison meta-analysis. Drug Alcohol Depend. 2010;108:110.
37. Gowing L, Ali R, White JM, Mbewe D. Buprenorphine for managing opioid withdrawal. Cochrane Database Syst Rev. 2017;(2):CD002025.
38. Donroe JH, Holt SR, Tetrault JM. Caring for patients with opioid use disorder in the hospital. Can Med Assoc J. 2016;188:1232.
39. Berg ML, Idrees U, Ding R, Nesbit SA, Liang HK, McCarthy ML. Evaluation of the use of buprenorphine for opioid withdrawal in an emergency department. Drug Alcohol Depend. 2007;86(2–3):239–44.
40. Ling W, Amass L, Shoptaw S, Annon JJ, Hillhouse M, Babcock D, et al. A multi-center randomized trial of buprenorphine-naloxone versus clonidine for opioid detoxification: findings from the National Institute on Drug Abuse Clinical Trials Network. Addiction. 2005;100(8):1090–100.
41. Gowing L, Ali R, White J, Mbewe D. Buprenorphine for managing opioid withdrawal. Cochrane Database Syst Rev. 2017;(2):CD002025. https://doi.org/10.1002/14651858.CD002025.pub5.
42. Gorodetzky CW, Walsh SL, Martin PR, Saxon AJ, Gullo KL, Biswas K. A phase III, randomized, multi-center, double blind, placebo controlled study of safety and efficacy of lofexidine for relief of symptoms in individuals undergoing inpatient opioid withdrawal. Drug Alcohol Depend. 2017;176:79–88.
43. Marsch LA. The efficacy of methadone maintenance interventions in reducing illicit opiate use, HIV risk behavior and criminality: a meta-analysis. Addiction. 1998;93(4):515–32.

44. Weiss R, Potter J, Fiellin D, et al. Adjunctive counseling during brief and extended buprenorphine-naloxone treatment for prescription opioid dependence. Arch Gen Psychiatry. 2011;68:1238–46.
45. Kakko J, Dybrandt Svanborg K, Jeanne Kreek M, Heilig M. 1-year retention and social function after buprenorphine-assisted relapse prevention treatment for heroine dependence in Sweden: a randomised, placebo-controlled trial. Lancet. 2003;361(9358):662–8.
46. Dunlap B, Cifu AS. Clinical management of opioid use disorder. JAMA. 2016;316:338–9.
47. Kampman K, Jarvis M. American Society of Addiction Medicine (ASAM) national practice guideline for the use of medications in the treatment of addiction involving opioid use. J Addict Med. 2015;9(5):358–67. Available from: http://content.wkhealth.com/linkback/openurl?sid=WKPTLP:landingpage&an=01271255-201510000-00003.
48. Schwarz R, Zelenev A, Bruce RD, Altice FL. Retention on buprenorphine treatment reduces emergency department utilization, but not hospitalization, among treatment-seeking patients with opioid dependence. J Subst Abus Treat. 2012;43(4):451–7.
49. Lo-Ciganic WH, Gellad WF, Gordon AJ, Cochran G, Zemaitis MA, Cathers T, et al. Association between trajectories of buprenorphine treatment and emergency department and in-patient utilization. Addiction. 2016;111(5):892–902.
50. Rubin R. As overdoses climb, emergency departments begin treating opioid use disorder. JAMA. 2018;319(21):2158–60.
51. D'onorfio G, O'Connor P, Pantalon M, et al. Emergency department–initiated buprenorphine/naloxone treatment for opioid dependence: a randomized clinical trial. JAMA. 2015;313(16):1636–44.
52. D'Onofrio G, Chawarski MC, O'Connor PG, Pantalon MV, Busch SH, Owens PH, et al. Emergency department-initiated buprenorphine for opioid dependence with continuation in primary care: outcomes during and after intervention. J Gen Intern Med. 2017;32(6):660–6.
53. Busch SH, Fiellin DA, Chawarski MC, Owens PH, Pantalon MV, Hawk K, et al. Cost-effectiveness of emergency department-initiated treatment for opioid dependence. Addiction. 2017;112(11):2002–10.
54. Sordo L, Barrio G, Bravo M, et al. Mortality risk during and after opioid substitution treatment: systemic review and meta-analysis of cohort studies. BMJ. 2017;357:j1550.
55. Trowbridge P, Weinstein ZM, Kerensky T, Roy P, Regan D, Samet JH, et al. Addiction consultation services – linking hospitalized patients to outpatient addiction treatment. J Subst Abus Treat. 2017;79:1–5.
56. ACOG. Opioid use and opioid use disorder in pregnancy. Obstet Gynecol. 2017;130(2):e81–94.
57. Samuels EA, Dwyer K, Mello MJ, Baird J, Kellogg AR, Bernstein E. Emergency department-based opioid harm reduction: moving physicians from willing to doing. Acad Emerg Med. 2016;23:455–65.
58. Dwyer K, Walley A, Langlois B, Mitchell P, Nelson K, Cromwell J, et al. Opioid education and nasal naloxone rescue kits in the emergency department. West J Emerg Med [Internet]. 2015;16(3):381–4. Available from: http://escholarship.org/uc/item/3kk3k7jk.
59. Drainoni ML, Koppelman EA, Feldman JA, Walley AY, Mitchell PM, Ellison J, et al. Why is it so hard to implement change? A qualitative examination of barriers and facilitators to distribution of naloxone for overdose prevention in a safety net environment. BMC Res Notes. 2016;9(1):1–14.
60. Standing orders [Internet]. Available from: http://naloxoneinfo.org/case-studies/standing-orders.
61. Brady JE, DiMaggio CJ, Keyes KM, Doyle JJ, Richardson LD, Li G. Emergency department utilization and subsequent prescription drug overdose death. Ann Epidemiol. 2016;25(8):613–9.
62. Rowe C, Santos GM, Behar E, Coffin PO. Correlates of overdose risk perception among illicit opioid users. Drug Alcohol Depend. 2016;159:234–9.
63. Pavarin RM, Berardi D, Gambini D. Emergency department presentation and mortality rate due to overdose: a retrospective cohort study on nonfatal overdoses. Subst Abus. 2016;37(4):558–63.

64. Ellison J, Walley AY, Feldman JA, Bernstein E, Mitchell PM, Koppelman EA, et al. Identifying patients for overdose prevention with ICD-9 classification in the emergency department, Massachusetts, 2013–2014. Public Health Rep. 2016;131(5):671–5.
65. CDC/NCHS, National Vital Statistics System, Mortality. CDC WONDER. Atlanta: US Department of Health and Human Services, CDC; 2018.

Chapter 2
Alcohol and Sedative Use Disorders and Related Emergencies

Curtis Wittmann, Abigail L. Donovan, and Mladen Nisavic

Introduction

Physical and psychiatric sequelae from alcohol and sedative use disorders are common factors in many ED presentations [1]. In the United States in 2016, 136.7 million people (50.7% of the adult population) were current alcohol users, and 16.3 million people (6% of the adult population) met criteria for an alcohol use disorder (AUD) [2]. The 12-month prevalence for an AUD was 13.9%, and the lifetime prevalence was 29.1% [3]. The high prevalence of AUDs has a significant impact on the emergency healthcare system. Between 2006 and 2014, the number of ED visits involving alcohol use increased by 61.6%, with an estimated annual cost of 15.3 billion dollars [4]. Acute alcohol intoxication is an important factor in accidents, exposure to violence, and self-harm, in addition to representing a potential medical emergency itself. Chronic alcohol use is associated with a range of medical and

C. Wittmann
Massachusetts General Hospital, Department of Psychiatry, Boston, MA, USA

Harvard Medical School, Boston, MA, USA

Acute Psychiatry Service, Massachusetts General Hospital, Boston, MA, USA

A. L. Donovan (✉)
Massachusetts General Hospital, Department of Psychiatry, Boston, MA, USA

First Episode and Early Psychosis Program, Massachusetts General Hospital, Department of Psychiatry, Boston, MA, USA

Harvard Medical School, Boston, MA, USA

Acute Psychiatry Service, Massachusetts General Hospital, Boston, MA, USA
e-mail: aldonovan@partners.org

M. Nisavic
Massachusetts General Hospital, Department of Psychiatry, Boston, MA, USA

Harvard Medical School, Boston, MA, USA

A. L. Donovan, S. A. Bird (eds.), *Substance Use and the Acute Psychiatric Patient*, Current Clinical Psychiatry, https://doi.org/10.1007/978-3-319-23961-3_2

psychiatric illnesses, including other substance use disorders, mood disorders, anxiety disorders, heart disease, liver disease, and malnutrition. Alcohol is the leading risk factor for premature death and disability among people aged 15–49 years worldwide [5]. In addition, withdrawal from alcohol or sedatives can be a medical emergency with significant morbidity and mortality. At least half of all patients with an AUD will experience alcohol withdrawal, and more severe complications, such as seizures or alcohol withdrawal delirium (delirium tremens), may occur in 3–5% of those patients [6]. Withdrawal is a potentially lethal condition, and, historically, mortality rates were as high as 35% in patients with alcohol withdrawal delirium [7]. Mortality from alcohol withdrawal delirium has decreased markedly since aggressive management with benzodiazepine replacement and intensive medical care have become standard, and current mortality is approximately 1–4% [7].

Alcohol has effects on multiple neurotransmitter systems within the central nervous system (CNS), including GABA (the major inhibitory neurotransmitter) and glutamate (the major excitatory neurotransmitter). Alcohol is a GABA agonist, causing CNS depressant effects, including behavioral disinhibition. Chronic use causes brain changes in response to excessive and ongoing GABA activation, including a decrease in GABA receptors, decreased GABA production, and decreased binding affinity to the GABA receptor complex. Alcohol also inhibits glutamate N-methyl-D-aspartate (NMDA) receptors, and chronic alcohol use leads to upregulation of these receptors. In withdrawal, the sudden decrease in GABA agonism and the increased endogenous glutaminergic tone are largely responsible for the development of complicated alcohol withdrawal [8–10].

Alcohol use is a major source of healthcare and societal expenditures both directly (i.e., costs related to the management of the alcohol use disorder) and indirectly (costs related to comorbid medical illnesses and accidents occurring while intoxicated). In 2010, the total national cost of excessive alcohol use was 249 billion dollars, exceeding the 2010 estimated national cost of depression of 210 billion dollars [11]. The majority of this expense was attributable to the economic consequences of binge drinking, largely due to lost workplace productivity. Medical expenses related to excessive alcohol use accounted for roughly 28 billion dollars [11]. In the United States in 2005, 65,000 deaths, over 1 million years of life lost, and over 3.5 million disability-adjusted life years were attributable to AUDs [12]. There are additional societal costs due to lost employment, frayed relationships, and disengagement from social and civic life that are much more difficult to measure but are nevertheless very important consequences of these disorders.

Sedative use disorders have many similarities to AUDs but are a less common cause of ED presentations. Sedatives are a diverse class of drugs, including benzodiazepines and barbiturates, with the final common effect of inducing sedation. Benzodiazepines, given their relatively high frequency of misuse, will be the primary focus of this chapter's discussion of sedative use disorders. There is significant overlap in the physiological effects of alcohol and benzodiazepines but also important differences in the risk of toxicity and associated medical comorbidities. Benzodiazepines also act via GABA agonism and have parallel effects as alcohol. Benzodiazepines are used non-medically by 2.3% of the US population annually, and 9.8% of this group meets diagnostic criteria for a benzodiazepine use disorder [13]. Benzodiazepine use disorders also represent a unique diagnostic challenge since many patients have active prescriptions for benzodiazepines and toxicology screening often fails to identify which benzodiazepine (the prescribed agent or another) was used by the patient. Barbiturates and other benzodiazepine receptor agonists, such as zolpidem, are also potential drugs of abuse, though both are misused less frequently than either alcohol or benzodiazepines. Barbiturates have historically been more associated with respiratory depression, compared to alcohol or benzodiazepines.

Most of the co-occurring psychiatric disorders associated with alcohol and sedative use disorders are discussed in detail elsewhere within this book; however, it is important to describe briefly some of the most notable connections between alcohol and sedative use and psychiatric illness. In addition to other substance use disorders, alcohol and sedative use disorders can play an important role in the course of many other psychiatric conditions, including anxiety, mood, psychotic, post-traumatic stress, and personality disorders. Having an AUD doubles the risk of having a major depressive disorder [14]. Among people with an AUD, the lifetime prevalence of any anxiety disorder is 47%, another drug use disorder is 43%, and any affective disorder is 41% [15]. AUD is also highly comorbid with PTSD, with rates as high as 41.8% being reported [16]. In addition, the presence of an alcohol or sedative use disorder can exacerbate the symptom severity of comorbid psychiatric disorders and make the underlying condition more challenging to treat. Reasons for this phenomenon include medication non-adherence, impaired efficacy of medication (even when taken correctly), and the potential social consequences of use, including decreased availability of social supports and financial resources. Alcohol and sedative use disorders are also important risk factors for both suicide [17, 18] and violence. Patients with AUDs have a six times higher rate of suicide than the baseline population, and, in one recent US study, alcohol was detected in nearly 36% of men and 28% of women who committed suicide [18].

Caring for ED patients with alcohol and sedative use disorders can be challenging due to a number of factors, including complex comorbid illnesses with significant mortality, limited resources for treatment and disposition, and negative feelings that may arise in both patients and providers from repeated ED presentations. Given these circumstances, a sophisticated understanding of alcohol's and sedatives' effects, associated medical and psychiatric issues, and recommended treatment options is essential for safely treating patients suffering from alcohol- and sedative-related illnesses.

Emergency Department Presentation

Patients with alcohol and/or sedative intoxication can have a variety of clinical presentations, depending on when and how much of the substance was consumed and the tolerance of the patient. Common signs and symptoms of alcohol intoxication include slurred speech, impaired cognition, impaired decision making, impaired balance and coordination (creating a fall risk), and disinhibition (increasing the risk of aggression and agitation). Patients who use alcohol chronically may develop significant tolerance and may not exhibit obvious signs of intoxication until higher blood alcohol levels. Patients can present with alcoholic hallucinosis, a condition marked by primarily auditory or visual hallucinations or paranoia. Alcoholic hallucinosis is most commonly seen with reduction of use or during early withdrawal, but it can also occur in the severely intoxicated patient following a prolonged period of heavy drinking. The clinical presentation of sedative intoxication is very similar to alcohol intoxication, but may also include excessive sedation, depending on the specific drug ingested, its half-life, and the total amount ingested.

Patients may also present to the ED with alcohol or sedative withdrawal syndromes, including a wide variety of symptoms mediated by excess rebound activation of the sympathetic nervous system. This activation is related to the imbalance between excessive GABA signaling caused by heavy drinking, countered by increased glutamatergic tone, and the presence of other excitatory neurotransmitters, such as norepinephrine and dopamine, which are then unopposed when alcohol intake is stopped. In early stages of withdrawal, anxiety is a prominent feature and may be accompanied by mild tremulousness and physical discomfort, including headaches and nausea. As the withdrawal syndrome progresses, vital sign abnormalities, such as tachycardia and hypertension, and physical signs, such as diaphoresis and coarse tremor, arise. If untreated, alcohol or sedative withdrawal may progress to severe withdrawal delirium, also called delirium tremens (DTs) with confusion, hallucinations, and inattention. This illness occurs in roughly 3–5% of patients admitted to a hospital for alcohol withdrawal [19], and it is defined by the presence of both alcohol withdrawal and delirium in a patient who recently stopped drinking. It is important to monitor the intoxicated patient's mental status, vital signs, and physical exam for findings of withdrawal and not to dismiss odd behavior as merely the product of intoxication. Any sign of impaired attention, awareness, memory, or orientation, autonomic instability, or the onset of hallucinations should prompt immediate consideration for alcohol withdrawal delirium. Alcohol withdrawal delirium typically occurs within 3 days of cessation of alcohol use and can last from 1 to 8 days [19] with mortality rates of 1–4% [7]. Patients with DTs require intensive medical monitoring and treatment, with aggressive management of alcohol withdrawal, and attention to rehydration and correction of nutritional deficiencies.

In addition to acute intoxication or withdrawal, many alcohol- or sedative-using patients present to the ED for other ostensible causes, and it is only through careful history taking that the contributory role of alcohol or sedatives is revealed. Specific examples include trauma (car accidents, assaults), accidents (falls), anxiety or panic attacks, insomnia or depression, gastrointestinal bleeding, liver failure, cardiac complications, or problems associated with use of other substances.

Medical Evaluation

A thorough medical evaluation is required for all patients with alcohol or sedative use disorders presenting to the ED, including history of presenting illness, review of systems, and physical examination. Alcohol and sedative use disorders increase the risk for a variety of medical problems, as well as physical trauma. Obtaining an accurate history may be difficult when patients present with an altered level of consciousness, making a careful physical exam, including vital signs, essential. Patients who are "found down" may require head imaging if there is concern for head trauma or if an altered level of consciousness does not improve over time. Medical evaluation of the patient with an alcohol-related presentation should assess for evidence suggesting chronic alcohol use, such as signs of liver failure, cardiac abnormalities, nutritional deficiency (including thiamine, folate, fat-soluble vitamins, B12), gastrointestinal bleeding, peripheral neuropathy, as well as any signs of trauma. Patients suspected of chronic alcohol use are at high risk for multiple vitamin deficiencies. They should receive IV thiamine to decrease the risk of Wernicke's encephalopathy and a multivitamin and folic acid to address other consequences of poor nutrition. Optimal dosing of thiamine remains poorly defined, but at least 100 mg should be provided IM or IV three times a day for the first 3 days of treatment before transitioning to an oral regimen [20].

Chronic alcohol use increases the likelihood of multiple medical conditions, including serious cardiovascular, hematologic, and gastrointestinal illnesses. Particularly for patients who are unable to provide a reliable review of systems, laboratory evaluation assists with screening for the presence of these conditions. Liver function tests may reveal transaminitis; PT/PTT may reveal signs of synthetic dysfunction; a CBC may reveal anemia, neutropenia, or thrombocytopenia; and a metabolic panel may reveal numerous abnormalities including hyponatremia, hypokalemia, and an elevated anion gap. Obtaining a patient's blood alcohol level, either through a breathalyzer or serum level, can provide information about how much alcohol someone has ingested and the current level of intoxication, although patients who regularly use large amounts of alcohol may appear clinically sober despite elevated serum alcohol levels. In the United States, an alcohol level of 80 mg/dl corresponds with "legal" intoxication (meaning it is not legal to drive a vehicle at or above this level), and, in many patients, levels above 400 mg/dl may lead to coma and even death [21]. However, patients with chronic alcohol use may present to the ED with levels as high as 700 mg/dl and, in very rare cases, even higher. At levels between these extremes, such as 200 or 300 mg/dl, the clinical presentation depends on multiple factors including the history of use and tolerance, but these levels are typically associated with decreased coordination, depressed level of consciousness, slurred speech, impaired judgment, and distorted perception. While the presence of an elevated alcohol level may confirm the diagnosis of alcohol intoxication, a negative test is important as well, because it signals the need to broaden the differential diagnosis of altered mental status and consider other etiologies, such as intoxication from a different substance, trauma, infection, stroke, and sepsis. Quantitative benzodiazepine levels are rarely useful, although detecting their absolute presence or absence through a urine toxicology screen can be helpful. It is appropriate to obtain a urine toxicology screen when there is concern that other substances, such as opioids, may be contributing to a clinical presentation.

Occult alcohol or sedative use should be considered even in patients who present to the ED for other reasons, as patients may omit or minimize information about their use. A careful screening history, physical examination, and review of available laboratory studies allow clinicians both to detect and discuss this possibility with patients in a neutral and non-judgmental manner and to monitor and treat potential alcohol or sedative withdrawal during the ED visit. Despite providers' best efforts, some patients' alcohol or sedative use history will be missed by or hidden from the ED treatment team. Thus, alcohol and sedative withdrawal should be high on any differential diagnosis for a patient who develops an acute change in vital signs, in addition to other signs of alcohol or sedative withdrawal, such as diaphoresis, anxiety, tremulousness, or seizures.

Psychiatric Evaluation

In addition to a thorough medical assessment, the initial emergency evaluation of the intoxicated patient should include an assessment of the risk for harm to self and others. Patients presenting with intoxication from alcohol or sedatives may experience acute dysphoria and suicidality, which can impact their ability to be safe in the ED. All patients presenting with intoxication, and particularly those with a history of prior suicidality or psychiatric illness, should be screened for current suicide risk. It is difficult to predict which patients may become behaviorally dysregulated based on the degree of intoxication alone, but any patient who exhibits impaired judgment and coordination should be considered potentially at risk for agitation and/or aggression.

In addition to an early assessment of safety risks, many patients with alcohol or sedative use will benefit from a more thorough psychiatric assessment during their ED visit, particularly those with co-occurring depression, anxiety, or other psychiatric conditions. Psychiatric consultation can be helpful to ED management when there is psychiatric comorbidity, particularly if acute safety concerns are identified or when the psychiatric symptom burden is significant and clearly impairing function. Whether performed by a primary clinician, a consulting service, or both, the psychiatric evaluation should include a thorough substance use history for all substances used by the patient, including duration of use; pattern of use; details regarding most recent use; history of extended periods of past sobriety and how they were attained; history of withdrawal and complicated withdrawal (e.g., seizure or delirium tremens); social losses related to use (e.g., job loss, relationship difficulties, legal difficulties); psychiatric complications related to use, including anxiety, depression, and psychosis; and history of suicidality or violence related to, or co-occurring with, substance use. It is always helpful to assess patients' strengths, including social and treatment supports, such as friends, family, and outpatient providers, as well as motivation for treatment. This assessment should ideally include collateral information from family members and/or treaters, given that patients may be unable or unwilling to clearly report the details and consequences of their own substance use. Although some pertinent information may be obtained while a patient is still intoxicated, critical portions, particularly a definitive assessment of safety issues, need to be completed when the patient is clinically sober.

Both the psychiatric and medical evaluation of the ED patient using alcohol or sedatives should also include an assessment of risk factors for severe alcohol or sedative withdrawal. Risk factors for severe alcohol withdrawal include history of previous alcohol withdrawal, history of complicated withdrawal (i.e., alcohol withdrawal complicated by seizures or delirium tremens), and heavy recent alcohol use, as measured by a blood alcohol level above 200 mg/dl [22]. The Prediction of Alcohol Withdrawal Severity Scale (PAWSS) [22] can be helpful in identifying high-risk patients (see Table 2.1).

Risk factors for benzodiazepine withdrawal similarly include higher frequency, duration, and intensity of use, although a specific threshold for use is unknown. Regular use of benzodiazepines with shorter half-lives, such as lorazepam and alprazolam, is likely to lead to withdrawal symptoms earlier after discontinuation, compared to agents with longer half-lives, such as diazepam. There is a higher risk for withdrawal seizures related to benzodiazepine use compared to alcohol. Considering such risk factors is important in determining a patient's risk for withdrawal, but accurate assessment can be challenging, particularly during the early period of a patient's ED visit. Intoxication may preclude a patient from providing an accurate history and, at severe levels of impairment, may even prevent an accurate determination of the patient's identity, limiting the use of prior medical records or collateral sources of history to establish these facts. Patients often underreport the amount of alcohol or sedatives they use, as well as minimize symptoms or social consequences associated with use. This common occurrence may be due to incor-

Table 2.1 Prediction of Alcohol Withdrawal Severity Scale (PAWSS)

Part A: Threshold criteria	(1 point either)
1. Have you consumed any amount of alcohol (i.e., been drinking) within the last 30 days? Or did the patient have a "+" BAL upon admission? *If* the answer to either is *yes*, proceed with test:	______
Part B: Based on patient interview	(1 point each)
2. Have you ever experienced previous episodes of alcohol withdrawal?	______
3. Have you ever experienced alcohol withdrawal seizures?	______
4. Have you ever experienced delirium tremens or DTs?	______
5. Have you ever undergone alcohol rehabilitation treatment?	______
6. Have you ever experienced blackouts?	
7. Have you combined alcohol with other "downers" like benzodiazepines or barbiturates during the last 90 days?	______
8. Have you combined alcohol with any other substance of abuse during the last 90 days?	______
Part C: Based on clinical evidence (1 point each)	
9. Was the patient's blood alcohol level (BAL) on presentation >200?	______
10. Is there evidence of increased autonomic activity? (e.g., HR >120 bpm, tremor, sweating, agitation, nausea)	______

Notes: Maximum score = 10. This instrument is intended as a screening tool. The greater the number of positive findings, the higher the risk for the development of alcohol withdrawal syndromes (AWS). A score of greater than or equal to 4 suggests *high risk* for moderate to severe AWS: prophylaxis and/or treatment may be indicated

rect recollection, denial, or a deliberate attempt to obfuscate use patterns that are associated with social disapprobation. Obtaining collateral information from any available sources (e.g., primary care physicians, medical records, family members, friends, etc.), within the bounds of HIPAA and confidentiality, can be critical for safe clinical management.

As noted above, alcohol and sedative use disorders often occur with other psychiatric conditions, and acute complaints of depression, anxiety, or psychosis are common in ED patients. Psychiatric consultation to assess these symptoms can occur in the context of clearly identified intoxication or withdrawal states or in the absence of any known substance use, as in the case of an occult alcohol or sedative use disorder. Collateral information and history regarding the onset and course of psychiatric symptoms relative to periods of substance use and sobriety are helpful in determining whether patients meet criteria for primary vs. substance-induced diagnoses. For example, although depressive episodes are common in patients with AUD, less than one-half of these represent primary major depression observed outside the context of active drinking and intoxication [6].

A key component of the psychiatric evaluation is the risk assessment. Alcohol and sedative use have a significant impact on a patient's risk for both self-harm and violence. The increased risk for self-harm appears to be true both for patients who have an AUD and for patients who do not meet criteria for an AUD, but who engage in binge drinking. In the latter group, acute intoxication likely decreases behavioral control over negative impulses or self-destructive thoughts, including suicidal ideation. Patients with active AUDs have an increased rate of both suicide attempts and completions, and the suicide rate for patients with AUDs is as high as six times the baseline population rate [17, 18]. This finding may be mediated by an increased risk for mood disorders or mood episodes or may be attributable to more direct effects on mental status, such as behavioral disinhibition and/or impaired judgment during states of intoxication. Numerous studies have documented a link between acute alcohol use and suicidal behavior with widely varying estimates of co-occurrence. A recent study attempted to determine the increase in suicide attempt risk by dose of alcohol and determined that each alcoholic drink resulted in a relative risk of 1.3, suggesting a 30% increased risk of a suicide attempt with each drink [23]. Though there is less evidence related to benzodiazepine use and suicide risk, a recent review of 17 studies found that, in the majority, there was an increased risk for suicide in patients who were prescribed benzodiazepines. Further research is needed to better understand this relationship and clarify whether it also applies to patients who are using illicit benzodiazepines [24].

An accurate safety assessment must be completed when the alcohol- or sedative-using patient is clinically sober. Mood, cognition, and suicidal symptoms often differ significantly during the intoxicated vs. sober state, as does the patient's ability and/or willingness to provide an accurate report of current suicidal ideation or other risk factors. Of note, some patients are more willing to disclose suicidal thinking when intoxicated and may appear more guarded upon sobering; therefore, suicidal statements made while intoxicated should not be ignored, but must be carefully evaluated within the clinical context and reassessed over time. Obtaining collateral information whenever possible is critical to verify a patient's report; gain a clearer understanding of recent symptoms, functioning, and safety; and determine disposition.

Management of Alcohol and Sedative Intoxication

Acute intoxication leading to an ED presentation generally requires close monitoring. The most significant medical complications of acute alcohol or sedative intoxication overlap significantly and include traumatic falls, over-sedation, and respiratory depression, as well as the risk of alcohol or sedative withdrawal. Patients should be assessed for their ability to walk during the physical examination, and, if they are unsteady, they should be placed on fall precautions. Level of consciousness should be assessed, and patients who are obtunded need close monitoring. Benzodiazepine overdose has a higher risk of respiratory depression and arrest when compared to alcohol and requires close monitoring. There is an available reversal agent, flumazenil, that antagonizes benzodiazepines; however, given the severity and frequency of adverse events associated with flumazenil (including seizures and arrhythmias), there are very limited circumstances when using this agent would be preferable to intubation and supportive management.

Some patients may present with agitation in the setting of intoxication (or withdrawal), putting themselves and others at imminent risk of injury. Attempts to prevent agitation, such as placing the patient in a low-stimulation environment, verbal de-escalation, addressing physical comfort, and offering medication when appropriate, are critical. Patients who escalate despite such interventions may require mechanical restraints to protect themselves and others, as well as consideration of emergency medication to assist with regaining behavioral control. Antipsychotic medications can help to decrease rage, fear, and agitation. Haloperidol is largely preferred due to less sedation and a long history of safe and effective use in the ED. In the setting of suspected or known alcohol or benzodiazepine intoxication, administering additional benzodiazepines to manage isolated agitation should generally be avoided, given that both agents bind to GABA receptors which are likely fully saturated during periods of intoxication. Giving additional benzodiazepines will not improve behavior and may cause unwanted respiratory suppression. It is also important to be aware that as intoxication wanes and risk of withdrawal increases, vital signs and assessment for emerging signs of withdrawal should be monitored at regular intervals.

The risk for self-destructive or suicidal behavior is markedly increased in the setting of alcohol or sedative intoxication. Patients who are identified as being at increased risk for immediate self-harm should be placed on suicide precautions, including, but not limited to, placement in a safe space devoid of dangerous objects or environmental hazards (such as ligature points), constant observation from a clinical monitor, and removal of personal belongings (which could contain weapons or additional substances). Additional safety interventions can also be implemented depending on the needs of the specific patient, any history of self-harm, and current clinical presentation. These interventions may include a higher level of monitoring for patients who have attempted to harm themselves in healthcare settings previously or additional security presence for patients who have a known history of aggression or violence during previous ED encounters. Patient-specific acute care plans can be helpful in guiding safe care of such high-risk patients.

Management of Alcohol and Benzodiazepine Withdrawal

Acute alcohol withdrawal occurs in the setting of chronic alcohol use with abrupt discontinuation. History of prior withdrawal, including complicated withdrawal, delirium, and seizures, carries the highest risk for reemergence of withdrawal complications, as does history of heavy, sustained alcohol use for prolonged periods of time (weeks to months or longer). The exact amount and duration of alcohol use resulting in withdrawal symptoms upon discontinuation vary significantly from person to person and cannot reliably predict risk. Likewise, blood alcohol level on admission may offer some sense of withdrawal risk, but may not reliably predict complications – in fact, even at relatively high but decreasing blood alcohol levels, chronic alcohol users may experience symptoms of withdrawal.

Alcohol withdrawal is commonly associated with signs of adrenergic excess, such as elevated heart rate or blood pressure, diaphoresis, tremor, and anxiety (see Table 2.2). Withdrawal symptoms usually begin between 6 and 24 hours after a patient's last drink, and anxiety and irritability are initially most prominent. These symptoms then progress to changes in the autonomic nervous system, including

Table 2.2 *Diagnostic and Statistical Manual of Mental Disorders,* Fifth Edition (DSM-5), criteria for alcohol withdrawal syndrome [6]

A. Cessation of or reduction in alcohol intake, which has previously been prolonged/heavy
B. Criterion A, plus any two of the following symptoms developing within several hours to a few days:
Autonomic hyperactivity
Worsening tremor
Insomnia
Vomiting and nausea
Hallucinations
Psychomotor agitation
Anxiety
Generalized tonic-clonic seizures
C. The above symptoms cause clinically significant distress or impairment in social, occupational, or other important areas of functioning
D. The above symptoms are not attributable to other causes, for example, another mental disorder, intoxication, or withdrawal from another substance
Specify if hallucinations (usually visual or tactile) occur with intact reality testing or if auditory, visual, or tactile illusions occur in the absence of a delirium

elevated heart rate and blood pressure, tremulousness, and nausea. Cardiac arrhythmias of several different types may also occur during this phase. Alcohol withdrawal seizures most commonly occur between 24 and 48 hours after cessation of alcohol use and are best addressed by benzodiazepine replacement rather than antiepileptic medication. Finally, alcohol withdrawal delirium, marked by disorientation, confusion, and hallucinations, most commonly occurs between 24 and 72 hours after cessation of alcohol use. This timeline can help distinguish withdrawal delirium from alcoholic hallucinosis, which typically occurs 12–24 hours after stopping drinking and resolves within 48 hours. In addition, alcoholic hallucinosis is not accompanied by clouding of sensorium, and vital sign abnormalities are uncommon. No specific symptom constellation is pathognomonic for alcohol withdrawal, and it is critical to consider alternative explanations of symptoms in individuals at risk for withdrawal (e.g., non-adherence with anti-hypertensive medications causing increased blood pressure or dehydration causing tachycardia); however, when taken in concert with a patient's alcohol use history and clinical presentation, alcohol withdrawal should be easily recognized. Some patients may exaggerate common symptoms of withdrawal, such as tremor in the extremities, in order to obtain medication (especially benzodiazepines). In cases when such behavior is suspected, objective signs, including elevated vital signs and physical findings that are hard to feign, such as tongue fasciculations, can be useful for corroborating that a patient is in true withdrawal.

Alcohol withdrawal is treated with benzodiazepines and may be managed either with a fixed-dose approach or a symptom-triggered model. A symptom-triggered approach is often guided by the use of a structured tool, such as the Clinical Institute Withdrawal Assessment for Alcohol – Revised (CIWA-AR) (see Table 2.3).

The CIWA scale is an evidence-based tool, which is not copyrighted and may be reproduced freely. It is designed to be administered at regular intervals by nursing staff to quantify the presence of signs and symptoms of alcohol withdrawal. The CIWA can be administered in approximately 5 minutes and consists of ten areas of questions. The total score is placed into an algorithm to determine appropriate benzodiazepine dosing. The maximum score is 67, and patients scoring less than 10 do not usually need additional medication for withdrawal [25]. The use of a structured instrument standardizes the treatment of withdrawal, minimizing the risk of over- or undertreating patients. Using the CIWA for a symptom-triggered protocol can significantly improve the care of patients in withdrawal, including using a smaller total benzodiazepine dose [26] and decreasing ED length of stay [27]. An alternative, fixed-dose approach attempts to estimate, based on the degree of alcohol or benzodiazepine use, how much benzodiazepine replacement a patient will require. After the benzodiazepine requirement has become clear over the first 24 hours, the total dose can then be gradually decreased and divided regularly throughout the day. The advantage of this approach is its simplicity for management; however, there is a risk of over- or underdosing the amount required, and close monitoring is necessary to ensure that withdrawal is being adequately managed. There is a version of the CIWA designed for use in benzodiazepine withdrawal, but it has not been as extensively evaluated.

Even in the absence of a structured rating scale, it is critical that patients at risk for alcohol or sedative withdrawal have close medical monitoring, with regular

Table 2.3 CIWA-AR [25]

Nausea and vomiting **Ask: "Do you feel sick to your stomach? Have you vomited?"** **Observation** 0 no nausea and no vomiting 1 mild nausea with no vomiting 2 3 4 intermittent nausea with dry heaves 5 6 7 constant nausea, frequent dry heaves, and vomiting	*Tactile disturbances* **Ask: "Do you have any itching, pins-and-needles sensations, burning, or numbness; or do you feel bugs crawling on/ under your skin?"** **Observation** 0 none 1 very mild itching, pins and needles, burning, or numbness 2 mild itching, pins and needles, burning, or numbness 3 moderate itching, pins and needles, burning, or numbness 4 moderately severe hallucinations 5 severe hallucinations 6 extremely severe hallucinations 7 continuous hallucinations
Tremor **Arms extended and fingers spread apart** **Observation** 0 no tremor 1 not visible, but can be felt fingertip to fingertip 2 3 4 moderate with patient's arms extended 5 6 7 severe, even with arms not extended	*Auditory disturbances* **Ask: "Are you more aware of sounds around you? Are they harsh? Do they frighten you? Are you hearing anything that is disturbing to you? Are you hearing things you know are not there?"** **Observation** 0 not present 1 very mild harshness or ability to frighten 2 mild harshness or ability to frighten 3 moderate harshness or ability to frighten 4 moderately severe hallucinations 5 severe hallucinations 6 extremely severe hallucinations 7 continuous hallucinations
Paroxysmal sweats **Observation** 0 no sweat visible 1 barely perceptible sweating, palms moist 2 3 4 beads of sweat obvious on forehead 5 6 7 drenching sweats	*Visual disturbances* **Ask: "Does the light appear to be too bright? Is its color different? Does it hurt your eyes? Are you seeing anything that is disturbing to you? Are you seeing things you know are not there?"** **Observation** 0 not present 1 very mild sensitivity 2 mild sensitivity 3 moderate sensitivity 4 moderately severe hallucinations 5 severe hallucinations 6 extremely severe hallucinations 7 continuous hallucinations

Table 2.3 (continued)

Anxiety **Ask: "Do you feel nervous?"** **Observation** 0 no anxiety, at ease 1 mildly anxious 2 3 4 moderately anxious or guarded, so anxiety is inferred 5 6 7 equivalent to acute panic state as seen in severe delirium or acute schizophrenic reaction	***Headache, fullness in head*** **Ask: "Does your head feel different? Does it feel like there is a band around your head?" Do not rate for dizziness or lightheadedness. Otherwise, rate severity.** 0 not present 1 very mild 2 mild 3 moderate 4 moderately severe 5 severe 6 very severe 7 extremely severe
Agitation **Observation** 0 normal activity 1 somewhat more than normal activity 2 3 4 moderately fidgety and restless 5 6 7 paces back and forth during most of the interview or constantly thrashes about	***Orientation and clouding of sensorium*** **Ask: "What day is this? Where are you? Who am I?"** 0 oriented and can do serial additions* 1 cannot do serial additions or is uncertain about date 2 disoriented for date by no more than 2 calendar days 3 disoriented for date by more than 2 calendar days 4 disoriented for place and/or person *Serial additions: Ask patient to add by 7s

clinical assessments at least every 2 hours, including vital signs. Typically, ED nursing staff performs these evaluations; and it is imperative that even subtle abnormalities, such as anxiety, tremor, or diaphoresis, are communicated to the ED provider. Given the significant risks associated with undertreatment, which include seizures, cardiac arrhythmias, and DTs, it is far better to begin treatment for withdrawal early, than to miss evidence of early withdrawal, delay treatment, and fall behind in management.

Numerous medications can be safely used to treat alcohol withdrawal, but benzodiazepines are the most widely used class, due in large part to the relative ease and safety of their use, efficacy, and wide range of available agents, with varying pharmacologic characteristics. Both alcohol and benzodiazepines primarily affect the GABA system, and, due to cross-reactivity, any benzodiazepine can be used to treat alcohol withdrawal. The most frequently used benzodiazepines include diazepam, lorazepam, chlordiazepoxide, and oxazepam. Each differs in terms of time of onset of action, elimination half-life, available formulations, and metabolism (see Table 2.4). Clinical decision making about which agent to use is based on these pharmacologic factors. For example, lorazepam or diazepam may be used when rapid onset of action

Table 2.4 Benzodiazepines

Agent	Half-life	Metabolism	Onset of action	Formulations
Lorazepam	12–14 hours	Renal	Rapid	PO/IM/IV
Diazepam	48 hours	Renal, hepatic	Rapid	PO/IM/IV
Chlordiazepoxide	48 hours (with metabolites)	Renal, hepatic	Slow	PO/IM
Oxazepam	~8 hours	Renal	Moderate	PO

is needed, lorazepam or oxazepam may be chosen when a patient's liver function is impaired, or chlordiazepoxide or diazepam may be given when there is clinical need for a long-acting agent.

There are several specific factors favoring the use of lorazepam in the ED management of alcohol withdrawal. Lorazepam can be administered orally, sublingually, intravenously, or intramuscularly, allowing for use when a patient may not be able to accept oral medications, when onset of action needs to be extremely rapid, or when a patient may be refusing treatment in the setting of delirium or agitation. Its metabolism is extra-hepatic, and it has no active metabolites, making it useful for patients with impaired hepatic function or when the status of hepatic function is unknown. It also has a relatively short half-life of 12–14 hours, which has both advantages and disadvantages. A shorter half-life decreases risk of over-sedation, and, in the case of excessive administration, adverse effects will wear off more quickly than with longer-acting agents. However, because the ED setting is often overburdened and provider resources may be stretched thin, this short half-life can also be problematic. A short half-life requires more frequent administration of medication, and in the absence of close monitoring between doses, withdrawal symptoms may reemerge and go unnoticed, with the risk of withdrawal progressing to an advanced state.

Diazepam, routinely used to manage alcohol withdrawal in the ED, has its own potential advantages and disadvantages. Like lorazepam, there are oral, intravenous, and intramuscular formulations of diazepam. Diazepam has a relatively rapid onset of action, which is valuable when a patient acutely develops severe alcohol withdrawal. However, unlike lorazepam, diazepam has a long half-life of approximately 48 hours, and active metabolites extend this half-life even further. Historically, in ED practice, diazepam was administered to patients leaving the ED without further treatment or even to those staying in the ED, for longer-term protection against reemerging alcohol withdrawal. While there is an intuitive appeal in using an agent in this way, a long half-life does not guarantee that a patient will be adequately treated by the first dose administered, nor does it negate the need for ongoing monitoring and management of withdrawal. Further, diazepam's long half-life can be a disadvantage if excessive medication is given. In this case, over-sedation, and other effects of benzodiazepine intoxication, may last for multiple days, potentially even requiring prolonged ED stay or medical admission.

Other benzodiazepines may also be used to manage withdrawal, including chlordiazepoxide. The advantages of chlordiazepoxide include a long half-life of up to 48 hours, similar to diazepam, which may allow for easier management of withdrawal when a patient is monitored closely. However, it is only available in an oral formulation, and its time to onset of action is significantly longer than lorazepam and diazepam. Therefore, it is a reasonable agent to use in the earliest stage of mild alcohol withdrawal, and, at times, it may even be used in a prophylactic manner, but it is a less optimal agent with moderate or severe alcohol withdrawal, given its time to onset of action.

While benzodiazepines remain the primary agent of choice for managing alcohol withdrawal, there are other classes of medication that can be effective. Barbiturates, specifically phenobarbital, were once a mainstay of treatment for alcohol withdrawal, but were supplanted for a variety of reasons, most prominently the benzodiazepines' favorable safety profile and ease of use. More recently, there has been a resurgence in the use of phenobarbital in the management of alcohol withdrawal, although phenobarbital has typically been used in settings outside of the emergency department, including inpatient medical and surgical services. There are notable advantages to using phenobarbital in inpatient services, including the opportunity for induction of treatment via a loading dose in high-risk patients to minimize or manage complicated withdrawal. While existing literature is heterogeneous, and only few emergency room-based studies are available, phenobarbital has been generally shown to be comparable in effectiveness to conventional benzodiazepine treatment. One small research study comparing phenobarbital to lorazepam for the management of moderate alcohol withdrawal in the ED found that both treatments had similar efficacy, length of stay, and admission rates [28]. Another small study suggested that phenobarbital might be superior to diazepam for patients already in severe alcohol withdrawal in the medical hospital [29]. While the overall effectiveness of the two medication classes appears comparable based on available data, there is some evidence to indicate that phenobarbital may offer a feasible alternative treatment choice in patients in the medical hospital with severe alcohol withdrawal who cannot tolerate and/or are refractory to benzodiazepine treatment [30]. Protocols for phenobarbital use in severe alcohol withdrawal have yet to be standardized, but an example approach is included in Table 2.5. This approach was developed in a large academic medical center with on-site respiratory therapy, ED pharmacy consultation, and available intensive care units. This protocol does not apply to withdrawing patients who are intubated.

Though phenobarbital remains a treatment option and may be necessary for some patients, there are disadvantages to starting phenobarbital in the ED. Patients receiving phenobarbital require intensive medical monitoring, including cardiac monitoring with continuous oxygen saturation measurement to monitor for respiratory suppression and the need for intubation. Phenobarbital should only be given to ED patients for whom medical admission is planned.

Insufficiently treated alcohol withdrawal can result in seizure activity in up to ~3% of patients. Generally, in the absence of clinical findings suggestive of another etiology, patients do not require imaging or further neurologic work-up if the history and presentation is consistent with alcohol withdrawal. Continued seizures after appropriate treatment of withdrawal necessitate consideration of a

Table 2.5 An approach to phenobarbital for management of severe alcohol withdrawal syndrome

For severe alcohol withdrawal syndrome **(for CIWA >15 plus two or more of the following: heart rate >110, SBP >140, diaphoresis, tongue fasciculations)**
Intravenous administration is only recommended for treatment of severe alcohol withdrawal syndrome
If patient has received <10 mg of lorazepam (or equivalent) in the last 2 hours:
Loading dose is 10 mg/kg (based on ideal body weight (IBW)) to a max of 650 mg, mixed in 100 mL of sodium chloride 0.9% and administered over 30 minutes
After 30 minutes, reassess, and if CIWA is < or = 15, proceed to PO maintenance taper over 6 days. If CIWA is >15, administer phenobarbital 130 mg IVP over 3 minutes
Notify respiratory therapy for repeated IV doses
After 30 minutes, reassess, and if CIWA is < or = 15, proceed to PO maintenance taper over 6 days. If CIWA is >15, administer phenobarbital 260 mg IVP over 5 minutes
After 30 minutes, reassess, and if CIWA >15, may repeat phenobarbital 260 mg IVP over 5 minutes
Stop at max dose of 20 mg/kg IBW and assess other delirium etiologies
If patient has received > or = 10 mg of lorazepam (or equivalent) in the last 2 hours:
Administer phenobarbital 130 mg IVP over 3 minutes
After 30 minutes, reassess, and if CIWA is < or = 15, proceed to PO maintenance taper over 6 days. If CIWA is >15, administer phenobarbital 260 mg IVP over 5 minutes
Notify respiratory therapy for repeated IV doses
After 30 minutes, reassess and if CIWA is < or = 15, proceed to PO maintenance taper over 6 days. If CIWA >15, may repeat phenobarbital 260 mg IVP over 5 minutes
Stop at max dose 20 mg/kg IBW and assess other delirium etiologies

broader differential diagnosis. Patients experiencing seizures in the setting of alcohol withdrawal do not require treatment with antiepileptic medication and are most properly managed with GABAergic agents, such as benzodiazepines or phenobarbital.

Withdrawal delirium is one of the most severe complications of untreated or insufficiently treated alcohol or benzodiazepine withdrawal. Alcohol withdrawal occurs in roughly 50% of people with an AUD who discontinue alcohol abruptly, and withdrawal delirium or seizures occur in roughly 3–5% of AUD patients experiencing withdrawal symptoms [19]. Alcohol withdrawal delirium is defined by the presence of delirium (an alteration in consciousness, attention, orientation, perception, cognition, and other cognitive domains) and the presence of alcohol withdrawal. Alcohol withdrawal delirium usually occurs approximately 3 days after cessation of alcohol use, with a typical duration of 2–3 days. 1–4% of patients who experience withdrawal delirium in a hospital setting die, typically from arrhythmias, hyperthermias, or complications from withdrawal seizures [7]. Treatment of withdrawal delirium generally takes place in an ICU setting. Patients require supportive care, including IV fluids, cardiac monitoring, and electrolyte repletion. The goal of light sedation should be achieved using benzodiazepine replacement therapy to keep the patient arousable, but calm. When patients are experiencing agitation or hallucinations, haloperidol, administered intramuscularly or intravenously, should be given. In cases when patients remain symptomatic or if haloperidol is contraindicated, additional agents, such as propofol or dexmedetomidine, may be used [19].

Nutritional deficiencies are common among patients with alcohol use disorders. Through a combination of poor absorption and limited nutritional intake during periods of heavy drinking, patients with severe AUD are at risk for medical complications secondary to malnutrition. Weight loss, muscle wasting, edema, and loss of hand strength are all possible indicators of malnutrition; and complaints of neuropathy, depression or other mood changes, sensory deficits (such as loss of position sense), glossitis, myelopathy, and hair loss are additional symptoms of vitamin deficiency that may require further assessment. The specific types of potential alcohol-related deficiencies can be broad, but early attention to possible deficiencies in thiamine, folate, and other B vitamins is the most critical. Patients with thiamine deficiency may not exhibit clinical signs until fairly late and, if not treated, may develop Wernicke-Korsakoff syndrome, a devastating and typically irreversible neurological condition marked by encephalopathy, gait ataxia, and nystagmus, as well as anterograde amnesia and confabulation. To prevent Wernicke's syndrome, alcohol-dependent patients should be treated with IV thiamine and PO folic acid during the course of their ED stay.

The clinical presentation of benzodiazepine withdrawal is very similar to alcohol withdrawal, typically including anxiety, diaphoresis, tachycardia, and other signs of adrenergic excess, although grand mal seizures occur more commonly than in patients with alcohol withdrawal, in as many as 20–30% of untreated patients. It is less clear how frequently delirium occurs in benzodiazepine withdrawal. There are no structured instruments for rating benzodiazepine withdrawal, but standard assessment protocols include frequent monitoring of vital signs and frequent patient assessments to evaluate for potential withdrawal. It is important to recognize that the time from last use to onset of withdrawal symptoms varies more widely with benzodiazepines, given the wide variability in the half-lives of different agents. Generally, agents with shorter half-lives tend to be associated with earlier onset of withdrawal syndromes, and agents with longer half-lives are associated with more delayed onset of withdrawal syndromes. It is important to note that with very long-half-life agents, such as diazepam or chlordiazepoxide, symptoms of withdrawal may not occur until 2–3 weeks after cessation. In general, withdrawal can be avoided by gradually tapering the dose that a patient is taking. Benzodiazepine withdrawal is managed by administering a sufficient dose of benzodiazepines to prevent or stop withdrawal symptoms and then proceeding with a gradual taper over multiple days. If it is possible to accurately quantify the daily amount of a patient's benzodiazepine use, it is reasonable to begin treatment for withdrawal by providing that dose on day 1 (or while in the ED) and then tapering over several days. There is generally significant cross-reactivity among different benzodiazepine medications (meaning that a patient who is using one benzodiazepine can be safely managed with a taper of a different benzodiazepine), but patients with mild withdrawal can also be treated with a gradual taper of the same agent that they have been using chronically. More severe benzodiazepine withdrawal is generally treated with a longer-acting agent [31], such as diazepam, which can initially be given IV and titrated for effective symptom control while optimally avoiding over-sedation or respiratory depression. Once withdrawal symptoms are controlled, the benzodiazepine dose should be slowly tapered to manage residual symptoms, which often last for weeks to months.

Provider Affect

Patients with substance use disorders may generate a range of challenging emotions within providers. Providers may believe that patients with alcohol and sedative use disorders (and other substance use disorders) are actively choosing to use substances and that they have, and should exercise, control over their use behavior. Due to the chronic and relapsing nature of substance use disorders, providers often see the same patients repeatedly presenting to the ED, with no sign of clinical improvement or even a worsening of their substance use disorder. These experiences can lead to caregiver fatigue and a nihilistic attitude about treatment. In addition, even typically polite individuals may become belligerent or frankly abusive when intoxicated, and such behaviors can engender frustration and anger within providers, who may then respond to patients with less interest in providing careful and compassionate treatment. Some patients recurrently present to the ED despite repeated referrals for outpatient treatment. Providers may come to know patients well through repeated visits, and treatment resources (such as detoxification, motivational interviewing, or other outpatient referrals) may cease to be provided, particularly when providers have been rebuffed numerous times and then assume patients are not interested in treatment. It is therefore essential that providers monitor their own feelings about patients and assess how their treatment recommendations may be influenced by these feelings. It is also useful to be aware of the reactions of other ED staff, both to monitor any impulses that may come from another provider's fatigue or other negative emotional states and to minimize the likelihood of a similar reaction in oneself. Particularly challenging cases can always benefit from peer consultation with professional colleagues and especially those with expertise in treating patients with SUDs.

Disposition

The immediate need for assessment and treatment of alcohol and sedative use disorders, particularly intoxication and withdrawal, is often the primary focus of ED providers, and, as described above, it is critical from the standpoint of minimizing medical risk. However, this essential initial treatment is only the beginning of a patient's treatment; while substantive long-term recovery work occurs after the ED visit, the foundation for that work can be set during a successful ED encounter. Management of acute intoxication and withdrawal provides a platform for further treatment that may include inpatient detoxification, residential rehabilitation, and ongoing outpatient care. Patients can engage in motivational interviewing to assess and/or increase their readiness for change. Patients can also receive critical education, provided in a non-judgmental way, about the physical and psychological consequences of their substance use. In addition, many EDs now employ people with lived experience with SUDs (e.g., recovery coaches) who can provide valuable peer support or interventions.

A patient's disposition from the ED is determined by numerous factors, including their medical stability, psychiatric stability, risk factors, willingness to engage in treatment, and availability of and access to treatments.

Patients with severe alcohol or benzodiazepine withdrawal may require medical admission, either for comorbid medical issues or for safe management of more severe or complicated withdrawal, including seizures, uncontrolled vital sign abnormalities, lack of response to or being unable to take oral medication, or withdrawal delirium. The presence of any of these conditions generally indicates the need for admission to a general hospital, rather than admission to a free-standing detoxification facility.

Another key factor in determining a patient's disposition is the psychiatric risk assessment. As previously discussed, patients with alcohol and sedative use disorders have an increased risk for harm to self and others. A psychiatric risk assessment should include an assessment of a patient's substance use; psychiatric symptoms; socioeconomic background; medical condition; suicidal, violent, or homicidal ideation; history of violence; and history of self-harm. Much of this information may be collected as soon as a patient is able to answer questions, but completion of the risk assessment, particularly questions about self-harm or harm to others, must be done when the patient is clinically sober. In difficult or unclear cases, contact with the patient's friends or family, as well as treaters, should inform the risk assessment. Patients with high risk of harm to self and/or others will likely require admission to a locked psychiatric unit so that their safety can be maintained while they are receiving intensive treatment.

In addition to increased risk of harm to self and others, acute alcohol or sedative intoxication can compromise self-care, raising concern about the patient's ability to remain safe in the community, secondary to impaired judgment or motor function. Evaluating the capacity for basic self-care is a distinctly different type of risk assessment than the assessment for violence or self-harm. It requires clinicians to evaluate patients' judgment and decision-making ability, as well as physical coordination (ability to safely ambulate or, when relevant, drive) in deciding if a patient is safe to leave the ED or even remain in the ED unmonitored. It is highly recommended that providers assess a patient's ability to walk steadily and to exhibit reasonable judgment, such as being able to describe a plan for transport to the patient's home or shelter, prior to discharge. For patients who lack ability or capacity in either domain, steps should be taken to ensure the patient does not leave the ED. In extreme circumstances, particularly for the grossly intoxicated patient insisting on discharge, providing adequate protection may require the use of physical restraints. While a patient's blood alcohol level provides some information that may be useful, the determination of a patient's sobriety or safety for discharge is a clinical one and should not be based on the lab value.

Most states allow for involuntary commitment to treatment for patients with suicidality and/or homicidality due to psychiatric illness. Most states also have statutes around the use of involuntary commitment for a primary substance use disorder (in the absence of another psychiatric disorder), although these vary more widely. While each jurisdiction's laws must be considered, a pattern of severe consequences related to substance use and a demonstrated inability or unwillingness to pursue or sustain treatment are essential elements in assessing the need for involuntary SUD treatment. ED providers will benefit from familiarity with the laws in their state of practice.

Most patients presenting to the ED with alcohol or sedative use disorders will not meet criteria for involuntary treatment. Patients may have limited motivation for longer-term substance use disorder treatment, but the ED encounter represents an important opportunity for interventions to achieve and maintain sobriety. Brief interventions that focus on motivational interviewing can increase the chance that a patient may be willing to accept referral for further substance use disorder treatment. Numerous studies have demonstrated that SBIRT (Screening, Brief Intervention, and Referral to Treatment) is effective in decreasing the short-term consequences of alcohol use, including decreased alcohol intake, lower ED utilization, and fewer physical injuries [32]. SBIRT typically takes between 5 and 10 minutes and is feasibly performed in the emergency setting. SBIRT starts with screening for a substance use disorder, which is then followed by a period of motivational interviewing and, for receptive patients, a referral to further treatment.

Multiple treatment options exist for patients who present to the ED seeking treatment for alcohol or sedative use disorders. Referral to an inpatient detoxification center (detox unit) is often necessary as a first step for patients presenting with evidence of physical dependence on alcohol or sedatives but not in need of inpatient medical admission to a general hospital. The capacity for managing comorbid SUDs or medical problems varies between facilities, and understanding potential limitations of various programs is critical to make safe referrals. Most detox facilities manage alcohol and sedative withdrawal by gradually tapering the total dose of benzodiazepines needed over a short course of several days. Typically, they also offer programming designed to increase a patient's readiness for change and abstinence from drinking or substance use. Typical inpatient detox programs do not have the ability to assess or manage comorbid psychiatric illnesses, such as depression or anxiety. The length of stay in these programs is generally less than a week, but they can often refer patients for long-term care when medically stable for discharge.

Rehabilitation programs (or residential settings) are a common referral from detoxification centers. It is theoretically possible for patients to go from an ED to a rehabilitation center, but this disposition is extremely uncommon, because rehabilitation programs do not have the capability to manage acute withdrawal. Rehabilitation programs are longer-stay facilities where patients may stay for weeks to months while maintaining sobriety and working to understand and manage their chronic alcohol or sedative use disorder. These programs may combine medication for co-occurring psychiatric illness, treatment groups focused on managing substance use, and sometimes traditional 12-step programs. There are a range of options for disposition at the end of this treatment, and what a patient chooses to do will vary based on resources available and treater recommendations.

Some ED patients may require treatment for both a substance use disorder and a co-occurring psychiatric condition. When there is severe psychiatric illness or concern for suicidality or homicidality, these patients should be referred to dual-diagnosis inpatient units. Factors suggestive of the need for dual diagnosis rather than detox admission include acute safety concerns or significant functional impairment related to the psychiatric condition (i.e., prominent suicidality, psychosis, aggression), significant depression, mania or anxiety, or clinical judgment that treatment of the primary psychiatric condition is essential in order to treat the substance use disorder successfully (e.g., a patient with untreated anxiety who is using excessive amounts of benzodiazepines or alcohol to "self-medicate").

Some ED patients may have less severe alcohol or sedative use disorders that may not necessitate a detoxification or inpatient dual-diagnosis treatment. These patients may be more appropriate for outpatient treatment, including partial hospital programs, intensive outpatient programs, and outpatient psychiatric or substance use disorder programs. The available resources are dictated by health insurance benefits, as well as program availability within the hospital and larger community. Intensive outpatient programs or partial hospitalization programs, which provide treatment for anywhere from a few hours to a full day, 2–5 days a week, are appropriate referrals for motivated patients who are unlikely to withdraw from alcohol or sedatives. These programs are typically focused on group psychotherapy work, stress management skills, and medication management for comorbid psychiatric disorders or for the primary substance use disorder, if appropriate. They are designed to assist patients in abstaining from substance use by identifying potential areas of vulnerability around relapse. They typically last 1–3 weeks and then transition patients into less-intensive outpatient modes of treatment. Follow-up referrals for ongoing care to an outpatient psychiatrist or substance use disorder specialist can be facilitated. This type of referral can be helpful if a patient is likely to need medications, either for co-occurring psychiatric illness or for assistance in abstinence. There are several medications that may be helpful in abstinence, although a complete review of these is beyond the scope of this chapter. Naltrexone, either as an injection or taken orally, as well as oral acamprosate, can decrease cravings in patients with alcohol use disorders. Disulfiram works differently by causing significant physical discomfort if a patient drinks after taking it, thus discouraging alcohol use.

One of the most prominent modes of treatment, familiar to both providers and patients, is 12-step programs; Alcoholics Anonymous is the most well-known of these programs. Patients often report reluctance to attend these types of programs, which may stem from denial of illness or stigma about being identified as having an alcohol or sedative use disorder or from misinformation about what these programs are like. Despite the long history of 12-step programs, evidence is still divided on how effective they are in helping patients maintain sobriety. Given the advantages of accessibility, low cost, and opportunities for frequent support, a referral to a 12-step program is reasonable to include in the discharge plan for any patient being discharged from the ED with an alcohol or sedative use disorder.

Conclusion

Alcohol and sedative use disorders are the most common serious substance use disorders that emergency providers face. Competent clinicians need a thorough, systematic approach to providing care to these ED patients. Many treatment challenges exist in caring for people suffering from these illnesses, including the physical effects of intoxication and withdrawal, associated medical and psychiatric conditions, as well as common barriers to accessing effective treatment following an ED visit. Individuals with alcohol and sedative use disorders are among the most vulnerable ED patients, and despite the challenges involved, each ED encounter with a patient suffering from these conditions is an opportunity to positively intervene, both to appropriately manage the patients' acute medical and psychiatric needs and to assist patients in accessing further treatment.

References

1. McDonald AJ, Wang N, Camargo CA. US emergency department visits for alcohol-related diseases and injuries between 1992 and 2000. Arch Intern Med. 2004;164:531–7.
2. Quality CfBHSa: 2016 National survey on drug use and health: detailed tables, Substance dependence or abuse in the past year among persons aged 18 or older, by demographic characteristics: numbers in thousands, 2015 and 2016; p. 170419 SAMHSA 2017. 5.8A.
3. Grant BF, Goldstein RB, Saha TD, Chou SP, Jung J, Zhang H, et al. Epidemiology of DSM-5 alcohol use disorder: results from the national epidemiologic survey on alcohol and related conditions III. JAMA Psychiat. 2015;72(8):757–66.
4. White AM, Slater ME, Ng G, Hingson R, Breslow R. Trends in alcohol-related emergency department visits in the United States: results from the nationwide emergency department sample, 2006–2014. Alcohol Clin Exp Res. 2018;42(2):352–9.
5. GBD 2016 Alcohol Collaborators. Alcohol use and burden for 195 countries and territories, 1990–2016: a systematic analysis for the Global Burden of Disease Study 2016. Lancet. 2018;392:1015–35.
6. American Psychiatric Association. Diagnostic and statistical manual of mental disorders. 5th ed. Washington, DC: American Psychiatric Publishing; 2013. DSM-5.
7. Long D, Long B, Koyfman A. The emergency management of severe alcohol withdrawal. Am J Emerg Med. 2017;35:1005–11.
8. Hoffman PL, Grant KA, Snell LD, Reinlib L, Iorio K, Tabakoff B. NMDA receptors: role in ethanol withdrawal seizures. Ann N Y Acad Sci. 1992;654:52–60.
9. Tsai G, Gastfriend DR, Coyle JT. The glutamatergic basis of human alcoholism. Am J Psychiatry. 1995;52:332–40.
10. Victor M, Adams RD. The effect of alcohol on the nervous system. Res Publ Assoc Res Nerv Ment Dis. 1953;32:526–73.

11. Greenberg PE, Fournier AA, Sisitsky T, Pike CT, Kessler RC. The economic burden of adults with major depressive disorder in the United States (2005 and 2010). J Clin Psychiatry. 2015;76(2):155–62.
12. Rehm J, Dawson D, Frick U, Gmel G, Roerecke M, Shield KD, Grant B. Burden of disease associated with alcohol use disorders in the United States. Alcohol Clin Exp Res. 2014;38(4):1068–77.
13. Becker WC, Fiellin DA, Desai RA. Non-medical use, abuse and dependence on sedatives and tranquilizers among U.S. adults: psychiatric and socio-demographic correlates. Drug Alcohol Depend. 2007;90(2–3):280–7.
14. Boden JM, Fergusson DM. Alcohol and depression. Addiction. 2011;106(5):906–14.
15. Kelly JF, Renner JA. Alcohol-related disorders. In: Stern TA, Fava M, Wilens TE, Rosenbaum JF, editors. Massachusetts General Hospital Comprehensive Clinical Psychiatry. 2nd ed. Philadelphia: Elsevier; 2016. p. 270–89.
16. Pietrzak RH, Goldstein RB, Southwick SM, Grant BF. Prevalence and Axis I comorbidity of full and partial posttraumatic stress disorder in the United States: results from Wave 2 of the National Epidemiologic Survey on Alcohol and Related Conditions. J Anxiety Disord. 2011;25:456–65.
17. Hung GC, Cheng CT, Jhong JR, Tsai SY, Chen CC, Kuo CJ. Risk and protective factors for suicide mortality among patients with alcohol dependence. J Clin Psychiatry. 2015;76(12):1687–93.
18. Kaplan MS, Huguet N, McFarland BH, Caetano R, Conner KR, Giesbrecht N, Nolte KB. Use of alcohol before suicide in the United States. Ann Epidemiol. 2014;24(8):588–592.e1–2. https://doi.org/10.1016/j.annepidem.2014.05.008.
19. Schuckit MA. Recognition and management of withdrawal delirium (delirium tremens). N Engl J Med. 2014;371(22):2109–13. https://doi.org/10.1056/NEJMra1407298.
20. Latt N, Dore G. Thiamine in the treatment of Wernicke encephalopathy in patients with alcohol use disorders. Intern Med J. 2014;44(9):911–5.
21. Olson KN, Smith SW, Kloss JS, Ho JD, Apple FS. Relationship between blood alcohol concentration and observable symptoms of intoxication in patients presenting to an emergency department. Alcohol Alcohol. 2013;48(4):386–9.
22. Maldonado JR, Sher Y, Ashouri JF, Hills-Evans K, Swendsen H, Lolak S, Miller AC. The "Prediction of Alcohol Withdrawal Severity Scale" (PAWSS): systematic literature review and pilot study of a new scale for the prediction of complicated alcohol withdrawal syndrome. Alcohol. 2014;48(4):375–90.
23. Borges G, Cherpitel CJ, Orozco R, Ye Y, Monteiro M, Hao W, Benegal V. A dose-response estimate for acute alcohol use and risk of suicide attempt. Addict Biol. 2017;22(6):1554–61. https://doi.org/10.1111/adb.12439.
24. Dodds TJ. Prescribed benzodiazepines and suicide risk: a review of the literature. Prim Care Companion CNS Disord. 2017;19(2).
25. Sullivan JT, Sykora K, Schneiderman J, Naranjo CA, Sellers EM. Assessment of alcohol withdrawal: the revised Clinical Institute Withdrawal Assessment for Alcohol scale (CIWA-Ar). Br J Addict. 1989;84:1353–7.
26. Eberly ME, Lockwood AG, Lockwood S, Davis KW. Outcomes after implementation of an alcohol withdrawal protocol at a single institution. Hosp Pharm. 2016;51:752–8.
27. Cassidy EM, O'Sullivan I, Bradshaw P, Islam T, Onovo C. Symptom-triggered benzodiazepine therapy for alcohol withdrawal syndrome in the emergency department: a comparison with the standard fixed dose benzodiazepine regimen. Emerg Med J. 2012;29(10):802–4. https://doi.org/10.1136/emermed-2011-200509.
28. Hendey GW, Dery RA, Barnes RL, Snowden B, Mentler P. A prospective, randomized, trial of phenobarbital versus benzodiazepines for acute alcohol withdrawal. Am J Emerg Med. 2011;29(4):382–5.
29. Kramp P, Rafaelsen OJ. Delirium tremens: a double-blind comparison of diazepam and barbital treatment. Acta Psychiatr Scand. 1978;58(2):174–90.

30. Mo Y, Thomas MC, Karras GE. Barbiturates for treatment of alcohol withdrawal syndrome: a systematic review of clinical trials. J Crit Care. 2016;32:101–7.
31. Puening SE, Wilson MP, Nordstrom K. Psychiatric emergencies for clinicians: emergency department management of benzodiazepine withdrawal. J Emerg Med. 2017;52(1):66–9.
32. Barata IA, Shandro JR, Montgomery M, Polansky R, Sachs CJ, Duber HC, et al. Effectiveness of SBIRT for alcohol use disorders in the emergency department: a systematic review. West J Emerg Med. 2017;18(6):1143–52. https://doi.org/10.5811/westjem.2017.7.34373.

Chapter 3
Stimulant Use Disorders and Related Emergencies

Amanda S. Green

Introduction

Patients who present to the emergency department (ED) due to stimulant use can include the anxious assistant professor who complains of insomnia and then discloses that he has been snorting Adderall; the disorganized woman with elevated vital signs who just used methamphetamine and, only after being asked directly, acknowledges that she has two young children but can't remember where she left them; the violent, disorganized, naked man with no identification who assaults multiple bystanders after using synthetic cathinones and requires ten police officers to restrain him; the college football player who complains of chest pain after a cocaine binge and is having a myocardial infarction; and the paranoid man who calls 911 from a gas station to report that he is being followed by a secret organization that wants to kill him, is furious when the police bring him to the hospital, and insists that the methamphetamine he used 3 days prior has nothing to do with his current presentation.

Stimulant use, both prescribed and illicit, has been on the rise over the past several decades. As the availability and use of stimulants grow, emergency departments increasingly serve as the front lines for managing the significant medical and psychiatric comorbidities that result from their use [1]. According to the results from the 2016 National Survey on Drug Use and the National Survey on Drug Use and Health by SAMHSA, in any 1-month period in 2016, there were approximately 1.7 million people over the age of 12 who used non-prescribed pharmaceutical amphetamines, 0.7 million people over the age of 12 who used methamphetamine, and an additional 1.9 million people over the age of 12 who used cocaine [2]. In total, over 4 million people in the United States used an illicit stimulant during any 1-month

A. S. Green (✉)
Central Texas Veterans Health Care System, Temple, TX, USA
e-mail: Amanda.Green5@va.gov

A. L. Donovan, S. A. Bird (eds.), *Substance Use and the Acute Psychiatric Patient*, Current Clinical Psychiatry, https://doi.org/10.1007/978-3-319-23961-3_3

period in 2016. This rate has been gradually increasing since 2005 [3]. Patterns of illicit stimulant use, like most drugs of abuse, vary nationwide and depend in large part on availability, price, manufacturing sites, and trafficking routes, all of which are subject to change. Regardless, stimulants are the second most widely used class of illicit drugs worldwide after cannabis, and all emergency department clinicians will encounter medical and psychiatric emergencies due to stimulant use [4].

Although stimulants play an important role in treating some medical and psychiatric illnesses, the potential side effects of both licit and illicit use pose significant challenges to an emergency department clinician. The stimulant-intoxicated patient can rapidly develop life-threatening complications that include cardiac arrhythmias and ischemia, hypertension, severe hyperthermia, rhabdomyolysis leading to acute kidney failure, seizures, and ischemic and hemorrhagic stroke [5, 6]. Furthermore, these patients are often highly agitated, paranoid, and violent. As such, they can pose significant dangers to themselves, to other patients, and to emergency department staff, making it difficult to provide timely medical treatment and severely taxing emergency department resources. Emergency departments also find themselves managing the public health consequences of widespread stimulant abuse, which include domestic violence, physical and sexual assaults, traumatic injuries, and the abuse and neglect of children [7–11]. In sum, emergencies that result from stimulant use present unique challenges to the ED clinician, due in part to (1) the high frequency of these cases, (2) the serious acute medical comorbidity that often results from stimulant use, and (3) the serious psychiatric sequelae of stimulant use, including severe agitation and psychosis that can be difficult to stabilize and manage in an ED setting.

Stimulants are used illicitly for many reasons. They are used to experience euphoria or "to get high." The appetite-suppressive properties of stimulants make them appealing to some; and this effect may account, in part, for the relatively high rates of use in women of child-bearing age. In addition, many "natural" weight loss products contain poorly labeled stimulants, and people can be unaware that they are even ingesting stimulants when they use these products [12, 13]. Stimulants are used to enhance sexual desire and performance; however, particularly for men, chronic stimulant use impairs sexual performance [6]. Stimulants are used to increase confidence, wakefulness, or energy. In some cases, stimulants are used to counter the effects of depressant drugs such as alcohol, opioids, or benzodiazepines. Stimulants are also used as "cognitive enhancers" in order to improve work or academic performance, although, in the absence of a legitimate diagnosis of ADHD, there is no clear evidence that stimulants improve performance and in some cases stimulants may worsen performance by increasing anxiety or worsening insomnia [14, 15]. Overall, there are many reasons why people illicitly use stimulants, and, thus, the demographics and presentations of stimulant-associated emergencies in the ED can vary widely.

In the DSM-5, stimulant use disorder is characterized by a pattern of use that leads to at least two signs of clinically significant impairment over a 12-month period [16]. Signs of this impairment include:

1. Using more of the stimulant or using it more frequently than intended
2. Inability to cut down or control use despite a desire to do so
3. Spending an excessive amount of time acquiring the stimulant, using the stimulant, or recovering from its use
4. Craving the stimulant
5. Inability to fulfill major role obligations at work, home, or school
6. Use continues despite persistent interpersonal or social problems that result from use
7. Using in situations that are physically dangerous
8. Use continues despite awareness of the problems associated with it
9. Withdrawal is experienced when the substance is stopped.

Stimulant intoxication, stimulant withdrawal, other stimulant-induced disorders, and unspecified stimulant-related disorders are also included in DSM-5. Although any stimulant can be misused and cause serious side effects, in this chapter, the focus will be on those stimulants that are most frequently implicated in psychiatric emergencies: amphetamines (including pharmaceuticals and methamphetamine), cocaine, and synthetic cathinones.

All stimulants work by acting directly on dopaminergic, adrenergic, and, to a lesser degree, serotoninergic pathways to increase available dopamine (DA), norepinephrine (NE), and serotonin (5-HT), respectively [17]. These monoamines play a vital role in regulating and modulating much of our day-to-day behaviors. Dopamine plays a key role in modulating cognition, reward, motivation, and movement, in part by activating the brain's reward circuit. Stimulants prevent the re-uptake of dopamine at the pre-synaptic terminals and in some cases, such as with methamphetamine, also increase the release of dopamine at these terminals. Increased levels of dopamine result in feelings of pleasure, well-being, and even euphoria. Excess dopamine also drives the paranoia, hallucinations, and uncomfortable motor effects observed in a stimulant-intoxicated patient. Repeated activation of the reward circuit plays a key role in the reinforcement of drug-seeking behaviors, paving the way to further drug use [18, 19].

Norepinephrine controls our "fight-or-flight" response, as well as more generally modulating arousal, learning, attention, and mood [20]. Stimulants are sympathomimetic drugs that cause the rapid release of norepinephrine into both peripheral and central pathways, activating the sympathetic nervous system and rapidly increasing heart rate, constricting blood vessels, releasing glucose, and stimulating bronchodilation. This adrenaline surge leads to feelings of increased energy, confidence, wakefulness, and heightened emotion. In excess, it drives many of the cardiac and neurological abnormalities observed with stimulant use.

Most stimulants, with the exception of MDMA (also known as "ecstasy"), have a less marked effect on serotonin levels. Serotonin modulates arousal, thermoregulation, mood, appetite, and sleep, and alterations in all these domains are seen with stimulant use [21]. Increased serotonin raises body temperature and leads to feelings of sexual arousal and well-being [22, 23]. Patients who use stimulants are at risk for serotonin syndrome, due to excessive serotonergic activity, characterized by altered mental status, autonomic instability, and neuromuscular excitability.

Stimulants include widely available over-the-counter substances such as nicotine, caffeine, and ephedrine; pharmaceuticals such as Ritalin and Adderall; and "street" drugs such as cocaine, methamphetamine, and "bath salts." In this chapter, stimulants will be organized into three subcategories: (1) "over-the-counter" stimulants, (2) pharmaceutical stimulants (that can be used both licitly and illicitly), and (3) "street" stimulants.

Over-the-counter stimulants are easily available and popular, especially among young people. For example, highly caffeinated drinks, "energy drinks," are implicated in an increasing number of emergency department visits. Specifically, emergency department visits that result from the consumption of energy drinks have doubled from 10,068 visits in 2007 to 20,783 visits in 2011, and one in ten of these visits results in a hospitalization [3]. Patients who have been overusing caffeine rarely present acutely psychotic as a result of caffeine ingestion, although patients with an underlying psychiatric illness, such as mania, psychosis, or anxiety, can find their psychiatric symptoms acutely worsened as a result of the ingestion, requiring emergency psychiatric management as a result. It is always important to screen for caffeine ingestion and other over the counter stimulant use in a patient who is reporting a recent worsening in these psychiatric symptoms.

Nicotine is another readily available over-the-counter stimulant; in excess, it can lead to nausea, vomiting, tachycardia, and then later diaphoresis, dizziness, and seizure. More severe poisonings are rare but can be fatal secondary to late-stage neuromuscular blockade resulting in hypotension and respiratory arrest [24]. Young children under the age of 6 are particularly vulnerable to severe poisoning due to accidental exposures, such as ingestion of a cigarette butt, dermal exposure, or ingestion of the liquid nicotine used in e-cigarettes. The liquid used in e-cigarettes contains highly concentrated (and sometimes sweet-smelling) nicotine that can be readily absorbed through the skin or accidentally ingested, and it is associated with more severe poisonings, as well as an increase in rates of nicotine poisoning overall [25, 26].

Pharmaceutical stimulants, such as methylphenidate (Ritalin, Concerta), amphetamine-dextroamphetamine (Adderall), dexmethylphenidate (Focalin), and dextroamphetamine (Dexedrine), are used to successfully treat a broad range of medical and psychiatric illnesses, including attention-deficit/hyperactivity disorder, major depressive disorder, narcolepsy, obesity, and respiratory problems. However, pharmaceutical stimulants can have serious side effects when used improperly and are also increasingly being used as drugs of abuse [27, 28]. Specifically, nonprescribed use of Adderall by 18–25-year-olds increased 67% between 2006 and 2011, and associated emergency department visits increased 156% during that period. While increasing numbers of people are being prescribed these pharmaceutical stimulants, in 2010, half of associated emergency room visits were due to their illicit use [3]. Even legitimately prescribed stimulants can be misused, either by overuse or by using alternative mechanisms of delivery, such as insufflation, rather than oral ingestion. Thus, it is important to ask about misuse of prescribed medication when clinically indicated. In addition, some prescription medications that are not classified as stimulants can have stimulant-like effects, and they can also be misused. For example, bupropion is an antidepressant medication that acts by increasing levels of norepinephrine and dopamine; some will insufflate crushed bupropion to potentiate its effects and when stimulants are not available [29].

"Street" stimulants, such as cocaine, methamphetamine, synthetic cathinones, and 3,4-methylenedioxymethamphetamine (MDMA), can cause serious medical and psychiatric morbidity and mortality. The reasons are multifactorial (i.e., co-ingestion with other drugs, presence of adulterants, faster mechanisms of delivery such as intravenous or insufflation, and unpredictable variability in purity and dosing), but, in no small part, the increased morbidity and mortality is due to the greater potency of these drugs. Since many of the effects with stimulants are dose related, it is not surprising these illicit substances, with their greater potency, are associated with the most severe psychiatric and medical emergencies.

Cocaine is the most commonly abused stimulant [2]. It can be formulated in two different ways, as a hydrochloride salt ("coke," "snow," "toot," "blow") that can be insufflated or injected or as a base form ("crack," "rock") that can be inhaled. Potency, dose, and route of administration all impact the effect of the drug. Generally, the time to peak effect for the injected and smoked forms is ~2–5 minutes and lasts for 30–60 minutes, and the time to peak effect for the insufflated form is ~15 minutes and lasts for 60–120 minutes. Cocaine users are at particularly high risk for serious cardiac and neurological emergencies, and cardiac complaints are the most common reason a cocaine user will present to the ED [30]. Cocaine, like all the stimulants, is a sympathomimetic, but it is also a class I anti-arrhythmic and a powerful vasoconstrictor, predisposing these patients to arrhythmias and ischemia [31]. Furthermore, cocaine, like many drugs, frequently has added adulterants, such as hydroxyzine, mannitol, diltiazem, strychnine, and procaine, leading to additional clinical effects [32]. For example, in 2009, the DEA reported that 69% of seized cocaine contained levamisole. Levamisole is a pharmaceutical with anthelmintic and immunomodulatory properties; there have been numerous reports of levamisole-induced complications in cocaine users, including vasculitis, soft tissue necrosis, and agranulocytosis [33–35].

Methamphetamine is the most commonly abused amphetamine. Methamphetamine has greater potency than the other amphetamines and cocaine due to the addition of a methyl group, making it lipophilic and allowing for greater penetration of the central nervous system. Methamphetamine can be formulated as a powder ("meth," "speed," "crank") which can be insufflated, smoked, injected, ingested, or inserted in the rectum or as a highly purified dextro-isomer crystalline form ("crystal," "ice," "tina") which can be smoked or injected. Regardless of its route of administration, methamphetamine has a half-life of ~12 hours, compared to cocaine's half-life of ~2 hours. Methamphetamine's longer half-life, combined with its lower cost than cocaine (it is sometimes called "poor man's cocaine") and its relative ease of manufacture, has contributed to its wide availability and popularity [36]. Methamphetamine's anti-arrhythmic and vasoconstrictive properties are not as strong as cocaine; however, the greater CNS penetration and longer half-life of methamphetamine make users much more prone to prolonged paranoia and frank psychosis than most other stimulants. In fact, the most common reasons for methamphetamine-related emergency department visits are mental health (18.7%), trauma (18.4%), skin infections (11.1%), and dental pathology (9.6%) [6, 37].

Synthetic cathinones (i.e., "bath salts," "white lightning," "flakka," "bloom," "vanilla sky") are becoming increasingly popular stimulants, in part because of their reputation as a "legal high." Synthetic cathinones can come in powder, liquid, tablet, or crystalline form and can be insufflated, ingested, inhaled, injected, or absorbed via mucous membranes [38, 39].Their half-life varies; but the psychoactive effects, which include everything from psychosis to an agitated delirium, can last for days to weeks. Synthetic cathinones comprise an ever-changing group of compounds that are derived from cathinone, a naturally occurring amphetamine analogue found in the khat plant [40]. For a long time, manufacturers could sell synthetic cathinones legally through shops that also legally sold paraphernalia for cannabis use (although not cannabis itself), also known as "head shops," and over the internet by labeling the synthetic cathinones as "not for human consumption" and touting them as "bath salts" or "jewelry cleaner." However, since 2011, the DEA has designated an increasing number of these compounds as schedule I drugs, cutting down, but not eliminating, their ready availability. Manufacturers continue to modify the chemical structure of these agents to avoid regulation and detection. Most frequently, the psychoactive substances in these cathinones are methylenedioxypyrovalerone (MDPV), methedrine, or methylene, although many other compounds are possible [41–44]. Clinical reports are concerning for a high degree of bizarre, violent, and delusional behaviors in patients who use bath salts. Alpha-pyrrolidinopentiophenone (a-PVP, "flakka," "flakes," "gravel") warrants special mention, as it is a particularly potent cathinone and has been implicated in multiple instances of extremely violent and dangerous behaviors since it appeared in 2015.

3,4-Methylenedioxymethamphetamine (MDMA) is both a stimulant and a hallucinogen. It was originally available as a tablet ("ecstasy," "x," "club drug," "disco biscuits," "roll"), but due to concerns about high rates of adulterants, some users prefer to use its crystalline form ("Molly," "Mandy") because it is thought to have fewer adulterants. These crystals can be swallowed whole or crushed and then either insufflated or dissolved in liquid and ingested. However, studies have shown that the crystalline form of MDMA is frequently contaminated with adulterants and, in some cases, doesn't contain MDMA at all, but rather other substances, such as synthetic cathinones ("bath salts"). Emergency room visits due to MDMA (or assumed MDMA) consumption rose 128% for people under age 21 from 4460 to 10,176 between 2005 and 2011 [45].

Intoxication

Patients acutely intoxicated on stimulants can be restless, irritable, euphoric, hypersexual, paranoid, delusional, disorganized, or outright violent. They typically arrive in the emergency department in a "fight-or-flight" mode, with signs of adrenergic excess, such as tachycardia, hypertension, diaphoresis, hyperglycemia, and mydriasis. The confused, agitated, diaphoretic patient with hyperthermia, tachycardia, and hypertension has a broad medical differential, including alcohol withdrawal, systemic infection, central nervous system infection, seizure, neurological injury, or other toxidromes, such as salicylate or anticholinergic overdoses. Thus, an ED clinician can find it challenging to distinguish stimulant intoxication from other medical emergencies. Toxicology tests are not particularly helpful in these cases because many widely used medications, such as bupropion, selegiline, trazodone, or ephedrine, can cause a false-positive result for amphetamines due to cross-reactivity on the rapid testing immunoassay that is utilized in the emergency room (Table 3.1). Gas chromatography/mass spectrometry testing can be more accurate but can still provide false-positive results. For example, gas chromatography/mass spectrometry fails to distinguish between the isomers l-methamphetamine, which is commonly found in nasal inhalers and has no psychoactive properties, and d-methamphetamine, which is the central nervous system stimulant found in some illicit drugs including methamphetamine [46]. Furthermore, the synthetic cathinones are not tested for on most standard immunoassay toxicology screens, and waiting for the results of more specialized testing can take hours to days and, therefore, is not clinically feasible in an emergency setting [47]. Thus, an ED clinician needs to have a high level of suspicion for stimulant use, because detailed history or definitive laboratory tests are often not available in the emergency setting. At the same time, many stimulant users are at high risk for serious medical emergencies independent of stimulant use, such as infection, traumatic injury, cardiac or neurological emergencies, and other toxic ingestions, and these possible life-threatening etiologies must always be considered when clinically appropriate.

Although stimulants can impact all the organ systems via ischemia secondary to vasospasm and demand dysregulation of the body's thermo-control, direct toxicity, and activation of clotting systems, the most common and important organ systems impacted in the stimulant-intoxicated patient are the heart, kidneys, and brain. Barring clinical evidence otherwise, these are the organ systems that should be examined and stabilized first. On initial presentation of a patient who is agitated and suspected of using stimulants, a clinician should first obtain vital signs and fingerstick blood glucose to rule out hypoglycemia as the etiology of agitation. Initial labs can include complete blood count, complete metabolic panel including blood urea nitrogen and creatinine, magnesium, liver function tests, blood glucose, pregnancy

Table 3.1 False Positive for Amphetamines on Urine Drug Screen

Antipsychotics	Chlorpromazine, promethazine, aripiprazole
Antidepressants	Trazodone, bupropion
Antibiotics	Ofloxacin
Others	Metformin, ranitidine
Decongestants/ antihistamines	Over-the-counter nasal decongestants, brompheniramine, phenylpropanolamine
Energy supplements	Dimethylamylamine (DMAA)
Street drugs	*Cathinones*

test, creatinine kinase, urinalysis, and urine and serum toxicology screens. Although most drug screens do not ordinarily test for synthetic cathinones, toxicology laboratories can often be asked to test for the most common cathinones. Head, lung, or other imaging and EEG may be appropriate depending on the clinical presentation.

All patients suspected of being on stimulants, or having used stimulants in the past several days, should get an electrocardiogram, as stimulants can prolong QTc, cause cardiac ischemia, and initiate cardiac arrhythmias. Patients should be carefully screened for chest pain, dyspnea, severe headache, evidence of infection, or focal neurological symptoms. Cocaine users are at particularly high risk for serious cardiac and neurological abnormalities, such as malignant arrhythmias, cardiac ischemia, aortic dissection, hypertensive crises, and stroke. Many patients use more than one illicit drug at a time, and the combination of cocaine and ethanol is a common and particularly cardiotoxic mixture. Ethanol decreases cocaine metabolism and elimination, increases cocaine absorption, and leads to the formation of cocaethylene, a cardiotoxic metabolite [48]. Thus, there can be toxic effects from lower doses of cocaine than expected when combined with ethanol, and these patients are at particularly high risk for cardiac or neurological emergencies, even when using doses of cocaine that they have otherwise tolerated in the past [30, 31, 49].

Sinus tachycardia and hypertension in stimulant intoxication are caused by central adrenergic excess and are extremely common, even with mild intoxication; decisions about whether to treat either will depend on clinical condition and medical comorbidity [49]. There has been a great deal of controversy about the use of beta-blockers, such as propranolol, in cocaine-intoxicated patients with cardiovascular complications. Stimulants are sympathomimetic drugs that increase both alpha-adrenergic and beta-adrenergic tones. Treating tachycardia or hypertension with medications that only (such as propranolol) or predominantly (such as labetalol) decrease beta-adrenergic tone can result in unopposed alpha-adrenergic tone, which can worsen vasoconstriction and lead to worse cardiac and neurological outcomes [31, 32].This risk is also applicable to other stimulants. Thus, in the emergency department, beta-blockers and medications with significantly more beta-adrenergic blockade than alpha should be avoided. Since most cardiac irregularities due to stimulant use are thought to be due to increased centrally mediated sympathetic tone, an important part of first-line treatment for cardiac complaints, including chest pain, is benzodiazepines. Alpha-adrenergic antagonists, such as phentolamine, can be used as second-line treatment for severe or refractory hypertension or chest pain due to stimulant use [31, 50, 51].

Hyperthermia is less common, and it is an ominous sign in a stimulant-intoxicated patient [52]. In areas where stimulant use is widespread, the naked agitated patient picked up by EMS after he was found running naked up the middle of the street is a relatively common presentation to emergency departments. "Agitation" and "nakedness" together in a patient should immediately cause an ED clinician to think "stimulants" and "hyperthermia." Hyperthermia is a marker for severity of the toxidrome, and it is independently associated with increased risk of morbidity and mortality. Hyperthermia worsens neurotoxicity, increases risk for seizure and end-organ damage, leads to clotting dysregulation, and worsens metabolic acidosis and risk for sudden death. The hyperthermia caused by stimulant intoxication is mediated both centrally and peripherally [53]. Increased levels of serotonin, dopamine, and norepinephrine disrupt thermoregulation centrally by acting on the hypothalamus, and increased norepinephrine causes excess motor activity and vasoconstriction that raises body temperature peripherally [53]. Thus, decreasing adrenergic tone and vasoconstriction and calming excess motor activity while also externally cooling the patient may be necessary [52]. Medications that can potentially worsen hyperthermia—such as beta-blockers, neuroleptics, or anticholinergics—should be avoided if clinically possible [54]. Benzodiazepines can play an important role in sedating the patient and, thus, decreasing motor activity that contributes to hyperthermia. Hyperthermic patients need to be medically managed and stabilized before any psychiatric needs can be assessed.

Stimulant-intoxicated patients are frequently dehydrated and undernourished and, thus, can have a host of electrolyte abnormalities that impact assessment and management. Special attention should be paid to creatinine kinase, creatinine, and urine analysis, as stimulant-intoxicated patients are at elevated risk for rhabdomyolysis and acute kidney failure. If there is concern for rhabdomyolysis or evidence of kidney injury, IV fluids should be initiated. Since stimulants can prolong the QTc interval, which can lead to cardiac arrhythmias, potassium and magnesium should be replenished aggressively. A complete blood count can help screen for infection, but it should be kept in mind that stimulants can cause demargination of white blood cells, resulting in an elevated white blood cell count without infection. Generally, in cases of demargination, the differential remains normal, versus infection, where an increase in neutrophil count is also noted. In addition, with demargination, a downward trend in the white blood cell count is seen, if serial complete blood counts are drawn. Pregnancy tests are important in guiding management in the stimulant-intoxicated female of child-bearing age. Stimulant use is associated with a host of perinatal morbidities for both mother and fetus, including placental abruption, hypertensive crises, and preterm labor. Furthermore, there is evidence that children exposed to stimulants in utero have higher rates of mood and behavioral difficulties. Methamphetamine's impact on the fetus is particularly concerning, due to its long half-life and extensive CNS penetration, as compared to other stimulants.

Methamphetamine and synthetic cathinone users are particularly challenging for the emergency clinician, because the high levels of agitation and paranoia in these patients, combined with the long half-lives of these substances, can delay potentially life-saving medical assessment and treatment and put the patient, other ED patients, and staff at risk. It is important to respond quickly and proactively when assessing and managing agitation, violence, and self-harm. Agitated behavior should be considered a symptom in a toxidrome, rather than "bad behavior." Clinicians need to screen early for paranoia, suicidality, and homicidality in these patients and be proactive about deescalating patients before they become aggressive. Restraints may be necessary to keep the patient and others safe. However, restraints can worsen hyperthermia and rhabdomyolysis and so should be used judiciously; patients should never be restrained without also receiving medication to treat their agitation. Stimulant-intoxicated patients who refuse initial interventions—including emergency medications, labs, and vitals—should be carefully screened by the physician for capacity to refuse emergency assessment and treatment; due to their psychosis, paranoia, or confusion, many of these patients do not have the capacity to refuse the emergency interventions while intoxicated.

Stimulant-induced agitation should be managed with high-dose benzodiazepines, rather than neuroleptics, whenever clinically possible. Although neuroleptics, such as haloperidol or olanzapine, are traditionally first-line treatments for agitation and psychosis, they should be used with caution in this population of patients [54, 55]. Stimulant intoxication can lead to seizures, malignant hyperthermia, and cardiac dysrhythmias in the setting of prolonged QTc. Since neuroleptics can lower the seizure threshold, interfere with a body's central thermoregulatory system, and prolong QTc, they should be used cautiously in this population. In some cases, however, a patient's agitation will be refractory to oral benzodiazepines, and alternative agents may be needed. If the patient has a normal body temperature and stable vitals, neuroleptics can be utilized to treat psychosis and agitation. In these cases, haloperidol is recommended, as it is very effective in the acute setting, can be administered as an intramuscular injection, and is commonly used with benzodiazepines, but is less likely to lower seizure threshold compared to other common neuroleptics [56, 57]. If a patient is severely hyperthermic or otherwise medically unstable, and agitation is severe and refractory to benzodiazepines and antipsychotics (or antipsychotics are not appropriate given the risk for worsening hyperthermia), sedation with midazolam or propofol and intubation may be necessary to be able to proceed safely and effectively with medical workup and treatment.

Even if they are not acutely agitated or violent, patients who have been using stimulants, particularly methamphetamine, are often frankly paranoid. Based on clinical experience, methamphetamine-intoxicated patients are frequently concerned that they are being followed or spied on or are about to be killed by a gang or cartel. In these cases, patients can become violent if they think hospital staff are not adequately protecting them or if they perceive staff or other patients are part of the conspiracy to harm or kill them. In some cases, the patient's concerns may be based on facts; collateral from police officers on scene or family members can provide important information to determine if a patient's concerns are delusional or reality-based, as there have been cases where real violence and threats directed at the patient can spill into the emergency room, putting patients and staff at risk. As with any paranoid patient, it is important to ask whether they have active homicidal or violent ideation or plans, whether they have specific suspicions or concerns about particular people, and whether they have possession of or access to weapons. These patients are also at high risk for elopement, and, if they meet criteria to be held involuntarily due to lack of decisional capacity secondary to intoxication or psychosis, they may need security to stand by, or another form of containment, to prevent elopement. Sometimes simple practical accommodations can help decrease a patient's anxiety, such as moving the patient away from a door or window if there are concerns about being stalked or asking security to stand either out of sight or in sight (depending on the patient's concerns). A clinician can acknowledge and empathize with the patient's very real anxiety and fear, without colluding with the patient's delusional belief system. Acknowledging a patient's terrifying experience while still being honest about the diagnosis and plan of care can often encourage cooperation from a very resistant, paranoid patient. Furthermore, in the absence of medical contraindications, an antipsychotic should be offered to psychotic patients, even if they are not overtly agitated, to relieve the acute suffering caused by their fear and paranoia.

The risk for suicide should always be assessed in the stimulant-intoxicated patient. Paranoid patients can be so frightened that they would rather kill themselves and "get it over with" than wait to see their fears realized. Patients can experience derogatory or command auditory hallucinations while stimulant-intoxicated or in early withdrawal, i.e., "crashing." Based on clinical experience, cocaine-intoxicated patients are particularly at risk of experiencing derogatory auditory hallucinations in the early withdrawal period. These auditory hallucinations can be command, telling the patient to harm himself, and the patients can be at elevated risk for suicide at this time. Patients also can have bizarre delusions, for example, about friends and family; and patients can attempt suicide out of despair, in the face of these frightening delusions. Overall, stimulants disinhibit patients and impair judgment, which heightens their risk for acting on delusional, violent, or suicidal thoughts.

Patients also sometimes report tactile hallucinations of bug infestations, known as formication. Patients will insist they see and feel bugs; they will often have extensive excoriations from scratching and picking at themselves and will be furious that they are being treated by a psychiatrist for delusions, rather than by the medical team for an infestation. There is some evidence that these hallucinations, if distressing enough, can be treated with neuroleptics; but these patients frequently have very little insight into the etiology of their symptoms [58].

Along with mental status changes, the acutely intoxicated patient can present with motoric symptoms, primarily due to dysregulation of dopamine. These symptoms include myoclonus, bruxism, transient chorea (also known as "crack dancing"), new tics or worsening of old ones, and repetitive non-goal-directed behaviors (also known as "punding") [59]. Aside from social stigma and discomfort, these motor symptoms usually self-resolve without intervention. The exception is in cases where motor symptoms are severe enough that they worsen rhabdomyolysis or hyperthermia, and, in those cases, benzodiazepines or even a paralytic may be necessary [60].

Children with guardians who misuse stimulants are at high risk for being neglected, suffering physical abuse or sexual abuse, or being the victim of homicide [61, 62]. All patients should be asked if they have children; and the custody, location, and safety of those children should be independently confirmed. There have been cases where a child has been confined to a home for years, due to a parent who is concerned that the child will share information about drug manufacturing and use in the home. Children are also at risk for accidental ingestion of drugs, and this risk is increased in the chaotic conditions in which many of these children live. Pediatric patients with accidental stimulant intoxication often present with nonspecific symptoms of crying, tachycardia, and restlessness, so an ED provider needs to have a high level of suspicion when clinically warranted. Children who live in homes where methamphetamine is being manufactured are at high risk of poisoning from the toxic precursors and by-products of methamphetamine production, as well as methamphetamine itself. In one study, 46% of children removed from homes that were methamphetamine production sites tested positive for methamphetamine [62]. Children who live in methamphetamine production sites are also at high risk for burn and inhalation injury.

Withdrawal

Stimulant withdrawal is not life-threatening, nor does it need to be medically monitored, although it can be very uncomfortable for patients and it is a high-risk time for relapse. The ED clinician should screen carefully for psychosis, severe mood symptoms, suicidality, and potential for violence in patients who are in stimulant withdrawal. Stimulant withdrawal can start within several hours after last use and generally lasts for hours to several days, although mild symptoms can be reported for months. Common symptoms include sleep disturbances, particularly hypersomnia and nightmares, as well as extreme fatigue, increased appetite, general aches and pains, intense drug cravings, anhedonia, irritability, dysphoria, paranoia, and even lingering psychosis. Underlying primary mood disorders, such as depression, may be acutely exacerbated during this period. Because of its longer half-life, methamphetamine users are likely to have more prolonged and severe withdrawal symptoms than other stimulant users. For example, after a methamphetamine binge, a patient may sleep for 24–36 hours. In these cases, an ED clinician may find that it is difficult or impossible to interview or discharge a patient during the early withdrawal period, because the patient is minimally interactive.

Chronic and high-dose use of stimulants is associated with increased risk for chronic psychosis, even after active metabolites have been eliminated from the body. This psychosis most commonly includes paranoia, delusions of persecution, tactile hallucinations, and derogatory auditory hallucinations. Patients who have been using cocaine frequently describe derogatory or threatening auditory hallucinations during the early withdrawal period, which last several hours and then resolve. It is not uncommon for patients to develop paranoia and hallucinations 2 or 3 days after their last methamphetamine use; in these cases, the psychosis is due to withdrawal rather than intoxication. Furthermore, the brain can become sensitized to the adverse effects of stimulants over time, including psychosis and paranoia. Thus, based on clinical experience, it is not uncommon for patients who have a history of decades of cocaine or methamphetamine use, without any psychosis or underlying primary psychiatric illness, to develop their first episode of substance-induced psychosis in their 50s.

Medications and medical monitoring are usually not necessary during simple stimulant withdrawal; reassurance and short-term observation, if indicated, are sufficient. Persistent psychosis can be extremely frightening and distressing for the patient and should be treated with a neuroleptic at this time; worsening of medical risks related to intoxication are no longer relevant, and benzodiazepines will not be effective, as the etiology of psychosis during stimulant withdrawal is not due to excessive sympathomimetic activity. If severe psychiatric symptoms do not resolve within 8–10 hours, and these symptoms put the patient at risk for harm to self or others, then inpatient admission for stabilization and treatment may be required [63]. Patients may retract suicidality once they are no longer in acute withdrawal, but this retraction may not be reliable or protective in cases of concerning and persistent suicidal behaviors during stimulant use or withdrawal, since patients are likely to use drugs again and return to the same high-risk mental state as soon as they leave the ED.

Pathological brain changes are seen with chronic stimulant use. Stimulants are directly toxic to the brain, damaging dopaminergic and serotonergic nerve terminals via oxidative stress, inflammation, excessive neuro-excitability, and depletion of dopamine stores. Hyperthermia has been shown to exacerbate this neurotoxicity [64]. These insults to the brain, over time, can result in cognitive deficits. The most frequently observed deficits are in episodic memory, executive functioning, and motor control, particularly fine motor control [9, 65]. Chronic stimulant users also often report chronic anhedonia after years of use, which may be due, in part, to damage to the dopaminergic reward system [66].

Medical Comorbidities

Common complications from stimulant use can result from the route of drug delivery. Insufflation of stimulants, particularly cocaine because of its strong vasoconstrictive properties, can cause necrosis of the septum. Inhalation of stimulants can cause serious pulmonary complications, including thermal lung injury and acute respiratory symptoms [67]. Intravenous use puts patients at risk for infections, including cellulitis, abscesses, endocarditis, HIV, and HCV. Illicit drugs are frequently contaminated, either purposefully or inadvertently. Bulking agents are substances that are added purposefully to a drug to increase apparent amount and potential profits from its sale. Common bulking agents in stimulants include talcum powder, hydroxyzine, procaine, levamisole, caffeine, and lidocaine. In some cases, a cheaper drug is substituted for a more expensive one, such as when synthetic cathinones are substituted for MDMA or methamphetamine or PCP is substituted for cocaine [68]. Contaminants, such as lead or mercury, can be present in improperly synthesized methamphetamine [69].

Common acute medical comorbidities of stimulant intoxication include cardiac emergencies such as myocardial infarction, arrhythmia, malignant hypertension, and aortic dissection. Patients who combine cocaine and alcohol are at particularly high risk for this cardiac toxicity. Neurological injury can also occur, including seizures and ischemic or hemorrhagic stroke. Seizures from stimulant use generally occur early in the intoxication period and are usually brief. If a patient has ongoing or prolonged seizures, other possible etiologies of seizures should be investigated, such as co-occurring stroke or infection. Furthermore, paroxysmal or atypical agitation in this population should prompt the clinician to consider nonconvulsive status epilepticus.

Rhabdomyolysis secondary to increased motor activity and hyperthermia can occur. Most patients who use stimulants will have some elevation in their creatinine kinase, but if the rhabdomyolysis is severe enough, acute kidney injury can occur. Clotting abnormalities, including disseminated intravascular coagulation (DIC), can occur. Ischemia from stimulant use can impact any organ system, and, in some cases, multiorgan failure can occur [70, 71]. Acute abdominal pain in the stimulant-intoxicated patient should raise suspicion for bowel ischemia.

Methamphetamine use, in particular, is associated with high rates of HIV. Methamphetamine is frequently used as an aphrodisiac; however, since its effects include impulsive and disinhibited behaviors, people are more likely to engage in risky sexual behaviors or to trade sex for money or drugs, leading to increased risk for infection [72, 73]. Stimulant users, particularly methamphetamine users, are at high risk for traumatic injuries, particularly secondary to motor vehicles' crashes and assault. This is likely due in part to methamphetamine's greater potency and CNS effect, which leads to greater disinhibition, paranoia, and agitation. Methamphetamine users are also at increased risk for dental caries, periodontal abscesses, and other dental pathologies ("meth mouth") due to poor hygiene and self-care, bruxism, xerostomia, and possibly gum ischemia.

Disposition Considerations

Disposition options for the stimulant user from the emergency department can appear frustratingly meager to the ED clinician (who can see patients present multiple times in the same week for stimulant toxicity). Because stimulant withdrawal does not require medical monitoring, most cases of stimulant misuse will be treated on an outpatient basis. Since most presentations of stimulant intoxication self-resolve, it is often prudent to hold a patient in the emergency room for 4–10 hours for observation when stimulant use is suspected, to avoid unnecessary hospitalization. However, if patients have prolonged psychosis or ongoing severe mood symptoms leading to suicidality or homicidality, an inpatient psychiatric admission is appropriate for safety and stabilization.

Most patients can be discharged safely home with referrals for outpatient care. If a patient's history is indicative of an underlying primary psychiatric disorder, independent of their drug use, then referrals for outpatient psychiatric care are appropriate. Unfortunately, at this time, there are no medications that have been shown to effectively decrease stimulant craving or misuse [74]. The best evidence for treatment of stimulant use disorders is either contingency management interventions [75, 76] or cognitive behavioral treatment [77–79]. Patients can also be provided with information for local recovery support groups.

Conclusion

Psychiatric and medical emergencies that result from stimulant use are increasingly common and pose significant diagnostic and management challenges for the emergency department physician. Stimulant-intoxicated patients are vulnerable to extreme paranoia and psychosis that can lead to behaviors that further endanger the patient, other patients, and emergency department staff. Stimulant-intoxicated patients are also at high risk for potentially life-threatening medical complications that can be difficult to manage due to agitation and paranoia. The stimulant-intoxicated patient may be actively suicidal due to paranoia or despair at another relapse, other people may have been injured by the patient, or children may have been neglected or harmed. The impulse when facing one of these patients in an emergency department setting can be to view agitated or paranoid behavior as "bad behavior." It is important to keep in mind the tremendous mortality, morbidity, and suffering—for the patient, for loved ones, and for dependents—that result from stimulant use disorders. Attention to safety for patients and staff is essential, so a physician should be proactive about treating agitation and paranoia with medication, reassurance, containment, and restraints if necessary. Benzodiazepines are preferred, but, when agitation is extreme, neuroleptics or even paralytics may be necessary. Patients should be assessed for acute suicidality, homicidality, and recent suicidal behaviors. Medical complications need to be addressed systematically, with a focus, barring clinical evidence otherwise, on stabilizing possible neurological, cardiac, and kidney dysfunction. Once acute issues have been addressed, subacute issues will need to be assessed, such as lingering psychosis, ongoing stimulant use, and chronic stimulant-related medical issues, and appropriate follow-up care and disposition will need to be arranged. The early recognition of this toxidrome to quickly and effectively manage it can be life-saving.

References

1. Fulde G, Forster S. The impact of amphetamine-type stimulants on emergency services. Curr Opin Psychiatry. 2015;28(4):275–9.
2. Substance Abuse and Mental Health Services Administration, Drug Abuse Warning Network, 2011: National estimates of drug-related emergency department visits. HHS Publication No. (SMA) 13-4760, DAWN Series D-39. Rockville: Substance Abuse and Mental Health Services Administration; 2013.
3. Center for Behavioral Health Statistics and Quality. Behavioral health trends in the United States: results from the 2014 National Survey on Drug Use and Health (HHS Publication No. SMA 15-4927, NSDUH Series H-50). 2015. Retrieved from http://www.samhsa.gov/data/.
4. United Nations Office on Drugs and Crime. World drug report. United Nations publication; 2014.
5. Vearrier D, Greenberg M, Miller S, Okaneku J, Haggerty D. Methamphetamine: history, pathophysiology, adverse health effects, current trends, and hazards associated with the clandestine manufacture of methamphetamine. Dis Mon. 2012;58(2):38–89.

6. Darke S, Kaye S, McKetin R, Duflou J. Major physical and psychological harms of methamphetamine use. Drug Alcohol Rev. 2008;27(3):253–62.
7. Stretesky P. National case-control study of homicide offending and methamphetamine use. J Interpers Violence. 2008;24(6):911–24.
8. Cartier J. Methamphetamine use, self-reported violent crime, and recidivism among offenders in California who abuse substances. J Interpers Violence. 2006;21(4):435–45.
9. Dawe S, Davis P, Lapworth K, McKetin R. Mechanisms underlying aggressive and hostile behavior in amphetamine users. Curr Opin Psychiatry. 2009;22(3):269–73.
10. Brecht M, Herbeck D. Methamphetamine use and violent behavior: user perceptions and predictors. J Drug Issues. 2013;43(4):468–82.
11. Sommers I, Baskin D, Baskin-Sommers A. Methamphetamine use among young adults: health and social consequences. Addict Behav. 2006;31(8):1469–76.
12. Ods.od.nih.gov. Office of Dietary Supplements – dietary supplements for weight loss. [online]. 2016. Available at: https://ods.od.nih.gov/factsheets/WeightLoss-HealthProfessional/.
13. Livescience.com. Untested stimulant drug found in 12 supplements. [online]. 2016. Available at: http://www.livescience.com/48191-dbma-stimulant-weight-loss-supplements.html.
14. Smith M, Farah M. Are prescription stimulants "smart pills"? The epidemiology and cognitive neuroscience of prescription stimulant use by normal healthy individuals. Psychol Bull. 2011;137(5):717–41.
15. Dance A. Smart drugs: a dose of intelligence. Nature. 2016;531(7592):S2–3.
16. Diagnostic and statistical manual of mental disorders. Washington, D.C.: American Psychiatric Association; 2013.
17. Courtney K, Ray L. Methamphetamine: an update on epidemiology, pharmacology, clinical phenomenology, and treatment literature. Drug Alcohol Depend. 2014;143:11–21.
18. Dichaira G, Bassereo V. Reward system and addiction: what dopamine does and doesn't do. Curr Opin Pharmacol. 2007;7(1):69–76.
19. Pierce R, Kumaresan V. The mesolimbic dopamine system: the final common pathway for the reinforcing effect of drugs of abuse? Neurosci Biobehav Rev. 2006;30(2):215–38.
20. Briley M, Chantal M. The importance of norepinephrine in depression. Neuropsychiatr Dis Treat. 2011;7:9.
21. Muller C, Homberg J. The role of serotonin in drug use and addiction. Behav Brain Res. 2015;277:146–92.
22. Rogers R. The roles of dopamine and serotonin in decision making: evidence from pharmacological experiments in humans. Neuropsychopharmacology. 2010;36(1):114–32.
23. Clarke H. Cognitive inflexibility after prefrontal serotonin depletion. Science. 2004;304(5672):878–80.
24. Lavoie F, Harris T. Fatal nicotine ingestion. J Emerg Med. 1991;9(3):133–6.
25. Bassett R, Osterhoudt K, Brabazon T. Correspondence: more on nicotine poisoning in infants. N Engl J Med. 2014;370:2249–50.
26. Kamboj A, Spiller HA, Casavant MJ, Chounthirath T, Smith GA. Pediatric exposure to E-cigarettes, nicotine, and tobacco products in the United States. Pediatrics. 2016;137(6):e20160041.
27. Nissen S. ADHD drugs and cardiovascular risk. N Engl J Med. 2006;354(14):1445–8.
28. Chen L, Crum R, Strain E, Alexander G, Kaufmann C, Mojtabai R. Prescriptions, nonmedical use, and emergency department visits involving prescription stimulants. J Clin Psychiatry. 2016;77:e297–304.
29. Ctvnews.ca. [online]. 2016. Available at: http://www.ctvnews.ca/health/healthheadlines/doctors-warn-of-potentially-fatal-abuse-of-wellbutrin-antidepressant-1.1383282.
30. Maraj S, Figueredo V, Lynn Morris D. Cocaine and the heart. Clin Cardiol. 2010;33(5):264–9.
31. Schwartz B, Rezkalla S, Kloner R. Cardiovascular effects of cocaine. Circulation. 2010;122(24):2558–69.
32. Cole C. Cut: a guide to adulterants, bulking agents, and other contaminants found in illicit drugs. [online]. 2010. Available at: http://www.cph.org.uk/wp-content/uploads/2012/08/cut-a-guide-to-the-adulterants-bulking-agents-and-other-contaminants-found-in-illicit-drugs.pdf.

33. Larocque A, Hoffman R. Levamisole in cocaine: unexpected news from an old acquaintance. Clin Toxicol. 2012;50(4):231–41.
34. Auffenberg C, Rosenthal L, Dresner N. Levamisole: a common cocaine adulterant with life-threatening side effects. Psychosomatics. 2013;54(6):590–3.
35. McGrath M, Isakova T, Rennke H, Mottola A, Laliberte K, Niles J. Contaminated cocaine and antineutrophil cytoplasmic antibody-associated disease. Clin J Am Soc Nephrol. 2011;6(12):2799–805.
36. Maxwell J, Brecht M. Methamphetamine: here we go again? Addict Behav. 2011;36(12):1168–73.
37. Hendrickson R, Cloutier R, John McConnell K. Methamphetamine-related emergency department utilization and cost. Acad Emerg Med. 2008;15(1):23–31.
38. Karila L, Weinstein A, Aubin H, Benyamina A, Reynaud M, Batki S. Pharmacological approaches to methamphetamine dependence: a focused review. Br J Clin Pharmacol. 2010;69(6):578–92.
39. Ross E, Reisfield G, Watson M, Chronister C, Goldberger B. Psychoactive "Bath salts" intoxication with methylenedioxypyrovalerone. Am J Med. 2012;125(9):854–8.
40. De Felice L, Glennon R, Negus S. Synthetic cathinones: chemical phylogeny, physiology, and neuropharmacology. Life Sci. 2014;97(1):20–6.
41. Karch S. Cathinone neurotoxicity. Curr Neuropharmacol. 2015;13(1):21–5.
42. Ross E, Watson M, Goldberger B. "Bath salts" intoxication. N Engl J Med. 2011;365(10):967–8.
43. Prosser J, Nelson L. The toxicology of bath salts: a review of synthetic cathinones. J Med Toxicol. 2011;8(1):33–42.
44. Baumann M, Solis E, Watterson L, Marusich J, Fantegrossi W, Wiley J. Baths salts, spice, and related designer drugs: the science behind the headlines. J Neurosci. 2014;34(46):15150–8.
45. Substance Abuse and Mental Health Services Administration, Drug Abuse Warning Network, 2011: National Estimates of drug-related emergency department visits. HHS Publication No. (SMA) 13-4760, DAWN Series D-39. Rockville: Substance Abuse and Mental Health Services Administration; 2013.
46. Moeller KE, Lee KC, Kissack JC. Urine drug screening: a practical guide for clinicians. Mayo Clin Proc. 2008;83(1):66–76.
47. Spiller H, Ryan M, Weston R, Jansen J. Clinical experience with and analytical confirmation of "bath salts" and "legal highs" (synthetic cathinones) in the United States. Clin Toxicol. 2011;49(6):499–505.
48. Farooq M, Bhatt A, Patel M. Neurotoxic and cardiotoxic effects of cocaine and ethanol. J Med Toxicol. 2009;5(3):134–8.
49. Won S, Hong R, Shohet R, Seto T, Parikh N. Methamphetamine-associated cardiomyopathy. Clin Cardiol. 2013;36(12):737–42.
50. McCord J, et al. Management of cocaine-associated chest pain and myocardial infarction: a scientific statement from the American Heart Association Acute Cardiac Care Committee of the Council on Clinical Cardiology. Circulation. 2008;117:1897–907.
51. Lange R, Hillis LD. Cardiovascular complications of cocaine use. N Engl J Med. 2001;345:351–8.
52. Callaway C, Clark R. Hyperthermia in psychostimulant overdose. Ann Emerg Med. 1994;24(1):68–76.
53. Eyer F, Zilker T. Bench-to-bedside review: mechanisms and management of hyperthermia due to toxicity. Crit Care. 2007;11(6):236.
54. Cabot R, Rosenberg E, Harris N, Shepard J, Cort A, Ebeling S, McDonald E, Benzer T, Nejad S, Flood J. Case 40-2013. N Engl J Med. 2013;369(26):2536–45.
55. Penders T. The syndrome of excited delirium following use of "bath salts". J Clin Psychiatry. 2013;74(5):518.
56. Hedges D, Jeppson K, Whitehead P. Antipsychotic medication and seizures: a review. Drugs Today (Barc). 2003;39(7):551–7.
57. Lertxundi U, Hernandez R, Medrano J, Domingo-Echaburu S, Garcia M, Aguirre C. Antipsychotics and seizures: higher risk with atypicals? Seizure. 2013;22(2):141–3.

58. Lepping P, Russell I, Freudenmann RW. Antipsychotic treatment of primary delusional parasitosis: systematic review. Br J Psychiatry. 2007;191:198–205.
59. Fasano A, Petrovic I. Insights into pathophysiology of punding reveal possible treatment strategies. Mol Psychiatry. 2010;15(6):560–73.
60. Deik A, Saunders-Pullman R, San Luciano M. Substance abuse and movement disorders: complex interactions and comorbidities. Curr Drug Abuse Rev. 2012;5(3):243–53.
61. Messina N, Jeter K, Marinelli-Casey P, West K, Rawson R. Children exposed to methamphetamine use and manufacture. Child Abuse Negl. 2014;38(11):1872–83.
62. Grant P, Bell K, Stewart D, Paulson J, Rogers K. Evidence of methamphetamine exposure in children removed from clandestine methamphetamine laboratories. Pediatr Emerg Care. 2010;26(1):10–4.
63. Marshall B, Galea S, Wood E, Kerr T. Injection methamphetamine use is associated with an increased risk of suicide: a prospective cohort study. Drug Alcohol Depend. 2011;119(1–2):134–7.
64. Cruickshank C, Dyer K. A review of the clinical pharmacology of methamphetamine. Addiction. 2009;104(7):1085–99.
65. Homer B, Solomon T, Moeller R, Mascia A, DeRaleau L, Halkitis P. Methamphetamine abuse and impairment of social functioning: a review of the underlying neurophysiological causes and behavioral implications. Psychol Bull. 2008;134(2):301–10.
66. Rusyniak D. Neurologic manifestations of chronic methamphetamine abuse. Neurol Clin. 2011;29(3):641–55.
67. Haim D, Lippmann M, Goldberg S, Walkenstein M. The pulmonary complications of crack cocaine. Chest. 1995;107(1):233–40.
68. Cut: a guide to adulterants, bulking agents and other contaminants found in illicit drugs. 2010. [ebook] Centre for Public Health Faculty of Health and Applied Social Sciences Liverpool John Moores University 5th Floor Kingsway House Hatton Garden. Available at: http://www.cph.org.uk/wp-content/uploads/2012/08/cut-a-guide-to-the-adulterants-bulking-agents-and-other-contaminants-found-in-illicit-drugs.pdf.
69. Broseus J, Gentile N, Esseiva P. The cutting of cocaine and heroin: a critical review. Forensic Sci Int. 2016;262:73–83.
70. Gurel A. Multisystem toxicity after methamphetamine use. Clin Case Rep. 2016;4(3):226–7.
71. Murray B, Murphy C, Beuhler M. Death following recreational use of designer drug "Bath salts" containing 3,4-methylenedioxypyrovalerone (MDPV). J Med Toxicol. 2012;8(1):69–75.
72. Buchacz K, McFarland W, Kellogg T, Loeb L, Holmberg S, Dilley J, Klausner J. Amphetamine use is associated with increased HIV incidence among men who have sex with men in San Francisco. AIDS. 2005;19(13):1423–4.
73. Colfax G, Shoptaw S. The methamphetamine epidemic: implications for HIV prevention and treatment. Curr HIV/AIDS Rep. 2005;2(4):194–9.
74. Karila L, Megarbane B, Cottencin O, Lejoyeux M. Synthetic cathinones: a new public health problem. Curr Neuropharmacol. 2015;13(1):12–20.
75. Roll J. Contingency management for the treatment of methamphetamine use disorders. Am J Psychiatr. 2006;163(11):1993.
76. Rawson R, McCann M, Flammino F, Shoptaw S, Miotto K, Reiber C, Ling W. A comparison of contingency management and cognitive-behavioral approaches for stimulant-dependent individuals. Addiction. 2006;101(2):267–74.
77. Vocci F, Montoya I. Psychological treatments for stimulant misuse, comparing and contrasting those for amphetamine dependence and those for cocaine dependence. Curr Opin Psychiatry. 2009;22(3):263–8.
78. Treatment for stimulant use disorders. Rockville: U.S. Dept. of Health and Human Services, Public Health Service, Substance Abuse and Mental Health Services Administration, Center for Substance Abuse Treatment; 2009.
79. Gonzales R, Mooney L, Rawson R. The methamphetamine problem in the United States. Annu Rev Public Health. 2010;31(1):385–98.

Chapter 4
Cannabis Use Disorders and Related Emergencies

S. Alex Sidelnik and Theodore I. Benzer

Introduction

Cannabis has been used both recreationally and therapeutically since early recorded history, with the earliest use of cannabis for medical purposes documented in a Chinese book of herbal remedies from about 2700 BC [1]. Evidence of cannabis use extends from these early reports to the modern day [1, 2]. Cannabis is a species of plant that has both psychoactive and non-psychoactive properties. There are two subspecies: sativa, commonly called hemp, which has few psychoactive properties but has been used extensively for fiber and rope production, and indica, which has a much higher concentration of psychoactive compounds.

Cannabis use is prevalent throughout the world and is thought to be the most commonly used illicit psychoactive substance. Estimates suggest that up to 4% of the adult population worldwide has used cannabis in the past year [3]. Its use does, however, vary widely in different geographic areas. Approximately 12% of the adult populations of North America and Africa use cannabis annually, compared to 0.6% of the population in South and East Asia [4]. At the time of this writing, the legal status of cannabis is in transition in the United States. Despite remaining an illegal substance under federal law, many states have legalized the therapeutic use of cannabis, and multiple states have legalized recreational use, including Colorado, California, Washington, Oregon, Alaska, Maine, Nevada, Vermont, and Massachusetts. The health impact of these changes remains to be seen.

S. A. Sidelnik (✉)
NYU School of Medicine, NYU Langone Health, Department of Psychiatry, New York, NY, USA
e-mail: alex.sidelnik@nyumc.org

T. I. Benzer
Harvard Medical School, Massachusetts General Hospital, Emergency Department, Boston, MA, USA

A. L. Donovan, S. A. Bird (eds.), *Substance Use and the Acute Psychiatric Patient*, Current Clinical Psychiatry, https://doi.org/10.1007/978-3-319-23961-3_4

The main psychoactive compound in marijuana is delta-9-tetrahydrocannabinol (THC), although the cannabis plant contains over 60 different cannabinols, some with psychoactive properties. THC is a partial agonist of endogenous cannabinoid receptors. There are two forms of the receptor: CB1, which is primarily found in the CNS, and CB2, which is found in immune tissue, as well as in the CNS. These proteins are G-protein-linked, inhibit adenylyl cyclase, and result in increased potassium conductance. The endogenous cannabinoid neurotransmitter is formed in the postsynaptic cell and released and then binds to presynaptic receptors, resulting in presynaptic inhibition [2]. The psychoactive effects of marijuana are mediated by THC binding to the endogenous cannabinoid receptor CB1 [5]. The other most abundant cannabinoid in marijuana is cannabidiol (CBD). CBD does not have the same psychoactive effects as THC. There is some emerging evidence suggesting CBD has both anxiolytic and antipsychotic properties [6, 7].

Other cannabis derivatives, such as synthetically derived cannabinoids, include a number of man-made compounds that interact with the endocannabinoid system. There are currently two FDA-approved synthetic cannabinoids, nabilone and dronabinol, which both act as THC analogs. Nabilone is approved for refractory chemotherapy-induced nausea and vomiting. Dronabinol is approved for AIDS-associated anorexia and chemotherapy-induced nausea and vomiting. Epidiolex, a plant-derived cannabidiol, has also been FDA approved for the treatment of seizures associated with Dravet syndrome and Lennox-Gastaut syndrome. Although the term "synthetic cannabinoids" technically refers to any man-made cannabinoids, the term often refers to illicit synthetic cannabinoids that are frequently abused. Recently, there has been a large increase in the production and illegal distribution of synthetic cannabinoids with psychoactive properties. These substances are primarily used for their cannabis-like psychoactive effects [8].

Cannabis is derived primarily from two sources. The first is marijuana, derived from the cannabis plant. There are many street names for marijuana, including pot, grass, dope, Mary Jane, weed, ganja, and hashish. Solvent-extracted concentrates of cannabis are called hash oil dabs, wax, and honey oil, among other names. Marijuana can be smoked, vaporized, or ingested. The dried flower heads can be smoked, or more concentrated preparations can be vaporized and inhaled. The onset of action is rapid, with psychotropic effects occurring within minutes and lasting about 2–3 hours. Alternatively, cannabis can be ingested for medicinal or recreational use. The psychoactive effects after oral ingestion are delayed compared to inhalation, with onset of action between 30 minutes and 3 hours, and duration up to 12 hours. The bioavailability of ingested cannabis is low because of extensive first-pass metabolism in the liver and inactivation by the acid environment in the stomach.

The second source of cannabis is synthetic cannabinoids. While technically outlawed by the Drug Abuse Prevention Act of 2012, cannabimimetic substances are often produced covertly, and legality is circumvented by altering the chemical compound slightly, thus making it a new substance not technically covered by the Drug Abuse Prevention Act. Typically, synthetic cannabinoids are dissolved in a solvent, applied to plant material, and smoked. They may be preferred over marijuana due to the relative ease of procurement, usually lower price, increased potency, limited detection in drug screening, and perceived safety of use [9, 10]. Street names for these products are numerous and include K2, Spice, White Rhino, Bliss, Blue Bombay, Genie, Zoh, or Scooby Snacks [11]. Illicit synthetic cannabinoids are largely potent agonists of CB1 receptors and are often far more dangerous than marijuana, with risks of severe tachycardia, hypertension, seizures, and acute kidney failure [12]. Synthetic cannabinoids are most often smoked and have a rapid onset of action. The duration of intoxication is variable, reflecting the large heterogeneity of synthetic cannabinoids, but it typically ranges from 1 to 24 hours [13].

Cannabis use disorders are comorbid with multiple psychiatric illnesses, including bipolar disorder, several personality disorders, and other substance use disorders [14]. Among patients with anxiety disorders, cannabis is the most commonly used substance [15]. Individuals with schizophrenia also have high rates of cannabis use, which has been associated with increased rates of psychotic symptoms [16]. Synthetic cannabinoids have been reported in subgroups of individuals with schizophrenia, including those in transitional housing shelters [9]. Cannabis use is also highly comorbid with tobacco use and is associated with increased risk of developing alcohol use disorder and worse clinical outcomes [17].

DSM-5 Criteria

In a discussion of cannabis use disorders, it is important to have a clear understanding of the diagnostic criteria. The DSM-5 includes three diagnoses related to cannabis with criteria listed below [18].

I. Cannabis intoxication:

- (i) Recent use of cannabis
- (ii) Clinically significant problematic behavioral or psychological changes that developed during or shortly after cannabis use
- (iii) At least two of the following signs developing within 2 hours of cannabis use:
    1. Conjunctival injection
    2. Increased appetite
    3. Dry mouth
    4. Tachycardia

II. Cannabis use disorder (mild, moderate, or severe):

- (i) Cannabis is often taken in larger amounts or over a longer period than was intended.
- (ii) There is a persistent desire or unsuccessful effort to cut down or control cannabis use.
- (iii) A great deal of time is spent in activities necessary to obtain cannabis, use cannabis, or recover from its effects.
- (iv) There is craving or a strong desire or urge to use cannabis.

(v) Recurrent cannabis use results in a failure to fulfill major role obligations at work, school, or home.
(vi) There is continued cannabis use despite having persistent or recurrent social or interpersonal problems caused or exacerbated by the effects of cannabis.
(vii) Important social, occupational, or recreational activities are given up or reduced because of cannabis use.
(viii) There is recurrent cannabis use in situations in which it is physically hazardous.
(ix) Cannabis use is continued despite knowledge of having a persistent or recurrent physical or psychological problem that is likely to have been caused or exacerbated by cannabis.
(x) There is tolerance, as defined by either (1) a need for markedly increased cannabis to achieve intoxication or desired effect or (2) markedly diminished effect with continued use of the same amount of the substance.
(xi) There is withdrawal, as manifested by either (1) the characteristic withdrawal syndrome for cannabis or (2) taking of cannabis to relieve or avoid withdrawal symptoms.
(xii) The severity of cannabis use disorder can be graded as mild with 2–3 symptoms, moderate with 4–5 symptoms, or severe with the presence of 6 or more symptoms.

III. Cannabis withdrawal:

(i) Cessation of cannabis use that has been heavy and prolonged (i.e., usually daily or almost daily use over a period of at least a few months)
(ii) Three (or more) of the following signs and symptoms develop within approximately 1 week after the above criteria:

1. Irritability, anger, or aggression
2. Nervousness or anxiety
3. Sleep difficulty (e.g., insomnia, disturbing dreams)
4. Decreased appetite or weight loss
5. Restlessness
6. Depressed mood

Cannabis Intoxication

The clinical manifestations of cannabis intoxication are broad and vary according to a number of clinical and substance-related factors, including formulation of cannabis, potency, method of administration, age of user, co-ingestion with other substances, and comorbid psychiatric illnesses.

Cannabis affects multiple organ systems with prominent neuropsychiatric effects, including changes in mood, cognition, perception, and psychomotor performance.

Cannabis can produce a euphoric effect that can be achieved at low dosages and is often described as the marijuana "high." Users may also report a feeling of decreased anxiety, decreased tension, and increased sociability [19]. Dysphoric reactions may occur with increases in anxiety or transient psychotic symptoms, including paranoia, thought broadcasting, hallucinations, and depersonalization. These symptoms generally occur at higher dosages, or in users with pre-existing psychiatric illnesses, such as psychotic or anxiety disorders. Cannabis can also heighten sensory experiences, making colors appear more vivid and tactile perceptions more intense [19]. Temporal perception may also be affected, with time appearing to progress more slowly. Cannabis intoxication has effects on cognition and psychomotor performance, including decreased concentration and impairment in reaction time and short-term memory. Long-term memory is not typically affected [20]. The cognitive effects of cannabis can lead to difficulty in completing tasks requiring divided attention, such as driving or operating heavy machinery [19, 21, 22].

Synthetic cannabis intoxication can cause different neuropsychiatric symptoms and medical complications. Clinical effects of synthetic cannabinoids are often unpredictable, due to inconsistent dosing, variable potency within each product, and wide variation in the specific chemical make-up of synthetic cannabinoids with differing cannabinoid receptor affinities. Users describe positive effects of relaxation, increased sociability, and increased laughter, while negative effects may include nausea, vomiting, aggression, hallucinations, chest pain, and palpitations [9]. Synthetic cannabinoids can also cause severe psychiatric effects, including agitation, delirium, and psychosis [12]. Conversely, CNS depression, lethargy, and disorientation have also been observed [23].

In some individuals, cannabis intoxication, either from marijuana or synthetic agents, can precipitate a substance-induced psychotic disorder in which psychotic symptoms persist beyond the acute intoxication period up to several months (see Chap. 7 for further details) [24]. In individuals with underlying psychotic disorders, the use of cannabis or synthetic cannabinoids can exacerbate symptoms or trigger recurrence of psychosis [25].

In children, intoxication most commonly occurs after accidental ingestion of edible forms of marijuana intended for adult use, including cookies, candies, or brownies, although direct administration from parents and caregivers has also been reported [26]. Symptoms of acute intoxication in children vary depending on the degree of exposure, but can include neurologic symptoms, such as lethargy, ataxia, and seizures [27, 28]. If large amounts of cannabis are ingested, prolonged lethargy, coma, or hypoxia may occur [29–31].

Withdrawal

While the syndrome of cannabis withdrawal has been supported by clinical observation and in research studies, it was first recognized as a distinct clinical syndrome only in the latest *Diagnostic and Statistical Manual of Mental Disorders* (DSM-5).

Cannabis withdrawal, as defined in DSM-5, is the development of at least three signs or symptoms within 1 week after cessation of heavy and prolonged cannabis use, including (1) irritability, anger, or aggression; (2) nervousness or anxiety; (3) sleep difficulty (e.g., insomnia, disturbing dreams); (4) decreased appetite or weight loss; (5) restlessness; (6) depressed mood; and (7) at least one of the following physical symptoms causing significant discomfort: abdominal pain, shakiness/tremors, sweating, fever, chills, or headache [18].

Acute cannabis withdrawal occurs most commonly in heavy users and has been observed in more than half of individuals presenting for the treatment of cannabis use disorder [32]. Symptoms of cannabis withdrawal typically emerge 1–3 days after cessation of use and peak after 2–6 days. Withdrawal symptoms typically last for 1–2 weeks, although symptoms can persist up to 4 weeks in some individuals [33]. Biologically, chronic cannabis use leads to a downregulation of CB1 receptors, due to increased agonist activation with exogenous cannabinoids. When cannabis use is discontinued, exogenous agonist activation is removed, leaving CB1 receptors in a hypoactive state, which presumably mediates withdrawal symptoms. As cessation from cannabis continues, CB1 receptors return to the pre-cannabis state within 4 weeks, and withdrawal symptoms abate [34].

Relative to other substance withdrawal syndromes, cannabis withdrawal is comparable to tobacco withdrawal in magnitude [35]. Although relatively mild, cannabis withdrawal can lead to functional impairments in daily activities and is associated with relapse of cannabis use [36]. Furthermore, cannabis withdrawal can serve as a negative reinforcement for sobriety, as attempts at abstinence are frequently followed by uncomfortable withdrawal symptoms [37].

Due to the psychiatric and neuro-vegetative symptoms associated with cannabis withdrawal, it can be challenging to differentiate symptoms from potentially co-occurring mood and anxiety disorders from those of the withdrawal state. Longitudinal history and observation over time can be useful in making this diagnostic distinction. Synthetic cannabinoids can have more severe withdrawal symptoms, with agitation, irritability, anxiety, mood swings, and insomnia, and may emerge as quickly as 15 minutes after use [38].

Medical Comorbidities of Cannabis Use

Presentations to the emergency department (ED) for symptoms associated with acute intoxication from cannabis alone are uncommon. Life-threatening complications are infrequent, although fatalities have been reported after cannabis use due to acute coronary syndrome and tachyarrhythmias [39]. Among patients who do present to the ED, common complaints or findings include agitation and aggressive behavior (22%), psychosis (20%), anxiety (20%), and vomiting (17%) [40].

Cannabis hyperemesis syndrome (CHS) is a cluster of symptoms characterized by cyclic vomiting, nausea, and abdominal pain, with no clear etiology, other than a presumed, paradoxical effect of chronic cannabis use. Symptoms typically improve with cessation of cannabis use or with hot showers and baths [41]. Acute treatment consists of administration of antiemetics, intravenous fluids, and benzodiazepines. In treatment refractory CHS, case reports indicate that using intravenous haloperidol at doses of 5 mg can be successful in reducing symptoms [42].

Patients using inhaled preparations of cannabis can develop pulmonary complications from the irritation of the inhaled smoke and increased intrathoracic pressures secondary to breath-holding during inhalation. Acute asthma exacerbation, bronchospasm, pneumothorax, and pneumomediastinum have all been reported after inhalation of marijuana. Unless obtained from an authorized dispensary, marijuana may contain contaminants, as well as other psychoactive compounds, and may induce allergic or bronchospastic reactions when the smoke is inhaled. In immunocompromised patients, inhalation of biologically contaminated marijuana may inadvertently lead to pulmonary infections [43].

Although rare, ischemic chest pain and myocardial infarction have been reported after marijuana use [39]. Again, if the preparation is contaminated with other compounds that are sympathomimetic, such as cocaine and methamphetamine, coronary ischemia can result from ingestion [44].

Children can present after cannabis ingestion with altered mental status that can progress to somnolence and coma. Depressed respirations and, in rare cases, apnea have been seen [27]. Accidental oral ingestions are more common in states where cannabis has been legalized for recreational use. These states have products available that mimic candies, cookies, and brownies, which children can ingest accidentally if the products are not carefully secured [45].

Patients who use synthetic cannabinoids are at risk of more serious medical complications. Synthetic preparations may be adulterated with other psychoactive chemicals, including amphetamines, cathinones, 3,4-methylenedioxymethamphetamine (MDMA), and other ingredients, all with significant sympathomimetic action. The most common complications from synthetic cannabinoid use include neuropsychiatric symptoms, including agitation, coma, psychosis, seizures, and delirium (66%); cardiovascular changes, including hypertension, tachycardia, or bradycardia (17%); and other systemic symptoms, including rhabdomyolysis (6%) and acute kidney injury (4%) [46].

Cannabis withdrawal is rarely life threatening; however, synthetic cannabinoid withdrawal may lead to seizures, kidney failure, and dyspnea [47, 48]. Synthetic cannabinoid withdrawal can also cause sympathetic autonomic hyperactivity, with associated hypertension, tachycardia, and diaphoresis. It may be difficult to differentiate if the physiologic effects are due to synthetic cannabinoid intoxication or withdrawal, as symptoms often overlap. Assessing for psychiatric symptoms of synthetic cannabinoid intoxication and determining time of last use may be helpful in differentiating the two.

Assessment and Management in the ED

The ED evaluation of the cannabis-using patient should clarify the history of cannabis use, including time of last use, chronicity and quantity of use, route of administration, formulation or type of cannabis, and co-ingestion with other substances.

The DSM-5 criteria previously discussed can help the clinician assess the potential presence and severity of a cannabis use disorder. Evaluation of psychotic, anxiety, or mood symptoms (either due to or comorbid with cannabis use) should also occur. All patients must be assessed for suicidality and homicidality. The mental status exam may be significant for conjunctival injection, odor of cannabis, disorganized thought process, persecutory delusions, thought broadcasting, referential thinking, anxiety, or euphoric mood. Collateral information from friends or family may be helpful, especially if the patient's ability to give a reliable history is compromised.

All patients presenting to the ED with cannabis-related complaints will benefit from a targeted medical evaluation. Obtaining vital signs, a physical examination, and routine laboratory studies, including urine toxicology screening, can aid in ascertaining medical stability.

In emergency settings, there are diagnostic challenges to identifying the patient who is using cannabis but not reporting it. Unfortunately, there is no readily available test for synthetic cannabinoids. The most commonly available urine toxicology screens are specific for THC and do not detect the other synthetic cannabinoids. In addition, for chronic cannabis users, a positive screen for THC can persist for days or weeks after use and long after the acute psychoactive effects have worn off. Thus, a patient's presenting symptoms may be attributed to cannabis use but, in fact, be unrelated. It is important to think critically about diagnosing a patient with cannabis intoxication based on a positive THC screen alone, especially when the clinical findings are atypical. A thorough history, physical exam, and observation over time may aid in clarifying acute intoxication versus prior cannabis exposure.

Laboratory Testing and Imaging

The most common screening tool for cannabis is the urine drug screen, consisting of an immunoassay to detect the metabolites of THC, primarily 11-*nor*-Δ-THC-9-carboxylic acid (THC-COOH). The detection time for cannabis in the urine is variable and is related to amount ingested, route of administration, frequency of use, THC content of cannabis, and cut-off value of the urine drug test. THC is highly lipophilic and can be stored in adipose tissue, where it is released into circulation over time. The mean detection time for smoking one marijuana cigarette is 1–2 days, while heavy users may be positive for THC up to 27 days [49]. As a result, a positive test may be helpful in identifying past use but does not always reflect recent cannabis exposure. False positives for cannabinoids with current immunoassays are typically rare but may include the synthetic cannabinoid dronabinol.

Detection of illicit synthetic cannabinoid exposure can be challenging, as synthetic cannabinoids do not typically share similar structures with THC or THC metabolites that are detected in standard immunoassays. While some immunoassays are available to detect common synthetic cannabinoids and their parent compounds, availability in most ED settings is limited [50]. As a result, the diagnosis of synthetic cannabinoid exposure is often based on clinical history.

If symptoms are atypical or if the diagnosis is unclear, evaluation for other medical or substance-related etiologies may be indicated. The differential diagnosis of patients presenting with signs and symptoms of acute cannabis intoxication is wide and can include blood sugar abnormalities (either hypoglycemia or hyperglycemia), metabolic disarray, CNS infection, carbon monoxide poisoning, other drug ingestions (sedatives, opioids, ethanol, etc.), or covert brain injury. Laboratory studies, including CBC, electrolytes, liver function tests, and urinalysis, can help exclude other medical etiologies. Imaging studies including head CT or MRI are not typically indicated, unless there is a suspicion for underlying neurologic injury.

Management of Intoxication

Cannabis intoxication rarely requires medical treatment. In more severe cases of intoxication, distressing psychiatric symptoms can occur and can lead to presentations for psychosis, mood disturbances, and anxiety symptoms. Management of the psychiatric effects of cannabis intoxication is largely supportive, and, depending on comorbidities, pharmacologic intervention is often unnecessary. If psychiatric symptoms are mild to moderate, behavioral and environmental interventions can be used, such as keeping the patient in a quiet environment with supportive reassurance.

More severe cases of intoxication with marked agitation or psychosis are more likely to be seen in emergency settings. In these cases, benzodiazepines or antipsychotics can be administered PO, IM, or IV for behavioral disturbances [51]. While there is a lack of vigorous clinical studies supporting a clear pharmacologic choice, benzodiazepines are generally preferred to antipsychotics for milder symptoms of anxiety or agitation, while antipsychotics are used to treat more overt psychotic symptoms or severe behavioral dysregulation. Psychotic symptoms associated with cannabis intoxication typically respond to low-dose first- or second-generation antipsychotics, including haloperidol, risperidone, or olanzapine. Hospital police and security presence can be helpful in managing violent behavior, and mechanical restraints can be used as a last resort to protect the safety of patients and others. If behavioral symptoms are severe and persist despite adequate trials of benzodiazepines and antipsychotics, sedation with other agents, including ketamine or dexmedetomidine, can be used with caution [52].

Management of Withdrawal

Cannabis withdrawal is rarely life threatening and does not usually require medical attention. In contrast, synthetic cannabinoid withdrawal can cause dyspnea, sympathetic autonomic hyperactivity with associated hypertension and tachycardia, seizures, and kidney failure [47, 48]. Medical management is dictated by the severity of the presenting symptoms.

Cannabis withdrawal can produce psychiatric symptoms of anxiety, insomnia, loss of appetite, irritability, and mood changes. Synthetic cannabinoids can have more severe withdrawal symptoms, with agitation, irritability, anxiety, mood swings, and insomnia. In the emergency setting, low-dose benzodiazepines can be used for withdrawal symptoms causing severe anxiety or distress.

Disposition Considerations

Cannabis intoxication or withdrawal by itself rarely requires inpatient admission. During periods of intoxication, patients may present with a variety of psychiatric concerns, including psychosis, mood disturbances, and anxiety symptoms, that typically resolve with sobriety. When clinically sober, the patient should be re-evaluated, to determine which, if any, symptoms remain, as these remaining symptoms will influence ultimate disposition. A thorough safety assessment should be performed prior to discharge in all patients presenting with suicidality, homicidality, psychosis, or significant behavioral disturbances. Furthermore, cannabis intoxication can affect cognition, psychomotor performance, and judgment and may affect the patient's ability to be safely discharged if driving a car or traveling alone [19, 21, 22]. The time needed to achieve sobriety can vary significantly and depends on a number of factors, including potency of cannabis product used, mode of ingestion, and co-ingestion with other substances.

Psychiatric admission should be considered for those unable to be safely discharged due to ongoing suicidality, homicidality, or persistent psychosis leading to inability to care for themselves. Additionally, if the patient had severe agitation requiring large amounts of sedating medications or restraints, psychiatric admission may be needed to ensure safety and further stabilization. For individuals with psychotic disorders, such as schizophrenia, worsening of psychosis can occur after cannabis or synthetic cannabinoid use. If acute psychotic symptoms persist beyond intoxication, psychiatric admission may be warranted. Cannabis withdrawal in the absence of other significant psychopathologies is largely managed in an outpatient setting. Admission for cannabis detoxification is rarely indicated.

When assessing the need for referral to outpatient treatment, a careful assessment of cannabis use and potential comorbid psychiatric illness should be performed. Individuals with cannabis use disorder or psychiatric illness can be provided with referrals to outpatient substance use disorder and/or psychiatric treatment. The referral should be appropriate to the patient's level of motivation and interest in treatment. Individuals with more severe cannabis use disorders can be referred to partial hospitalization or intensive outpatient programs for substance use disorder treatment where available. Information on self-help groups, such as Marijuana Anonymous or SMART Recovery, can be provided, although their effectiveness has not been rigorously studied.

Rarely do patients require hospital admission for medical complications of cannabis. Possible medical complications prompting admission may include myocardial infarction, cannabis hyperemesis, seizures, renal failure, and pneumothorax. In pediatric cannabis exposure, observation or medical admission may be necessary, given potential risks of coma, seizures, and hypoxia [28–31].

Conclusion

In summary, cannabis has a long history of human consumption, and it is thought to be the most commonly used illicit psychoactive substance worldwide. The cannabis plant is composed of a number of cannabinoids that interact with the body's endogenous cannabinoid system. The most abundant psychoactive cannabinoid in cannabis is THC, which is responsible for its psychoactive effects. Synthetic cannabinoids also interact with the endogenous cannabinoid system and have a variety of psychoactive and physiologic effects, reflecting the large heterogeneity in compounds. Intoxication with cannabis often produces euphoria, perceptual changes, but also distressing symptoms of anxiety, paranoia, or worsening of underlying psychiatric illness. In the ED, patients may present with the more distressing symptoms of intoxication, prompting psychiatric assessment. Intoxication with cannabis is often self-limited and improves with supportive treatment or limited use of benzodiazepines or antipsychotics. In some individuals, including those with psychotic disorders, cannabis or synthetic cannabinoid intoxication may lead to worsening of underlying psychiatric illness. Medical consequences of cannabis or synthetic cannabinoid intoxication are rare and not often life threatening. As the legal status of marijuana continues to be in transition, clinicians may begin to encounter an increasing number of individuals with cannabis intoxication and its related emergencies.

References

1. Pain S. A potted history. Nature. 2015;525(7570):S10–1.
2. Mechoulam R, Parker LA. The endocannabinoid system and the brain. Annu Rev Psychol. 2013;64:21–47.
3. Leggett T, United Nations Office on Drugs and Crime. A review of the world cannabis situation. Bull Narc. 2006;58(1):1–155.
4. United Nations Office on Drugs and Crime, World Drug Report 2016. Vienna United Nations.
5. Gomez-Ruiz M, Hernandez M, de Miguel R, Ramos JA. An overview on the biochemistry of the cannabinoid system. Mol Neurobiol. 2007;36(1):3–14.
6. McGuire P, Robson P, Cubala WJ, Vasile D, Morrison PD, Barron R, et al. Cannabidiol (CBD) as an adjunctive therapy in schizophrenia: a multicenter randomized controlled trial. Am J Psychiatry. 2018;175(3):225–31.
7. Blessing EM, Steenkamp MM, Manzanares J, Marmar CR. Cannabidiol as a potential treatment for anxiety disorders. Neurotherapeutics. 2015;12(4):825–36.
8. Gunderson EW, Haughey HM, Ait-Daoud N, Joshi AS, Hart CL. "Spice" and "K2" herbal highs: a case series and systematic review of the clinical effects and biopsychosocial implications of synthetic cannabinoid use in humans. Am J Addict. 2012;21(4):320–6.

9. Barnett BOM. Synthetic cannabinoid use in a transitional housing shelter: a survey to characterize awareness of risks and reasons for use. Am J Psychiatry Residents' J. 2016;11(10):4–6.
10. Every-Palmer S. Synthetic cannabinoid JWH-018 and psychosis: an explorative study. Drug Alcohol Depend. 2011;117(2–3):152–7.
11. 700 Street Names for Synthetic Marijuana (Spice, K2, etc.).
12. Monte AA, Calello DP, Gerona RR, Hamad E, Campleman SL, Brent J, et al. Characteristics and treatment of patients with clinical illness due to synthetic cannabinoid inhalation reported by medical toxicologists: a ToxIC database study. J Med Toxicol. 2017;13(2):146–52.
13. Tournebize J, Gibaja V, Kahn JP. Acute effects of synthetic cannabinoids: update 2015. Subst Abus. 2017;38(3):344–66.
14. Lev-Ran S, Le Foll B, McKenzie K, George TP, Rehm J. Cannabis use and cannabis use disorders among individuals with mental illness. Compr Psychiatry. 2013;54(6):589–98.
15. Conway KP, Compton W, Stinson FS, Grant BF. Lifetime comorbidity of DSM-IV mood and anxiety disorders and specific drug use disorders: results from the National Epidemiologic Survey on Alcohol and Related Conditions. J Clin Psychiatry. 2006;67(2):247–57.
16. Foti DJ, Kotov R, Guey LT, Bromet EJ. Cannabis use and the course of schizophrenia: 10-year follow-up after first hospitalization. Am J Psychiatry. 2010;167(8):987–93.
17. Subbaraman MS, Kerr WC. Simultaneous versus concurrent use of alcohol and cannabis in the National Alcohol Survey. Alcohol Clin Exp Res. 2015;39(5):872–9.
18. American Psychiatric Association. Diagnostic and statistical manual of mental disorders. 5th ed. Washington, D.C.: American Psychiatric Association; 2013.
19. Ashton CH. Pharmacology and effects of cannabis: a brief review. Br J Psychiatry. 2001;178:101–6.
20. Ranganathan M, D'Souza DC. The acute effects of cannabinoids on memory in humans: a review. Psychopharmacology. 2006;188(4):425–44.
21. Neavyn MJ, Blohm E, Babu KM, Bird SB. Medical marijuana and driving: a review. J Med Toxicol. 2014;10(3):269–79.
22. Rogeberg O, Elvik R. The effects of cannabis intoxication on motor vehicle collision revisited and revised. Addiction. 2016;111(8):1348–59.
23. Adams AJ, Banister SD, Irizarry L, Trecki J, Schwartz M, Gerona R. "Zombie" outbreak caused by the synthetic cannabinoid AMB-FUBINACA in New York. N Engl J Med. 2017;376(3):235–42.
24. Hurst D, Loeffler G, McLay R. Psychosis associated with synthetic cannabinoid agonists: a case series. Am J Psychiatry. 2011;168(10):1119.
25. Radhakrishnan R, Wilkinson ST, D'Souza DC. Gone to pot – a review of the Association between Cannabis and Psychosis. Front Psych. 2014;5:54.
26. Blackstone M, Callahan J. An unsteady walk in the park. Pediatr Emerg Care. 2008;24(3):193–5.
27. Wang GS, Roosevelt G, Heard K. Pediatric marijuana exposures in a medical marijuana state. JAMA Pediatr. 2013;167(7):630–3.
28. Bonkowsky JSD, Pomeroy S. Ataxia and shaking in a 2-year-old girl: acute marijuana intoxication presenting as seizure. Pediatr Emerg Care. 2005;21(8):527–8.
29. Appelboam A, Oades PJ. Coma due to cannabis toxicity in an infant. Eur J Emerg Med. 2006;13(3):177–9.
30. Boros CA, Parsons DW, Zoanetti GD, Ketteridge D, Kennedy D. Cannabis cookies: a cause of coma. J Paediatr Child Health. 1996;32(2):194–5.
31. Carstairs SD, Fujinaka MK, Keeney GE, Ly BT. Prolonged coma in a child due to hashish ingestion with quantitation of THC metabolites in urine. J Emerg Med. 2011;41(3):e69–71.
32. Bonnet U, Preuss UW. The cannabis withdrawal syndrome: current insights. Subst Abus Rehabil. 2017;8:9–37.
33. Budney AJ, Moore BA, Vandrey RG, Hughes JR. The time course and significance of cannabis withdrawal. J Abnorm Psychol. 2003;112(3):393–402.
34. Hirvonen J, Goodwin RS, Li CT, Terry GE, Zoghbi SS, Morse C, et al. Reversible and regionally selective downregulation of brain cannabinoid CB1 receptors in chronic daily cannabis smokers. Mol Psychiatry. 2012;17(6):642–9.

35. Vandrey RG, Budney AJ, Hughes JR, Liguori A. A within-subject comparison of withdrawal symptoms during abstinence from cannabis, tobacco, and both substances. Drug Alcohol Depend. 2008;92(1–3):48–54.
36. Allsop DJ, Copeland J, Norberg MM, Fu S, Molnar A, Lewis J, et al. Quantifying the clinical significance of cannabis withdrawal. PLoS One. 2012;7(9):e44864.
37. Levin KH, Copersino ML, Heishman SJ, Liu F, Kelly DL, Boggs DL, et al. Cannabis withdrawal symptoms in non-treatment-seeking adult cannabis smokers. Drug Alcohol Depend. 2010;111(1–2):120–7.
38. Macfarlane V, Christie G. Synthetic cannabinoid withdrawal: a new demand on detoxification services. Drug Alcohol Rev. 2015;34(2):147–53.
39. Aryana A, Williams MA. Marijuana as a trigger of cardiovascular events: speculation or scientific certainty? Int J Cardiol. 2007;118(2):141–4.
40. Dines AM, Wood DM, Galicia M, Yates CM, Heyerdahl F, Hovda KE, et al. Presentations to the emergency department following cannabis use – a multi-centre case series from ten European countries. J Med Toxicol. 2015;11(4):415–21.
41. Sun S, Zimmermann AE. Cannabinoid hyperemesis syndrome. Hosp Pharm. 2013;48(8):650–5.
42. Witsil JC, Mycyk MB. Haloperidol, a novel treatment for cannabinoid hyperemesis syndrome. Am J Ther. 2017;24(1):e64–e7.
43. Hamadeh R, Ardehali A, Locksley RM, York MK. Fatal aspergillosis associated with smoking contaminated marijuana, in a marrow transplant recipient. Chest. 1988;94(2):432–3.
44. Havakuk O, Rezkalla SH, Kloner RA. The cardiovascular effects of cocaine. J Am Coll Cardiol. 2017;70(1):101–13.
45. Monte AA, Zane RD, Heard KJ. The implications of marijuana legalization in Colorado. JAMA. 2015;313(3):241–2.
46. Riederer AM, Campleman SL, Carlson RG, Boyer EW, Manini AF, Wax PM, et al. Acute poisonings from synthetic cannabinoids – 50 U.S. Toxicology Investigators Consortium Registry Sites, 2010–2015. MMWR Morb Mortal Wkly Rep. 2016;65(27):692–5.
47. Cooper Z. Adverse effects of synthetic cannabinoids: management of acute toxicity and withdrawal. Curr Psychiatry Rep. 2016;18(5):52.
48. Sampson CS, Bedy SM, Carlisle T. Withdrawal seizures seen in the setting of synthetic cannabinoid abuse. Am J Emerg Med. 2015;33(11):1712.
49. Huestis MA, Mitchell JM, Cone EJ. Detection times of marijuana metabolites in urine by immunoassay and GC-MS. J Anal Toxicol. 1995;19(6):443–9.
50. Wohlfarth A, Scheidweiler KB, Castaneto M, Gandhi AS, Desrosiers NA, Klette KL, et al. Urinary prevalence, metabolite detection rates, temporal patterns and evaluation of suitable LC-MS/MS targets to document synthetic cannabinoid intake in US military urine specimens. Clin Chem Lab Med. 2015;53(3):423–34.
51. Leweke FM, Gerth CW, Klosterkotter J. Cannabis-associated psychosis: current status of research. CNS Drugs. 2004;18(13):895–910.
52. Leikin JB, Amusina O. Use of dexmedetomidine to treat delirium primarily caused by cannabis. Am J Emerg Med. 2017;35(3):524 e1–2.

Chapter 5
Management of Acute Substance Use Disorders: Hallucinogens and Associated Compounds

Mladen Nisavic and Melisa W. Lai-Becker

Introduction

Patients presenting with substance use disorders (SUDs) are a common occurrence in most emergency departments (ED), with Drug Abuse Warning Network (DAWN) and Substance Abuse and Mental Health Services Administration (SAMHSA) estimating over 5 million of the 136.3 million total emergency department visits in 2011 were related to drug use – a 100% increase compared to their 2004 estimate. Of these, nearly one half (about 2.5 million ED visits) were attributed to acute medical emergencies from incapacitating drug abuse [1, 2]. While opioids, cocaine, alcohol, and stimulants are most commonly seen, patients intoxicated with hallucinogens and various so-called club drugs present not infrequently.

Hallucinogens are a broad and markedly diverse class of drugs of abuse. Unlike most other substances discussed in this book, hallucinogens are grouped together not because of shared molecular structure or CNS-binding properties, but because of their intended mode of action – to produce a transient alteration in cognition, enhance emotional states, and alter sensation and reality perception. As such, this drug class includes a variety of compounds, ranging from plant-derived chemicals used to heighten religious experiences (e.g., peyote) to dissociative anesthetics (e.g., ketamine), to synthetic compounds designed as "club drugs" (e.g., lysergic acid diethylamide = LSD derivatives). While historical use of hallucinogens has been to potentiate mystical/religious experiences, most contemporary use in the

M. Nisavic (✉)
Massachusetts General Hospital, Department of Psychiatry, Boston, MA, USA

Harvard Medical School, Boston, MA, USA
e-mail: mnisavic@partners.org

M. W. Lai-Becker
Whidden Hospital Emergency Department, Division of Medical Toxicology, Whidden Hosptial Campus of Cambridge Health Alliance, Department of Emergency Medicine, Everett, MA, USA

A. L. Donovan, S. A. Bird (eds.), *Substance Use and the Acute Psychiatric Patient*, Current Clinical Psychiatry, https://doi.org/10.1007/978-3-319-23961-3_5

United States is for recreational purposes. Some estimated 1.2 million people have used hallucinogens in 2014, with this drug class accounting for approximately 7 percent of all drug-related ED visits in the United States [1, 2]. Although these drugs remain relatively uncommon in patients presenting to the ED with substance use issues – especially when compared to use of alcohol, cocaine, and opioids – familiarity with various hallucinogenic compounds' symptoms of acute intoxication and knowledge of acute management interventions are essential skills for ED physicians and consulting psychiatrists.

The following terms are commonly used by patients to refer to the acute intoxicating effects of hallucinogens, as well as their sequelae:

- "Tripping" is a term used to describe acute hallucinogen intoxication. A "bad trip" denotes intoxication marked by unintended side effects (e.g., fear, agitation, paranoia), while a "good trip" will describe a more pleasant experience for the user.
- Patients will often describe their experiences as "hallucinations," although they may commonly retain some awareness that these perceptions are not real. In fact, most of the sensory misperceptions induced by hallucinogens are better classified as illusions rather than frank hallucinations.
- "Flashbacks" resemble acute intoxication but are more transient phenomena and commonly occur months or years since last use of the drug. Most patients will describe visual misperceptions, including geometric shapes, objects in the periphery of vision, flashes of color, afterimages, halos, micropsia, macropsia, or increased color intensity, and will retain awareness that these experiences are not reality-based. Estimates of prevalence of flashbacks have varied across studies, and anywhere between 5% and 50% of all patients exposed to hallucinogens may experience at least one flashback after acute drug use. LSD is the best-studied, and also the most frequently implicated, hallucinogen associated with flashbacks. These are commonly not perceived as distressing, and most cases will remit spontaneously over the course of a few months [3].

The neurobiology of hallucinogens is complex, as befitting such a wide and diverse class of compounds, and thus beyond the scope of this chapter. Most of the compounds are believed to exert their clinical effect through modulating the availability of psychoactive neurotransmitters such as serotonin, dopamine, and glutamate. Effects of these chemicals on receptors outside the CNS may also lead to sympathomimetic effects throughout the rest of the body, causing mydriasis, hypertension, tachycardia, and hyperthermia, though generally to a lesser degree than stimulants, such as amphetamines and cocaine [4, 5].

A brief overview of the most commonly used hallucinogenic compounds is outlined below:

- *Lysergic acid diethylamide (LSD)*: Synthesized in 1938 by the Swiss scientist, Albert Hofmann Ph.D., LSD is the first and one of the best known hallucinogenic compounds. The drug was initially marketed as an anesthetic and enjoyed brief popularity as an adjunct for psychotherapy, before gaining notoriety as a psychedelic drug in the 1960s. By 1968, LSD was listed as a drug of abuse by the US government. Since then, the use of LSD has steadily diminished, as people turn to alternative compounds, including cannabinoids, other hallucinogens, and stimulants. LSD is most commonly available in liquid form (e.g., added to blotter paper) or, more rarely, as a pill.

- *Dextromethorphan (DXM)*: Technically part of the opioid class of drugs, DXM is a dextro-isomer of levorphanol (a codeine analogue) and is readily available as a cough suppressant in various over-the-counter cough remedies. Most DXM use is seen in adolescents, who ingest higher than recommended doses of the drug to produce a trancelike dissociative state or "high." Colloquially, this practice is also known as "Robo tripping" (derived from the drug's presence in Robitussin™-DM cough syrup) and "skittling" (due to the use of tablets of DXM that, when sold commercially in push packs, may look like pieces of the candy Skittles™ made by the Wrigley J. Company). As DXM is often combined with other compounds in cold remedies (e.g., acetaminophen, NSAIDs, antihistaminergics), all patients suspected of DXM intoxication should be evaluated for potential co-ingestions and related complications [6].
- *Mescaline*: Mescaline is found in the peyote cactus (*Lophophora williamsii*), a plant native to the southwest United States. The plant is commonly dried into "buttons" which can be ingested or used to produce a tea. Most people will use between 6 and 10 buttons to become intoxicated. Mescaline produces a psychedelic state similar (though generally milder) to that seen with LSD. Mescaline was historically used by Native Americans for religious purposes, and the members of Native American Church can still use the plant and its derivative for religious purposes without legal consequences. All other use of mescaline is considered illegal by the US government [7].
- *Psilocybin*: Psilocybin is a naturally occurring hallucinogenic compound found in a number of fungi species native to the Pacific Northwest and Southern United States. These mushrooms are known by their street names of "magic mushrooms" or "shrooms" and are commonly dried and ingested with food (as this minimizes the nausea and vomiting that may precede the high). Patients reporting use of hallucinogenic mushrooms are at risk for accidental ingestion of both toxic fungi (due to misidentification) and other hallucinogens (e.g., edible mushrooms laced with LSD) [7].
- *Salvinorin A*: Salvinorin A is found in the leaves of the *Salvia divinorum* plant, and it is not a federally controlled substance in the United States. Most people obtain the drug (as complete plant, leaves, or extracts) freely through the Internet. Compared to other hallucinogens, salvia has a relatively short duration of action (1–2 hours) and is perceived as a safer alternative by many users. Traditionally, salvia plant leaves were either chewed/swallowed outright or crushed and mixed with water to create a potable infusion. Nowadays, most recreational users smoke the dried plant leaves as this results in quicker onset of symptoms and shorter "high." [8]
- *Phencyclidine (PCP, angel dust)*: PCP is a noncompetitive antagonist of the N-methyl-D-aspartate (NMDA) receptor. This drug was initially developed as an anesthetic, but the use was abandoned due to its significant side-effect pro-

file. The drug is available in a variety of forms (e.g., capsules, tablets, powder) and can be used in a variety of modes, including insufflation, inhalation (often added to cannabis, tobacco, or other herbs), ingestion, or intravenous use. PCP is notorious among emergency medicine responders and is by far the most dangerous compound discussed in this chapter, in large part due to its toxidrome, which is marked by violent and bizarre behavior. Acute intoxication may result in an unpredictable "high" state marked by depersonalization, increased feeling of strength and invulnerability, reduced inhibition, and diminished pain response. Furthermore, individuals may experience sensory distortions or even frank hallucinations and may exhibit thought disorganization and paranoia. Occasionally, acutely intoxicated individuals may become violent, often with minimal provocation. Rare and bizarre reports of extreme violence, including self-mutilation and even cannibalism, have also been described with acute PCP intoxication. Much like LSD, PCP use reached its peak popularity in the 1960s and has since diminished in prevalence as users transition to safer and cheaper alternatives [9, 10].

- *Ketamine (special K)*: Structurally similar to PCP, ketamine also works through binding at the NMDA receptor as an antagonist. Ketamine is commonly used in hospital settings as a safe anesthetic for conscious sedation and analgesia, and there is growing research in the use of ketamine for treatment of refractory major depressive disorder. As a drug of abuse, ketamine is used to produce a trancelike dissociative state, not dissimilar to that seen with other hallucinogens. Unintended overdose may lead to coma; thus patients suspected of ketamine intoxication warrant careful medical monitoring.

Intoxication

Acute intoxication with hallucinogenic compounds will inevitably lead to neuropsychiatric sequelae. These include changes in emotional states (from euphoria and well-being to fear and paranoia), sensory misperceptions (e.g., colors perceived as brighter), frank hallucinations, distorted perception of time, and dissociative experiences. Ultimately, the patient's clinical presentation will depend on the specific combination of symptoms the patient is experiencing, the subjective level of distress, patients' awareness that the symptoms are drug-induced, and the specific profile of the drug used.

An acutely intoxicated patient that is experiencing a "good trip" may require little beyond containment and monitoring. At worst, these patients may resemble patients in an acute manic state, presenting as expansive and euphoric, with ideas of reference and vivid hallucinations. Patients may attempt to act on their grandiose and delusional thoughts and thus place themselves in danger inadvertently. A "bad trip" may present with a range of undesired effects, including overwhelming anxiety or panic, paranoia, and frightening hallucinations. In the absence of a clear history of drug use or psychiatric history, it may be difficult to differentiate hallucinogen intoxication from a primary psychotic disorder. The presence of visual phenomena, prominent dissociative experiences, and distorted sensory and time perception are all uncommon in primary psychosis and may instead indicate acute hallucinogen intoxication. These symptoms should gradually abate and resolve as the offending agent is metabolized and/or eliminated from the body. Depending on the drug and amount taken, residual effects of an exposure may last from hours to days or even weeks. Rarely psychosis may persist and one hypothesis is that hallucinogen use (similar to cannabis) may expose latent primary psychotic disorders in vulnerable individuals [11].

Most cases of mild hallucinogen intoxication should respond well to containment and destimulation (e.g., placement in a quieter area of the ED). Patients with prominent anxiety, fear, or even mild agitation can be treated with benzodiazepines, which will also address mild vital sign changes (e.g., tachycardia or hypertension) related to increased autonomic arousal. Lorazepam (e.g., 1–2 mg) or diazepam (5 mg) can be both administered parenterally and thus present reasonable options in the emergency department setting. Dopamine antagonists (e.g., haloperidol 5 mg IM or IV) can be used in conjunction with benzodiazepines to help manage symptoms of psychosis or more severe agitation. Clinicians should exercise caution when considering the use of dopamine blockers as these drugs may worsen pre-existing hyperthermia, catatonia, and extrapyramidal motor symptoms and can also reduce the seizure threshold in a hallucinogen-intoxicated patient. In our clinical practice, often the best results are achieved by administering benzodiazepines (e.g., IV lorazepam) with dopamine blockers (e.g., IV haloperidol), as the two drug classes work extremely well in combination – benzodiazepines provide additional tranquilizing effect not seen with haloperidol alone and will reduce risk for seizures, while the dopamine blockers will provide superior control of hallucinations and thought disorganization.

PCP intoxication is an important exception to the general explanation of the hallucinogen toxidrome described above. Although its primary effect is through NMDA receptor antagonism, PCP will also block reuptake of monoamines, including dopamine, norepinephrine, and serotonin, and act on the sigma receptors [12, 13]. This particular binding profile, specifically NMDA antagonism in the limbic system, neocortex, and basal ganglia, combined with a pro-dopaminergic and anticholinergic state, will contribute to the severe behavioral disturbances seen in patients who have used PCP. With low doses, patients present with dissociative symptoms, distorted sensory perceptions, and social withdrawal. With ingestion of higher doses, bizarre behavior becomes more prominent, and patients may exhibit hallucinations, delusional thinking, agitation, and significant violence. Furthermore, sensory misperceptions and altered sense of self become more prominent, including increased sensation of personal strength and power, as well as diminished pain awareness. Agitation appears to occur in 34–64% of PCP-intoxicated patients seen in hospital settings. As noted previously, cases of extreme violence have been described with PCP intoxication, including significant destruction of property and harm to others (estimated 13% of patients). At significant doses, patients may present with worsening stupor or even coma, and catatonia has also been described [9, 12].

Given the significant potential for violent behavior in PCP-intoxicated patients, ED staff should remain vigilant about safety when working with a patient with suspected PCP ingestion. Safety measures may include moving the patient to a quiet containment space within the emergency room devoid of excess sensory stimulation, ready access to medications to help with agitation and hyperarousal (such as benzodiazepines or antipsychotics), and utilization of locked door seclusion or physical restraints with severe violence. Frequent vital sign monitoring is essential, and many patients will show tachycardia (30–40%), hypertension (30–50%), and temperature changes (both hyperthermia and hypothermia have been described) [9, 12]. Initial laboratory workup of a suspected PCP ingestion should also include monitoring for electrolyte abnormalities, renal dysfunction, and rhabdomyolysis. Patients may have diminished pain perception and limited ability to provide history or may even present following a prehospital altercation, so trauma assessment and imaging studies should be considered. Nystagmus (horizontal and vertical) is a classic finding and is observed in 60–90% of all patients. Other neurologic findings, including dystonic reactions, tardive dyskinesia, ataxia, and seizures, may occur.

Withdrawal

Physiologic dependency has not been described with the hallucinogens mentioned in this chapter. Acute withdrawal or discontinuation symptoms are not a significant issue with most hallucinogens, and the majority of patients return to their usual level of functioning within 6–12 hours following drug ingestion.

Medical Comorbidities

With few notable exceptions, significant medical complications are uncommon with the use of most hallucinogens and, if present, should raise concerns for ingestion of another compound or for comorbid acute medical issues. Vital sign changes can occur, including, most commonly, elevated temperature, hypertension, and tachycardia. Hyperthermia may occur due to increased physical activity or psychomotor agitation and less commonly from serotonergic excess. Most cases of hyperthermia will respond well to supportive care, although patients should be monitored for potential medical complications including electrolyte abnormalities, occult fluid loss (leading to dehydration), rhabdomyolysis, and acute renal injury/failure. Tachycardia is a particularly consistent finding with DXM and PCP intoxication, but is generally less commonly seen with other hallucinogens. Hypertension, similarly, may reflect acute PCP intoxication and is less often seen with other drugs in this class.

Given the frequency of co-ingestion and overlapping clinical presentations from a variety of drug exposures, serum toxicology screening for acetaminophen, salicylates, and presence of ethanol is essential in all patients presenting with acute hallucinogen intoxication. ECG for QTc prolongation, CK monitoring, and chest x-ray (for aspiration pneumonia) should be considered in acutely intoxicated patients. Information from urine toxicology screening, which at most facilities screens for "street drugs" or "drugs of abuse" (e.g., THC, amphetamines, cocaine metabolites, opiates), can be helpful for post-acute-phase counseling, but acute clinical management should not be delayed in the service of obtaining a urine sample and awaiting its results.

Serotonin syndrome, presenting as altered mental status, CNS excitability (e.g., rigidity, hyperreflexia, and clonus), and autonomic hyperactivity, has been described with a number of hallucinogenic compounds, including LSD and DXM. Most commonly, this life-threatening reaction occurs in patients who use hallucinogens while also taking other serotonergic agents including SSRIs, MAOIs, linezolid, meperidine, or lithium. If serotonin syndrome is suspected, a psychiatric consultation should be strongly considered for assistance with diagnostic clarification and management, as a number of potentially life-threatening conditions may present similarly, including neuroleptic malignant syndrome (NMS) and catatonia. All serotonergic agents should be discontinued, and patients should be monitored for end-organ damage related to hyperthermia and other vital sign abnormalities (in particular hypertension and tachycardia) and may require intensive unit admission for further stabilization and monitoring. Additional treatment is largely supportive and can include the use of benzodiazepines for agitation or, more rarely, use of serotonin antagonists.

Ketamine, PCP, and DXM overdoses may all result in significant obtundation and coma, and patients suspected of using these substances should be carefully monitored, with intubation and admission to the ICU considered in more severe cases.

Some of the less common medical side effects related to the use of hallucinogenic compounds are primarily seen with ketamine. This drug has been associated with laryngospasm (especially in infants and children) that tends to be time-limited and short-lasting. It is also associated with increased salivation, which responds well to glycopyrrolate. Chronic ketamine use may lead to ketamine-induced ulcerative cystitis [14–16].

Disposition Considerations

Given significant variability in presenting symptoms, patients' ultimate disposition will depend on the severity and duration of their toxidrome, as well as any underlying comorbidities. Mild cases should be able to return to home following brief observation (6–8 hours) and resolution of acute intoxication. Severe cases of intoxication may warrant hospitalization for management and stabilization. As with other drugs of abuse, engagement of patients with addiction resources should begin as soon as possible. Psychiatric consultation should be considered both during acute intoxication, to assist with management of agitation or psychosis, and following resolution of symptoms, for assistance with referrals to addiction services and aftercare.

Conclusion

Hallucinogens include a diverse class of substances, unified by their intended effect rather than a shared chemical structure, or even receptor binding profile. Most of these drugs will seldom result in emergency department visits, but as these compounds can precipitate dramatic (or even violent) reactions, all emergency providers and consulting psychiatrists should have a degree of familiarity with hallucinogens. Most patients will respond to containment and supportive care and will be able to return to their lives following resolution of acute symptoms.

References

1. U.S. Department of Health and Human Services, Substance Abuse and Mental Health Services Administration, Center for Behavioral Health Statistics and Quality, 2011 *Drug Abuse Warning Network, 2011:National Estimates of Drug-Related Emergency Department Visits.* Last accessed: 12 June 2016.
2. United Nations Office on Drugs and Crime 2015 *World Drug Report 2015.* Report no. E.15. XI.6, Vienna.
3. Hermle L, Simon M, Ruschsow M, Geppert M. Hallucinogen-persisting perception disorder. Ther Adv Psychopharmacol. 2012;2(5):199–205.
4. Nichols DE. Hallucinogens. Pharmacol Ther. 2004;101:131.
5. Fantegrossi WE, Murnane KS, Reissig CJ. The behavioral pharmacology of hallucinogens. Biochem Pharmacol. 2008;75:17.
6. Boyer EW. Dextromethorphan abuse. Pediatr Emerg Care. 2004;20:858.
7. Halpern JH. Hallucinogens and dissociative agents naturally growing in the United States. Pharmacol Ther. 2004;102:131.
8. Hoover V, Marlowe DB, Patapis NS, et al. Internet access to *Salvia divinorum*: implications for policy, prevention, and treatment. J Subst Abus Treat. 2008;35:22.
9. McCarron MM, Schulze BW, Thompson GA, et al. Acute phencyclidine intoxication: incidence of clinical findings in 1,000 cases. Ann Emerg Med. 1981;10:237.
10. McCarron MM, Schulze BW, Thompson GA, et al. Acute phencyclidine intoxication: clinical patterns, complications, and treatment. Ann Emerg Med. 1981;10:290.
11. Halpern JH, Pope HG Jr. Do hallucinogens cause residual neuropsychological toxicity? Drug Alcohol Depend. 1999;53:247.
12. Akunne HC, Reid AA, Thurkauf A, et al. [3H]1-[2-(2-thienyl)cyclohexyl]piperidine labels two high-affinity binding sites in human cortex: further evidence for phencyclidine binding sites associated with the biogenic amine reuptake complex. Synapse. 1991;8:289.

13. Javitt DC, Zukin SR. Recent advances in the phencyclidine model of schizophrenia. Am J Psychiatry. 1991;148:1301.
14. Reich DL, Silvay G. Ketamine: an update on the first twenty-five years of clinical experience. Can J Anaesth. 1989;36:186.
15. Green SM, Li J. Ketamine in adults: what emergency physicians need to know about patient selection and emergence reactions. Acad Emerg Med. 2000;7:278.
16. Shahani R, Streutker C, Dickson B, Stewart RJ. Ketamine-associated ulcerative cystitis: a new clinical entity. Urology. 2007;69:810.

Part II
Management of Substance-Induced and Co-occurring Disorders

Chapter 6
Substance/Medication-Induced Mood Disorders and Co-occuring Mood and Substance Use Disorders: Evaluation and Management in Emergency Department and Psychiatric Emergency Service Settings

Lior Givon

Introduction

Substance/medication-induced mood disorders (S/MIMDs) and co-occuring mood and substance use disorders are common, complex, and heterogeneous syndromes that can be difficult to diagnose and treat appropriately. S/MIMDs include patients who experience clinically significant mood symptoms in the setting of substance intoxication or withdrawal. Co-occurring mood and substance use disorders, often called "dual diagnosis" disorders, represent the presence of both mental health and substance use disorders. Patients with these disorders frequently utilize emergency services and have overall poor outcomes, including severe symptoms and functional impairment [1, 2]. In addition, co-occurring mood and substance use disorders carry high risk for suicidal behaviors [3], as well as risk for involvement with the legal system [4].

It can be difficult to consistently characterize and distinguish S/MIMD and co-occurring mood and substance use disorders from each other, making appropriate treatment recommendations challenging. Obstacles to definitive diagnosis can include the lack of specificity of symptoms, unreliable history obtained from patients during periods of acute intoxication or withdrawal, and scarcity of available information regarding the course of the symptoms and the individual's prior episodes of care. Often, the temporal relationship between the use of substances and the onset of psychiatric symptoms is blurred and inaccurate, relying on subjective reports from patients, families, and first responders. In addition, substance use

L. Givon (✉)
Psychiatric Emergency Services, Cambridge Hospital, Cambridge Health Alliance, Department of Psychiatry, Cambridge, MA, USA
e-mail: lgivon@challiance.org

A. L. Donovan, S. A. Bird (eds.), *Substance Use and the Acute Psychiatric Patient*, Current Clinical Psychiatry, https://doi.org/10.1007/978-3-319-23961-3_6

may coincide with the onset of a primary mood disorder or exacerbate preexisting mood episodes, making it difficult to determine whether the acute mood symptoms are attributable primarily to the substance use or to an underlying non-substance-induced condition. In addition, S/MIMDs are mostly episodic and self-limited conditions and may present differently depending on the substance used and whether the patient is intoxicated or in withdrawal at the time of assessment.

Individuals with S/MIMD and co-occuring disorders often fail to recognize the effects of chronic patterns of substance use on their mood (and the impact of their mood on their substance use) and may resist engaging in substance use disorder or mental health treatments. They often present to healthcare providers with acute physical symptoms, such as respiratory, abdominal, neurological, cardiac, and pain complaints. Frequently, patients use multiple nonintegrated healthcare systems that do not exchange information, resulting in poorly coordinated care and failure to adequately address the mood and substance use disorders. When substance use and mood disorders become chronic, healthcare providers may feel helpless and discouraged in their ability to treat and change the trajectory of these conditions. Similarly, patients may feel that they will never be able to recover and maintain significant sobriety, abstinence, and mental stability.

DSM-5 Criteria for S/MIMD for Depression and Mania

The Diagnostic and Statistical Manual of Mental Disorders (DSM-5, 5th edition) [5] provides guidance for the diagnosis of substance-related disorders resulting from the use of tobacco, alcohol, caffeine, marijuana, hallucinogens, opiates, inhalants, sedatives, stimulants, and other substances, such as anabolic steroids. Substance use disorders imply a clinical continuum that no longer distinguishes “abuse” versus “dependence.” Mood is defined as “Bipolar and related disorders” and “Depressive disorders” [5] (pg. 232). The diagnostic criteria are:

A. The disorder represents a clinically significant symptomatic presentation of a relevant mental disorder.
B. There is evidence from the history, physical examination, or laboratory findings of both of the following:
    1. The disorder developed during or within 1 month of a substance intoxication or withdrawal or taking a medication.
    2. The involved substance/medication is capable of producing the mental disorder.
C. The disorder is not better explained by an independent mental disorder (i.e., one that is not substance- or medication-induced). Such evidence of an independent mental disorder could include the following:
    1. The disorder preceded the onset of severe intoxication or withdrawal or exposure to the medication.

2. The full mental disorder persisted for a substantial period of time (e.g., at least 1 month) after the cessation of acute withdrawal or severe intoxication or taking the medication.

D. The disorder does not occur exclusively during the course of a delirium.
E. The disorder causes clinically significant distress or impairment in social, occupational, or other important areas of functioning.

For depressive disorders, Criterion A requires, "a prominent and persistence disturbance in mood that predominates in the clinical picture and is characterized by depressed mood or markedly diminished interest or pleasure in all, or almost all activities" [5]. For substance-induced bipolar and related disorders, Criterion A indicates that "a prominent and persistent disturbance in mood that predominates in the clinical picture and is characterized by elevated, expansive, or irritable mood, with or without depressed mood, or markedly diminished interest or pleasure in all, or almost all, activities" [5]. Of note, the research published to date on this topic is based on DSM IV-TR [6] criteria for S/MIMD, although the criteria are not substantively different.

Epidemiology of Substance Use and Mood Disorders

It was estimated in 2014 that approximately 7.7 million adults in the United States had co-occurring disorders and those with any mental illness were more likely to experience alcohol and/or substance use disorders [7]. While the prevalence, co-occurrence, and comorbidity of mood and substance use disorders are well documented [8–10], those of S/MIMD are not.

Both major depression and bipolar disorder are heavily comorbid with substance use disorders. Comorbidity prevalence of major depressive disorder with alcohol use disorders was estimated at 21%, with lifetime comorbidity of 40% [11]. Youth having a major depressive episode in the past year were twice as likely than those without a major depressive episode to have used illicit drugs [12]. Comorbidity of any bipolar disorder (I and II) with alcohol use is estimated at 39–48% and drug abuse at 28–42%, with women with bipolarity having 7.3 times greater risk than men of having an alcohol use disorder [13–15]. Adolescents with mental disorders had elevated rates of both alcohol (10%) and illicit drug (15%) use [16].

Comorbid mental illness and substance use disorders are costly to society. Globally, in 2010, mental illness and substance use disorders were the leading causes of years lived with disability [17]. The burden of co-occurring mental illness and substance use on EDs is well documented. Nationally, the Agency for Healthcare Research and Quality reported that between 2000 and 2007, ED visits in the United States due to mental health or substance use more than doubled [12.5% in 2007, up from 5.4% in 2000] [18].

Mood Symptoms Induced by Substances and Medications

Diverse classes of prescribed/diverted medications, alcohol, and illicit substances can present with unique symptoms, necessitating expertise in recognizing the symptoms and signs of intoxication and withdrawal. Mood symptoms associated with substances or medications vary depending on the specific substance, concomitant use of multiple substances, whether the individual is intoxicated or withdrawing, the historical extent and pattern of substance use, the presence of tolerance, metabolic and excretion capacity, vulnerability to mood or other psychiatric disorders, and biological/genetic predisposition. While neither exhaustive nor exclusive, below is a summary of mood symptoms associated with the most commonly used substances and prescribed medications.

Substance/Medication-Induced or Co-occurring Depressive Disorders

The symptoms of substance/medication-induced or co-occuring depression manifest differently in different individuals, but may include depressed or irritable mood, hypersomnia or hyposomnia, lethargy and fatigue, social withdrawal, appetite changes, concentration changes, psychomotor changes, hopelessness, guilt, or suicidal thoughts [19]. Of concern, particularly to the emergency psychiatrist, are severe depressive symptoms that may increase the risk of suicide. Mood disorders, specifically depression and bipolar disorder, carry a high risk for suicidal behaviors [20–22], and the diagnoses of alcohol use disorder [23] and substance use disorders (cannabis, opiates, tobacco) further increase the risk for suicidal behaviors [24]. Data from the Nationwide Emergency Department Sample (2006–2013) showed that 83% of the patients who presented to EDs after a suicide attempt had a mental illness and/or substance use disorder. Those with mood disorders accounted for 42% of the presentations, substance-related disorders accounted for 12%, and alcohol-related disorders accounted for 9% [25]. The risks associated with co-occurring mood and substance use disorders, as well as S/MIMDs, present ED clinicians with the dilemma of when to involve a mental health professional emergently. For some patients, suicidality is associated solely with the intoxication phase and will resolve when the patient is sober, while for others, suicidality may be present even during sobriety. Additionally, patients who return to the ED multiple times with similar presentations of substance use, abnormal mood, and suicidality are frequently dismissed as "low risk" and often do not receive the mental health evaluation they deserve.

Substance/medication-induced depression is associated with many substances and classes of prescribed medications. The depressive effects of alcohol on mood are well established in adults [26–28]. Young adults and adolescents are also highly susceptible to the depressive effects of alcohol [29]. In addition, lifetime prevalence of cannabis use predicts a modest increase in the risk for a first major depressive episode (OR 1.62) and a greater risk for first bipolar episode (OR 4.98) [30], as well as suicidal tendencies, psychosis in vulnerable individuals, and, with prolonged use, neurocognitive impairment [31, 32]. Synthetic cannabinoid use has been associated with agitation and irritability, hallucinations and delusions, catatonia, and self-injurious behaviors [33]. The use of cocaine often accompanies acute psychiatric presentations. Cocaine users are susceptible to polysubstance use in order to "enhance the high" or treat withdrawal and are twice as likely to have symptoms of depressive or anxiety disorders.[19.] Cigarette smoking is more prevalent among patients with mental illness, twice as much for those with depression and three times as much for those with schizophrenia. While nicotine enhances dopamine and the sensation of euphoria, habitual cigarette smoking is associated with increased risk of new onset of mood and anxiety disorders in those between the ages 18 and 49 years [34].

Among prescribed medications with a potential to cause depression for the duration of the medication intake are antiviral medications [efavirenz, acyclovir], chemotherapeutic agents, immunologic agents [interferon-α, interferon-β], cardiovascular agents [reserpine, methyldopa, clonidine, propranolol, calcium-channel blockers, digitalis/digoxin], asthma medication [montelukast], dermatologic agents [retinoic acid derivatives], anticonvulsant medications [phenobarbital, levetiracetam, tiagabine, topiramate, vigabatrin, ethosuximide, methsuximide], antimigraine medication [triptans], hormonal-like agents [corticosteroids, GnRH agonists, tamoxifen, oral contraceptives], sedative-hypnotics [benzodiazepines], and smoking cessation agents [varenicline] [35–39]. Medications associated with an increase in suicidal thoughts and behaviors include interferon-α [40], anticonvulsant medications, specifically levetiracetam, gabapentin, lamotrigine, tiagabine and valproate [41–43], glucocorticosteroids [44], and anabolic steroids [45].

Substance or Medication-Induced or Co-occurring Mania

In the acute setting of the ED, it is hard to know whether a newly presenting patient with manic symptoms has an underlying bipolar disorder or whether the symptoms represent acute and transient intoxication. It is estimated that 30–50% patients with bipolarity (bipolar I or bipolar II) will develop a co-occurring substance use disorder, and co-occurring substance use is higher among those with bipolar disorder than with any other psychiatric disorder [46–48]. In addition, patients with comorbid bipolar disorder and alcohol use disorder are more likely to attempt suicide and be hospitalized, compared to patients with bipolar disorder alone [49].

Manic symptoms can present in acute settings as irritability or euphoria, agitation, distractibility, impulsivity, grandiosity, increased activity, sleep dysregulation, pressured speech, and racing thoughts [50]. Mania can be induced by antidepressant medications, such as SSRIs, tricyclic antidepressants, and MAOIs, in those patients with a diathesis for bipolarity [51–53]. Mania and hypomania can also be induced by stimulants (cocaine, amphetamines, and amphetamine derivatives), prescribed and/or illicit [54–56]. In addition, evidence exists for mania induced by the use of levodopa and associated pro-dopamine medications (mostly used as anti-Parkinson's agents) [50, 57, 58], corticosteroids [59–62], and anabolic steroids [63]. Thyroxine, iproniazid, isoniazid, sympathomimetics, chloroquine, baclofen, alprazolam, and captopril have also been associated with medication- or substance-induced mania [50, 64, 65] (Tables 6.1a and 6.1b).

Table 6.1a Substances inducing mood syndromes during intoxication and withdrawal

Substance	Intoxication	Withdrawal
Alcohol	Depressed/labile mood Suicidal ideation	Depressed mood Anxiety
Amphetamines/stimulants (cocaine, amphetamine, methamphetamine, prescribed psychostimulants)	Mania Psychosis Anxiety	Depressed mood
Caffeine	Manic symptoms Irritability Anxiety	Dysphoric/depressed mood Irritability
Cannabis	Dysphoric/depressed mood Anxiety Psychosis	Depressed mood Irritability Anxiety
Cannabinoids (including synthetic cannabinoids)	Psychosis Suicidal ideation	Anxiety
Hallucinogen (dextromethorphan, ecstasy, LSD, mescaline phencyclidine, psilocybin)	Anxiety Psychosis Depressed mood	Anxiety Depressed mood
Inhalants (volatile hydrocarbons: solvents, gasoline, gases, nitrites)	Psychosis	Irritability
Nicotine	Depressed mood Anxiety	Anxiety Depressed mood Irritability

Table 6.1b Prescribed and OTC medications inducing mood syndromes during intoxication and withdrawal

Antidepressant medications (SSRIs, SNRIs)	Agitation Anxiety Mania	Depressed mood Anxiety
Antidepressant medications (tricyclics)	Mania	Depressed mood Anxiety
Antidepressant medications (MAOIs)	Mania	Depressed mood Anxiety
Sedative-hypnotics (benzodiazepines)	Depressed mood Anxiety [paradoxical reaction]	Anxiety Depressed mood
Steroids (anabolic and sex steroids, steroidal anti-inflammatory)	Anxiety Depressed mood Mania Psychosis	Depressed mood Irritability

Assessment and Treatment of S/MIMD and Co-occurring Mood and Substance Use Disorders

Patients who present to the ED with symptoms suggestive of mood and substance use disorders first need a thorough medical evaluation. This medical evaluation should evaluate for signs and symptoms of acute medical illness, as well as for evidence of intoxication and/or withdrawal. The medical evaluation should include a physical exam, review of systems, and targeted neurological exam. Vital signs should be monitored throughout the ED stay. Specific medical evaluations based on substances used are described in other chapters.

Labs and imaging may include the following:

(i) Urine and serum toxicology screens
(ii) Chemistry: Complete blood count, complete metabolic panel (blood glucose, electrolytes, liver function tests), and, when indicated, amylase, lipase, CPK, HIV, RPR, thyroid-stimulating hormone, folate, and vitamin B12
(iii) Urine pregnancy test for reproductive age females
(iv) Electrocardiogram when the individual presents with cardiac symptoms or has a known cardiac history, following an overdose, or when the intoxication or withdrawal has potential cardiac sequelae
(v) Chest X-ray, if aspiration or pneumonia suspected
(vi) Head imaging when clinically indicated

Following a thorough assessment of the patient's medical complaints, signs, and symptoms, attention should be given to the acute substance use and mental health issues. The history should be obtained from the patient, if he/she is able to provide reliable information, and collateral information should be obtained from family members, co-workers, friends, healthcare providers, parole/probation officers, and electronic medical records.

For patients with S/MIMD or co-occuring disorders, the psychiatric evaluation should focus on the current mood symptoms, including depressive and manic symptoms, as well as recent substance use. In addition to assessing the quality and severity of the current mood symptoms, attempting to determine if the patient has a comorbid mood and substance use disorder or a S/MIMD can also be helpful for planning appropriate treatment recommendations. Cross-sectionally, it is nearly impossible to determine if a patient has a comorbid mood and substance use disorder or S/MIMD; therefore, elucidating a longitudinal history of symptoms is important. If possible, establishing a timeline for the onset of mood symptoms, and the relationship to substance intoxication or withdrawal, can be valuable in narrowing down this differential diagnosis. In addition, it is helpful to determine how sobriety has affected the patient's mood in the past. A patient with S/MIMD would be expected to have euthymic moods during periods of sustained sobriety, while a patient with comorbid mood and substance use disorders could experience persistent mood symptoms during periods of sobriety. In addition, it is important to consider if the substances used are known to cause the mood symptoms being reported. A patient using alcohol on a daily basis could be experiencing depression due to either a depressive disorder or the effects of alcohol, but alcohol triggering mania would be much less likely, raising suspicion for a primary bipolar disorder.

A detailed history of substance use includes the following elements:

(i) Assessment of acute intoxication or withdrawal: Type, quantity, and frequency of substance(s) being used recently, with particular attention to substances used immediately prior to ED presentation and current symptoms of intoxication or withdrawal.
(ii) Substance use history: For each class of substance used: age of use onset; periods of sobriety; pattern of use (binge, continuous); amount and frequency of use; route of substance administration (oral, intranasal, IV); physiological and psychological symptoms of intoxication and withdrawal (including history of severe or life-threatening withdrawal symptoms); psychological and physical signs of dependence (including tolerance and craving); physical, psychological, or social sequelae of use; history of intentional and unintentional overdoses; history of harm to self or others when intoxicated; past treatment (including dual diagnosis, detox, mandated treatment, IOP, outpatient, sober houses/residential facilities)
(iii) Psychological concomitants: Awareness of the substance use causing problems; history of trauma; protective and resilience factors; social, ethnic, and cultural factors affecting the patient; readiness for change

The remainder of the psychiatric assessment should include the standard elements. Specifically, the past psychiatric history should include prior diagnoses, hospitalizations, suicide attempts, episodes of violence, current treaters, and state agency involvement. A legal history should include both general legal problems and any substance-related legal problems. Family history should include not only psychiatric illness but also history of substance use disorders. Social history should include information about the impact of substances on the patient's social life and also a description of current functioning and social supports. The mental status exam may be initiated when the patient is intoxicated, but it is also necessary to evaluate the patient's mental status when clinically sober, in order to determine appropriate disposition.

The risk assessment is a critical part of the ED evaluation. The risk assessment may be initially performed upon presentation, but it cannot be completed until the patient is assessed when clinically sober. During triage, it is standard practice to assess suicidal ideation, plans, and intent, as well as risk of agitation or violence, so that the patient's safety may be appropriately monitored during the ED visit. Once the patient is sober, the patient should be evaluated again for suicidality and homicidality or aggression with a thorough history, including history of suicidal ideation, suicide attempts (including lethality and intention), history of self-injurious behaviors, family history of suicidality, history of violence and aggression, and access to weapons. The presence or absence of safety concerns will be a key factor in determining disposition.

Some EDs are using standardized screening tools to screen for suicidality and aggression. A Consensus Guide for Emergency Departments (2015) [66] recommends using the Decision Support Tool to assess which patients with suicide risk may need mental health evaluation while in the ED. The tool is a "yes/no" 6-item instrument that assesses present risk, past attempts, substance use, history of mental illness, and irritability, agitation, and aggression. Additional screening tools used in EDs are the Columbia-Suicide Severity Rating Scale [67] and Ask Suicide-Screening Questions for youth ages 10–24 years [68]. Patients who screen positive on these tools will require more in-depth psychiatric evaluation.

Management of S/MIMD and Co-occurring Mood and Substance Use Disorders in the ED

Management of Intoxication and Withdrawal: General Principles

Short-term management goals of ED patients with potential S/MIMDs or co-occurring mood and substance use disorders are to establish medical stability, address acute intoxication and withdrawal symptoms, reduce immediate cravings, and stabilize severe mood symptoms, agitation, and imminent risk to self or others. Treatment recommendations are based on the standard of care for acute intoxication and withdrawal of substances, in the context of "co-occurring" mood disorders. The management of intoxication and withdrawal for specific substances (without co-occurring mood symptoms) is well described in other chapters.

While the intoxication phase of most substances lasts from hours to a few days, withdrawal symptoms, including the psychiatric sequelae of withdrawal, can last for days, weeks, or months. Targeting the substance-induced symptoms, use patterns, and emerging mood disorder should be the preliminary focus of the management in the ED. In many instances, the substance or substances causing the mood symptoms should be discontinued. If a prescribed medication is causing mood instability, a consultation with the prescribing physician should be initiated, to discuss dose adjustment or discontinuation.

Antidepressant medications have not been found effective in alleviating substance-related symptoms in patients with mood and anxiety disorders in acute settings [69], but continued monitoring and behavioral containment was found to be helpful. In addition, some patients may benefit from the acute anxiolytic effects of oral benzodiazepine or antipsychotic medications. Management of agitation associated with mood instability includes the use of verbal de-escalation techniques, as well as decreasing physical and environmental stimuli. Use of emergency medications and restraints are recommended as a last resort when the patient is not responding to de-escalation. First- and second-generation antipsychotic medications, as well as benzodiazepines, are recommended to calm the acutely agitated patient in the ED [70].

There are no established guidelines for the treatment of acute substance-induced mania. However, the general principles of managing acute mania can apply to both substance- or medication-induced mania and mania comorbid with substance use. The goals of treating acute mania are to stabilize the patient and relieve the manic symptoms, including agitation, mood lability, hypersexuality, and impulsivity. In acute settings, antipsychotics (haloperidol, quetiapine, olanzapine, risperidone) and fast-acting benzodiazepines are effective in decreasing the levels of agitation, impulsivity, and psychosis, and restoring sleep [71]. For mania emerging from medications, such as psychostimulants, muscle relaxants [baclofen], antirejection agents [cyclosporine], Parkinson medications [carbidopa/levodopa], antidepressant medications, steroids, dopamine agonists, and theophylline, a short course of benzodiazepines, such as lorazepam, and antipsychotic medications should be administered, and the offending agent should be discontinued, if possible.

Treatment Planning and Disposition

While S/MIMD is often a brief and time-limited condition (unless use of the implicated substance is chronic), individuals with a diathesis for mood and substance use disorders may develop chronic depressive symptoms, as well as bipolarity, especially those with irritable and anxious temperaments who are at a particularly high risk for concomitant alcohol use [72]. Little information is available on prevention strategies for substance-induced depressive and manic episodes. Those with risk factors for developing prolonged mood episodes (past mood episodes, family history of mood disorders) should be aware of the effects of alcohol, substances, and medications in prolonging mood symptoms. Although sometimes time limited (e.g., heavy drinking during young adulthood), substance use disorders can evolve into insidious and chronic conditions, subject to frequent relapse. In this case, the most realistic expectation is that the disorder may be brought under control through a combination of psychological and pharmacological treatments tailored to the individual's needs. In ED settings, psychiatrists, psychologists, and social work clinicians should look at the patient's history, including collateral information from outpatient providers and family members, to verify the patient's history and tailor treatment to past successes. Determination of level of care is based upon many factors, including: information about periods of sobriety, willingness and readiness to engage in treatment, compliance with psychiatric outpatient care, history of successfully completing substance use programs, medical illness that may be exacerbated during relapse and early sobriety, the patient's resources and supports, and particularly any safety concerns.

In the acute setting of the ED/PES, the first step in treatment planning is assessing the patient's motivation and readiness for change. These can be assessed and potentially enhanced by using motivational interviewing strategies. These strategies utilize nonjudgmental interactions in an attempt to reduce stigmatization and shame, demonstrating acceptance of the possibility of ongoing use while encouraging safer use and consideration of abstinence. Strategies incorporate the principle of acceptance, acknowledging that substance use is part of our society and may have played a very important role in the patient's life. PES clinicians can engage the patient in an exploration of treatment alternatives in a noncoercive manner, empowering him/her by preserving autonomy when presenting treatment options and recognizing that social determinants and inequalities, such as poverty, race, social isolation, trauma, and gender discrimination, are intertwined with substance use and mental illness [73]. For those in the pre-contemplative stage (i.e., those who are not yet interested in changing their substance use pattern), harm reduction strategies are recommended. Harm reduction strategies are geared to reducing negative consequences associated with drug use and can include access to needle exchanges, carrying Narcan, and using substances with trusted peers. Individuals with substance and mood disorders can be encouraged to talk to family and trusted supports, associate with sober friends and colleagues, and seek support from community organizations such as Alcoholics Anonymous (AA) and Narcotics Anonymous (NA).

For those actively contemplating or seeking change and recovery, treatment for substance use can be initiated in the ED by referring the patient to an appropriate substance use disorder or mental health clinic. Educating at-risk individuals and their family members about the symptomatology of S/MIMD and co-occurring substance use and mental illness, and when and how to seek treatment, should be part of the treatment plan. Facilitating real-time access to appropriate programs can enhance acceptance and engagement with care.

Even in the absence of diagnostic clarity, patients with significant safety concerns, such as suicidality, homicidality, or impaired self-care, that do not resolve with sobriety will typically require inpatient psychiatric admission. Patients with severe or life-threatening withdrawal may require medical admission, while patients with less critical withdrawal syndromes may benefit from inpatient or outpatient detox. Patients with S/MIMD, without active safety or medical concerns, will benefit from treatment targeted to their substance use disorder, because when the substance use disorder is treated, the mood symptoms will improve and resolve. Patients can be referred back to their primary care clinic if they are otherwise psychiatrically stable and have good rapport with their providers. Patients with comorbid mood and substance use disorders will benefit from treatment targeted to both of their illnesses, which could include inpatient, partial hospital, or outpatient dual diagnosis treatment. Outpatient care, after initial detox, may include pharmacotherapy, individual therapy, and group therapy. If lingering and debilitating depression ensues as a consequence of substance use, a trial of antidepressant medications should be pursued. Similarly, mood stabilizers and antipsychotic medications are indicated for debilitating and lasting manic symptoms.

Social barriers to care for those with comorbid substance use disorder and mental illness include lack of integration between mental health and substance use treatments, inadequate availability of psychiatric prescribers in dedicated substance use programs, restrictions based on health insurance coverage, language and cultural barriers, and bias against those individuals with substance use and serious mental illness. Individuals with co-occurring substance use and mental illness who are in the criminal justice system often do not have access to adequate care while incarcerated and when released back to the community [74]. Emotional obstacles due to the chronicity of substance use and mental illness comorbidity include self-blame, shame and humiliation, emotional fatigue that emerges after multiple relapses, and chronic nonadherence with psychiatric care. Additionally, patients with co-occurring substance use and mental illness are vulnerable to trauma in the community and are reluctant to return to programs where they were mistreated, assaulted, or violated.

Conclusion

Little systematic research is available on substances (illicit and legal), as well as prescribed and OTC medications, causing acute onset of mood symptoms. Nationally, the prevalence of mood disorders and substance use is widespread and rampant, starting in mid-adolescence, with comorbid conditions developing in young adulthood. The ED presentation of patients with S/MIMDs and comorbid mood and substance use disorders is heterogeneous and complex. Often, it is unclear whether the clinical symptoms represent comorbid mood and substance use disorders or S/MIMD. Substance-induced psychiatric conditions range from mild dysthymia to profound depression, mood lability and irritability, manic-like symptoms, as well as anxiety and psychosis, depending on the substance(s) ingested. Polysubstance use can cause a complex psychiatric picture, making the diagnosis and treatment even more challenging.

S/MIMD and co-occurring mood and substance use disorders carry high morbidity and mortality, with lifetime challenges that include acute and chronic medical illnesses, multiple and prolonged hospitalizations, emergence of protracted and chronic mood disorders, suicidal and homicidal behaviors, aggression, victimization and trauma, socioeconomic decline, interpersonal problems, and involvement with the legal system. If individuals do not obtain treatment, they are at increased risk for relapse and worsening medical and psychiatric consequences. The longer the substance use and mood disorders go untreated, the greater the impact on the individual, the family, and larger community.

Treatment of S/MIMD and co-occurring mood and substance use disorders should be tailored to the individual's needs. Patients with ongoing or severe symptoms will require intensive treatment. Psychiatrists, EM physicians, other medical professionals, patients, and families should be made aware of the relationship between substance use, medications and mood instability, and the available treatment options for patients. Finally, more research is needed to establish guidelines for care of this population in the acute settings.

References

1. Drake RE, Essock SM, Shaner A, Carey KB, Minkoff K, Kola L, Lynde D, Osher FC, Clark RE, Rickards L. Implementing dual diagnosis services for clients with severe mental illness. Psychiatr Serv. 2001;52:469–76.
2. Davis LL, Frazier E, Husain MM, Warden D, Trivedi M, Fava M, Cassano P, McGrath PJ, Balasubramani GK, Wisniewski SR, Rush AJ. Substance use disorder comorbidity in

major depressive disorder: a confirmatory analysis of the STAR*D cohort. Am J Addict. 2006;15(4):278–85.
3. Carrà G, Bartoli F, Crocamo C, Brady KT, Clerici M. Attempted suicide in people with co-occurring bipolar and substance use disorders: systematic review and meta-analysis. J Affect Disord. 2014;167:125–35.
4. Balyakina E, Mann C, Ellison M, Sivernell R, Fulda KG, Sarai SK, Cardarelli R. Risk of future offense among probationers with co-occurring substance use and mental health disorders. Community Ment Health J. 2014;50(3):288–95.
5. Diagnostic and Statistical Manual of Mental Disorders (5th edition): Desk reference to the diagnostic criteria. Washington, D.C.: American Psychiatric Publishing; 2013.
6. Diagnostic and Statistical Manual of Mental Disorders (4th edition-TR). Washington, D.C.: American Psychiatric Association; 2000.
7. Co-occurring Disorders: The NSDUH Report, SAMHSA. Rockville; 2014. https://www.samhsa.gov/data/sites/default/files/NSDUH-SR200-RecoveryMonth-2014/NSDUH-SR200-RecoveryMonth-2014.htm
8. Kessler RC, Berglund P, Demler O, Jin R, Merikangas KR, Walters EE. Lifetime prevalence and age-of-onset distributions of DSM-IV disorders in the national comorbidity survey replication. Arch Gen Psychiatry. 2005;62(6):593–602.
9. Kessler RC, Chiu WT, Demler O, Walters EE. Prevalence, severity, and comorbidity of 12-month DSM-IV disorders in the national comorbidity survey replication. Arch Gen Psychiatry. 2005;62(6):617–27.
10. Swendsen JD, Merikangas KR. The comorbidity of depression and substance use disorders. Clin Psychol Rev. 2000;20(2):173–89.
11. Grant BF, Harford TC. Comorbidity between DSM-IV alcohol use and major depression: results of a national survey. Drug Alcohol Depend. 1995;39:197–206.
12. Hedden SL, Kennet J, Lipari R, Medley G, Tice P, Copllo EAP, Krouti LA. Behavioral health trends in the United States: results from the 2014 National Survey on Drug Use and Health. Rockville; 2015.
13. Merikangas KR, Akiskal HS, Angst J, Greenberg PE, Hirschfeld RMA, Petukhova M, Kessler RC. Lifetime and 12-month prevalence of bipolar spectrum disorder in the National Comorbidity Survey replication. Arch Gen Psychiatry. 2007;64(5):543–52.
14. Frye MA, Altshuler LL, McElroy SL, Suppes T, Keck PE, Denicoff K, Nolen WA, Kupka R, Leverich GS, Pollio C, Grunze H, Walden J, Post RM. Gender differences in prevalence, risk, and clinical correlates of alcoholism comorbidity in bipolar disorder. Am J Psychiatry. 2003;160(5):883–9.
15. Cassidy F, Ahearn EP, Carroll BJ. Substance abuse in bipolar disorder. Bipolar Disord. 2001;3:181–8.
16. Conway KP, Swendsen J, Husky MM, He JP, Merikangas KR. Association of lifetime mental disorders and subsequent alcohol and illicit drug use: results from the National Comorbidity Survey-Adolescent supplement. J Am Acad Child Adolesc Psychiatry. 2016;55(4):280–8.
17. Whiteford HA, Degenhardt L, Rehm J, Baxter AJ, Ferrari AJ, Erskine HE, Charlson FJ, Norman RE, Flaxman AD, Johns N, Burstein R, Murray CJ, Vos T. Global burden of disease attributable to mental and substance use disorders: findings from the Global Burden of Disease Study 2010. Lancet. 2013;382(99D4):1564–74.
18. McKenna M. The growing strain of mental health care on emergency departments: few solutions offer promise. Ann of Emerg Med. 2011;57(6):18A–20A.
19. Meador P. Substance or medication induced depressive disorder DSM-5 (ICD-9-CM and ICD-1O-CM). https://www.theravive.com/therapedia/substance-or-medication-induced-depressive-disorder-dsm%2D%2D5-(icd%2D%2D9%2D%2Dcm-and-icd%2D%2D1o%2D%2Dcm).
20. Goodwin FK, Jamison KR. Suicide in manic-depressive illness. New York: Oxford University Press; 1999.
21. Miret M, Ayuso-Mateos JL, Sanchez-Noreno J, Vieta E. Depressive disorders and suicide: epidemiology, risk factors, and burden. Neurosci Behav R. 2013;37:2372–4.

22. Beck AT, Steer RA. Clinical predictors and eventual suicide: a 5- to 10-year prospective study of suicide attempters. J Affective Disord. 1989;17(3):203–9.
23. Randall RE. Alcohol and suicide. Subst Alcohol Actions Misuse. 1983;4(2–3):121–7.
24. Gates ML, Turney A, Ferguson E, Walker V, Staples-Horne M. Associations among substance use, mental health disorders, and self-harm in a prison population: examining group risk for suicide attempt. Int J Environ Res Public Health. 2017;14(3):1–16.
25. Canner JK. Visits for attempted suicide and self-harm in the USA: 2006-2013. Epidemiol Psychiatr Sci. 2016;7:1–9.
26. Raimo E, Schuckit MA. Alcohol dependence and mood disorders. Addict Behav. 1998;23(6):933–46.
27. Boden JM, Fergusson DM. Alcohol and depression. Addiction. 2011;106:906–14.
28. Lynskey MT. The comorbidity of alcohol dependence and affective disorders: treatment implications. Drug Alcohol Depend. 1998;52:201–9.
29. Deykin EY, Levy JC, Wells V. Adolescent depression, alcohol and drug abuse. AJPH. 1987;77(2):178–82.
30. Van Laar M, Van Dorsselaer S, Monshouwer K, de Graaf R. Does cannabis use predicts the first incidence of mood and anxiety disorders in the adult population? Addiction. 2007;102:1251–60.
31. Karila L, Roux P, Rolland B, Benyamina A, Reynaud M, Aubin HJ, Lançon C. Acute and long-term effects of cannabis use: a review. Curr Pharm Des. 2014;20(25):4112–8.
32. Buckner JD, Keough ME, Schmidt NB. Problematic alcohol and cannabis use among young adults: the roles of depression and discomfort and distress tolerance. JAMA. 2010;303(14):1401–9.
33. Mills B, Yepes A, Nugent K. Synthetic cannabinoids. Am J Med Sci. 2015;350(1):59–62.
34. Mojtabai R, Crum RM. Cigarette smoking and onset of mood and anxiety disorders. Am J Public Health. 2013;103(9):1656–65.
35. Kandel DB, Huang FY, Davies M. Comorbidity between patterns of substance use dependence and psychiatric syndromes. Drug Alcohol Depend. 2001;64:233–41.
36. Preda A. Substance-induced mood disorder. Medscape reference: drugs, diseases and procedures. 2012. http://emedicine.medscape.com/article/286885-overview.
37. Patten SB, Love EJ. Can drugs cause depression? A review of the evidence. J Psychiatry Neurosci. 1993;18(3):92–102.
38. Patten SB, Barbui C. Drug-induced depression: a systematic review to inform clinical practice. Psychother Psychosom. 2004;73(4):207–15.
39. Botts S, Ryan M. Depression. In: Tisdale J, Miller DA, editors. Drug induced diseases: prevention, detection, and management. Bethesda: American Society of Health System Pharmacists, Inc.; 2010.
40. Janssen HL, Brouwer JT, Van der Mast RC, Schalm SW. Suicide associated with alpha-interferon therapy for chronic viral hepatitis. J Hepatol. 1994;21(2):241–3.
41. FDA Public Health Advisory: suicidal thoughts and behavior: anticonvulsant. http://www.fda.gov/Drugs/DrugSafety/PostmarketDrugSafetyInformationforPatientsandProviders/ucm100195.htm.
42. Update on suicidal behavior and ideation and anticonvulsant drugs: Update May 5, 2009. http://www.fda.gov/Drugs/DrugSafety/PostmarketDrugSafetyInformationforPatientsandProviders/ucm100190.htm.
43. Patorno E, Bohn RL, Wahl PM, Avorn J, Patrick AR, Liu J, Schneeweiss S. Anticonvulsant medications and the risk of suicide, attempted suicide, or violent death. JAMA. 2010;303(14):1401–9.
44. Brauser D. Glucocorticoids linked to suicide. Neuropsychiatric disorders. 2012. http://www.medscape.com/viewarticle/759566.
45. Thiblin I, Runeson B, Rajs J. Anabolic androgenic steroids and suicide. Ann Clin Psychiatry. 1999;11(4):223–31.
46. Bauer MS, Altshuler L, Evans DR, Beresford T, Williford WO, Hauger R. Prevalence and distinct correlates of anxiety, substance, and combined comorbidity in a multi-site public sector sample with bipolar disorder. J Affect Disord. 2005;85:301–15.

47. Bizzarri JV, Sbrana A, Rucci P, Ravani L, Massei GJ, Gonnelli C, Spagnolli S, Doria MR, Raimondi F, Endicott J, Dell'Osso L, Cassano GB. The spectrum of substance abuse in bipolar disorder: reasons for use, sensation seeking and substance sensitivity. Bipolar Disord. 2007;9:213–20.
48. Chengappa KN, Levine J, Gershon S, Kupfer DJ. Lifetime prevalence of substance or alcohol abuse and dependence among subjects with bipolar I and II disorders in a voluntary registry. Bipolar Disord. 2000;2:191–5.
49. SAMHSA. Advisory: an introduction to bipolar disorder and co-occurring substance use disorders. HHS Publication. Rockville; 2016.
50. Peet M, Peters S. Drug-induced mania. Drug Saf. 1995;12(2):146–53.
51. Henry C, Sorbara F, Lacoste J, Gindre C, Leboyer M. Antidepressant-induced mania in bipolar patients: identification of risk factors. J Clin Psychiatry. 2001;62(4):249–55.
52. Goldberg JF, Whiteside JE. The association between substance abuse and antidepressant-induced mania in bipolar disorder: a preliminary study. J Clin Psychiatry. 2002;63(9):791–5.
53. Boerlin HL, Gitlin MJ, Zoellner LA, Hammen CL. Bipolar depression and antidepressant-induced mania: a naturalistic study. J Clin Psychiatry. 1998;59(7):374–9.
54. Barnhorst A, Xiong GL, Talavera F. Amphetamine-related psychiatric disorders. Medscape: Drugs, Diseases & Procedures. 2015. http://emedicine.medscape.com/article/289973-followup#e8.
55. Ross RG. Psychotic and manic-like symptoms during stimulant treatment of attention deficit hyperactivity disorder. Am J Psychiatry. 2006;163(7):1149–52.
56. Chakraborty KS. Methylphenidate-induced mania-like symptoms. Indian J Pharmacol. 2011;43(1):80–1.
57. Sidi H, Asiff M, Kumar J, Das S, Hatta NH, Alfonso C. Hypersexuality as a neuropsychiatric disorder: the neurobiology and treatment options. Curr Drug Targets. 2018;19(12):1391–401.
58. Beaulieu-Boire I, Lang AE. Behavioral effects of levodopa. Mov Disord. 2015;30(1):90–102.
59. Wada K, Yamada N, Suzuki H, Lee Y, Kuroda S. Recurrent cases of corticosteroid-induced mood disorder: clinical characteristics and treatment. J Clin Psychiatry. 2000;61(4):261–7.
60. Cerullo MA. Corticosteroid-induced mania: prepare for the unpredictable. Curr Psychiatr Ther. 2006;5(6):43–50.
61. Warrington TP, Bostwick JM. Psychiatric adverse effects of corticosteroids. Mayo Clin Proc. 2006;81(10):1361–7.
62. Zagaria MAE. Systemic corticosteroid–associated psychiatric adverse effects. US Pharm. 2016;41(7):16–8.
63. Wolkowitz OM. Prospective controlled studies of the behavioral and biological effects of exogenous corticosteroids. Psychoneuroendocrinology. 1994;19(3):233–55.
64. Verma R, Sachdeva A, Singh Y, Balhara YPS. Acute mania after thyroxin supplementation in hypothyroid state. Indian J Endocrinol Metab. 2013;17(5):922–3.
65. Sultzer DL, Cummings JL. Drug-induced mania – causative agents, clinical characteristics and management: a retrospective analysis of the literature. Med Toxicol Adverse Drug Exp. 1989;4(2):127–43.
66. A Consensus Guide for Emergency Departments: caring for adult patients with suicidal risk. Suicide Prevention Resource Center/Education Development Center; 2015.
67. Posner K, Brown GK, Stanley B, Brent DA, Yershova KV, Oquendo MA, Currier GW, Melvin GA, GA GL, Shen S, Mann JJ. The Columbia–Suicide Severity Rating Scale: initial validity and internal consistency findings from three multisite studies with adolescents and adults. Am J Psychiatry. 2011;168(12):1266–77.
68. Horowitz LM, Bridge JA, Teach SJ, Ballard E, Klima J, Rosenstein DL, Wharff EA, Ginnis K, Cannon E, Joshi P, Pao M. Ask Suicide-Screening Questions (ASQ): a brief instrument for the pediatric emergency department. Arch Pediatr Adolesc Med. 2012;166(12):1170–6.
69. Kelly TM, Daley DC, Douaihy AB. Treatment of substance abusing patients with comorbid psychiatric disorders. Addict Behav. 2012;37(1):11–24.
70. Foulds JA, Adamson SJ, Boden JM, Williman JA, Mulder RT. Depression in patients with alcohol use disorders: systematic review and meta-analysis of outcomes for independent and substance-induced disorders. J Affect Disord. 2015;185:47–59.

71. Vieta E. Acute and long-term treatment of mania. Dialogues Clin Neurosci. 2008;10(2):165–79.
72. Khazaal Y, Gex-Fabry M, Nallet A, Weber B, Favre S, Voide R, Zullino D, Aubry JM. Affective temperaments in alcohol and opiate addictions. Psychiatry Q. 2013;84(4):429–38.
73. Harm reduction coalition: principles of harm reduction. New York. http://harmreduction.org/about-us/principles-of-harm-reduction/.
74. Access to mental health care and incarceration. Mental Health America. Alexandria; 2017. http://www.mentalhealthamerica.net/issues/access-mental-health-care-and-incarceration.

Chapter 7
Substance-Induced Psychosis and Co-occurring Psychotic Disorders

Hannah E. Brown, Yoshio Kaneko, and Abigail L. Donovan

Introduction

Psychotic disorders and substance use disorders are common yet challenging presentations for the emergency department (ED) clinician. The areas where these disorders overlap, including substance-induced psychosis (SIP) and co-occurring substance use and psychotic disorders, offer particular clinical challenges. This chapter will discuss clinical presentations of SIP, differentiation between SIP and primary psychosis with and without co-occurring substance use, acute management of psychosis in the emergency setting, and associated disposition considerations. This chapter will focus on schizophrenia and non-affective psychoses; mood disorders, with and without psychosis, are covered primarily in Chap. 6.

H. E. Brown (✉)
Wellness and Recovery After Psychosis Program, Boston Medical Center, Boston, MA, USA

Boston University School of Medicine, Boston, MA, USA
e-mail: hannah.brown2@bmc.org

Y. Kaneko
First Episode and Early Psychosis Program, Massachusetts General Hospital, Department of Psychiatry, Boston, MA, USA

Harvard Medical School, Boston, MA, USA

Transitional Age Youth Clinic, Massachusetts General Hospital, Boston, MA, USA

Newton-Wellesley Hospital, Newton, MA, USA

A. L. Donovan
Massachusetts General Hospital, Department of Psychiatry, Boston, MA, USA

First Episode and Early Psychosis Program, Massachusetts General Hospital, Department of Psychiatry, Boston, MA, USA

Harvard Medical School, Boston, MA, USA

Acute Psychiatry Service, Massachusetts General Hospital, Boston, MA, USA

A. L. Donovan, S. A. Bird (eds.), *Substance Use and the Acute Psychiatric Patient*, Current Clinical Psychiatry, https://doi.org/10.1007/978-3-319-23961-3_7

As many as 30% of patients who present to the ED for psychiatric reasons have substance use disorders [1]. Moreover, estimates of the prevalence of schizophrenia and co-occurring substance use disorders range from 25% to 50% [2, 3], and approximately 30% of individuals with first-episode psychosis have a co-occurring substance use disorder [4]. In addition, many drugs of abuse can cause psychotic symptoms (i.e., a SIP) in an individual with no prior history of a psychotic disorder.

Differentiating between SIP and a primary psychotic illness, with or without co-occurring substance use, is important for clinical decision-making in the emergency setting. The Diagnostic and Statistical Manual of Mental Disorders, 5th edition (DSM-5), criteria for diagnosis of a substance-induced psychotic disorder include (1) clinical symptoms consistent with psychosis; (2) evidence from history, physical exam, and laboratory measures that the psychotic symptoms developed during or within 1 month of substance use (intoxication or withdrawal) and the substance in question is known to cause psychotic symptoms; (3) the psychotic symptoms are not better explained by another psychiatric illness; (4) the psychosis does not occur only during a delirious process; and (5) the psychosis causes significant distress and impairment in functioning. By contrast, a primary psychotic illness can only be diagnosed when "the disturbance is not attributable to the physiologic effects of a substance" [5]. Therefore, a primary psychotic illness with co-occurring substance use is diagnosed when a patient has an independent primary psychotic disorder, such as schizophrenia, and also separately meets diagnostic criteria for a substance use disorder. In this case, the substance use may exacerbate psychotic symptoms, though it is not the underlying cause of them. The situation is made even more complex longitudinally because early SIP may actually predict the later development of an independent psychotic disorder. For example, in a large 8-year cohort study, the cumulative risk of a schizophrenia spectrum disorder diagnosis was 46% after diagnosis of cannabis-induced psychosis; the risk was 30% after diagnosis with amphetamine-induced psychosis [6].

Substances Causing Psychotic Symptoms

Many different substances directly affect the central nervous system and can cause psychotic symptoms. Psychotic symptoms can occur during periods of intoxication, withdrawal, or both (see Table 7.1). Alcohol intoxication and withdrawal, benzodiazepine intoxication and withdrawal, and intoxication with cannabis, hallucinogens (including phencyclidine (PCP) and lysergic acid diethylamide (LSD)), inhalants, opioids, stimulants (including amphetamines and cocaine), and other substances (e.g., synthetic cannabinoids, bath salts) can all produce psychotic symptoms [5]. Some substances, such as PCP, amphetamines, and bath salts, can also cause severe agitation accompanying the psychotic symptoms. While the clinical presentations of these substance-induced psychoses are similar, several commonly used substances, including alcohol, benzodiazepines, stimulants, and cannabis, deserve further discussion.

Table 7.1 Psychotic symptoms present during intoxication or withdrawal

Substance	Intoxication	Withdrawal
Alcohol	√	√
Benzodiazepines	√	√
Cannabis	√	
Hallucinogens	√	
Opioids	√	
Amphetamines/cocaine	√	
Other		
Bath salts	√	
Synthetic cannabinoids	√	
γ–Hydroxybutyrate (GHB)	√	

Alcohol and Sedatives

Alcohol can cause psychotic symptoms during both intoxication and withdrawal. "Pathologic [alcohol] intoxication," though controversial and extremely rare, is characterized by intoxication from small amounts of alcohol, with subsequent behavioral manifestations including agitation, aggression, visual hallucinations and delusions, as well as complete amnesia for the event. The symptoms typically last for several hours, but, rarely, can last for a few days [7]. Alcohol withdrawal syndrome (AWS) usually develops between 6 and 24 hours after the cessation or decrease in chronic alcohol consumption and ranges in severity [8]. Alcohol withdrawal can be accompanied by perceptual disturbances, such as visual or auditory hallucinations, even in the absence of delirium. Alcoholic hallucinosis, or alcohol-induced psychotic disorder (AIPD), is a more severe form of this phenomenon, which is characterized by acute onset of severe auditory, visual, or tactile hallucinations, and/or persecutory delusions, with loss of insight and impaired reality testing, in the setting of a clear sensorium (e.g., NOT in the presence of a delirium) [9]. Alcoholic hallucinosis occurs in the context of chronic alcohol abuse, either in early withdrawal (12–24 hours after cessation of use) or in periods of decreased alcohol consumption during which alcohol levels are low relative to a chronic baseline [8]. Alcohol withdrawal delirium, the most severe stage of AWS, occurs in 5% of individuals with AWS and usually develops about 72 hours after the onset of symptoms of alcohol withdrawal. Withdrawal delirium can last from 1 day to more than 1 week and is characterized by co-occurring delirium (disorientation, impaired attention, agitation) and withdrawal symptoms, including autonomic instability and seizures. Auditory, visual, and tactile hallucinations are present as part of the delirious process, thus helping to differentiate withdrawal delirium from AIPD [10, 11]. Psychotic symptoms due to alcohol withdrawal are typically accompanied by other signs or symptoms of substance withdrawal (such as vital sign changes, tremor, and diaphoresis) and typically remit with both treatment of the withdrawal syndrome and prolonged sobriety.

Benzodiazepines and barbiturates can cause visual and auditory hallucinations as a part of a delirium in cases of extreme intoxication, such as overdose. If the hallucinations occur only in the context of a delirious process, the diagnosis is not consistent with SIP. Psychotic symptoms are more common during sedative withdrawal. Benzodiazepine withdrawal can include perceptual changes and multimodal hallucinations [12]. As with alcohol withdrawal, psychotic symptoms due benzodiazepine withdrawal are typically accompanied by other signs or symptoms of substance withdrawal (such as vital sign changes, tremor, and diaphoresis) and they typically remit with treatment of the withdrawal syndrome.

Stimulants

Stimulant-induced psychosis (e.g., amphetamine-induced and cocaine-induced psychosis) can appear identical to an acute exacerbation of a primary psychotic disorder [13]. Symptoms include auditory hallucinations, hypervigilance, referential thinking, and paranoid delusional beliefs [14]. Up to 50% of cocaine users and up to 46% of methamphetamine users have reported transient psychotic symptoms during use [15, 16]. Stimulant-induced psychosis is often associated with additional physical symptoms including tachycardia, hypertension, pupillary dilation, perspiration, and formication psychosis. The extent of the physical symptoms will depend on the user's tolerance and amount consumed. Both cocaine-induced and amphetamine-induced psychosis may resolve within hours (although may still last the duration of the emergency room visit) or may persist for weeks to months in more chronic users [17–19]. In general, the effects of regular methamphetamine use may be more prolonged compared to those of cocaine [20]. Further risk factors for amphetamine-induced psychosis in chronic methamphetamine users include younger age of first amphetamine use, history of schizoid, schizotypal or antisocial personality traits, history of depression, and alcohol use disorder [21].

Cannabis

Psychosis induced by acute intoxication with either cannabis or synthetic cannabinoids typically includes auditory and/or visual hallucinations, paranoid delusions, and ideas of reference [22]. Additional psychotic symptoms can include depersonalization and derealization and disorganized thinking. Between 20% and 50% of cannabis users endorse transient psychotic symptoms during intoxication [23]. The presence of physical symptoms including conjunctival injection, increased appetite, dry mouth, and tachycardia should increase the suspicion for acute cannabis intoxication. In rare cases, the psychotic symptoms induced by cannabis use can persist for weeks, despite abstinence from cannabis [24–26]. Assessment is further complicated by the fact that chronic cannabis use, particularly in adolescence, is associated in a dose-dependent fashion with an increased risk of developing a persistent psychotic disorder [27]. Chronic cannabis use can also produce an "amotivational syndrome," with symptoms that mimic the negative symptoms of schizophrenia including blunted affect, apathy, lethargy, social withdrawal, and decreased ability to concentrate [23].

Keys to Differentiating SIP and a Primary Psychotic Disorder in the ED Setting

There are many challenges when differentiating between SIP and primary psychotic disorders in the emergency setting, and making an exact diagnosis can be difficult. A targeted medical workup, the details of which are beyond the scope of this chapter, should be initiated to exclude potential underlying medical etiologies to the psychosis. Determining a clear symptom timeline with any patient can be a challenge, one that is made even more complex with a psychotic, potentially intoxicated patient in the emergency room. Among substance-using first-episode psychotic patients who presented to an urban psychiatric emergency department, one-year follow-up revealed that of those individuals initially diagnosed with a primary psychotic disorder, 25% were subsequently determined to have SIP or no evidence of current, ongoing psychotic illness. Of the patients initially diagnosed with SIP, 21% were re-diagnosed with a primary psychotic disorder [28]. This diagnostic shift was most likely to occur within the first 6 months after the initial ED presentation in the setting of persistent psychotic symptoms independent of substance use. Yet, as challenging as it is for ED clinicians to make accurate diagnostic assessments of psychotic patients, doing so accurately has major implications for subsequent decision-making about treatment. Patients who receive an initial diagnosis of a primary psychotic disorder are more likely to be treated with mood stabilizing and antipsychotic medications, more likely to be hospitalized and more likely to be referred for outpatient psychiatry follow-up. In contrast, patients who receive an initial diagnosis of SIP are more likely to be referred for substance use treatment [28, 29]. At 2-year longitudinal follow-up, both groups (those with primary psychotic illness and those with SIP) had reduced psychotic symptoms, decreased rates of substance dependence, and improved social functioning [29].

Achieving diagnostic clarity, or at least attempting to do so, while in the emergency setting is also important for implementing appropriate treatment during the ED visit. For a substance-dependent patient, misdiagnosis in the ED puts patients at risk for untreated withdrawal symptoms if SIP is not recognized. Understanding whether a psychosis is primary or due to the effects of a substance can change the timing and focus of the clinical interview and influence the psycho-education given to the patient and family. Patients with a primary psychotic disorder with co-occurring substance use may benefit from understanding that substance use can cause worsening of baseline psychotic symptoms and lead to high-risk behaviors and hospitalizations, while patients with a SIP may benefit from understanding that the substance itself is causing the psychotic symptoms and that ongoing use carries the risk of more persistent psychosis. Disposition considerations are also significantly influenced by diagnosis. For example, a patient who is acutely psychotic due to an underlying primary psychotic disorder will require referral for long-term treatment with antipsychotic medication and other tailored psychosocial interventions (e.g., individual therapy, cognitive remediation, and vocational rehabilitation). While some of these referrals may not be made directly from the ED, patients and families can be educated about what types of treatments to seek on an outpatient basis. In contrast, an individual with a SIP may not require long-term antipsychotic medication treatment but may need referral for specialized substance abuse interventions. Individuals with both a primary psychotic disorder and a comorbid substance use disorder will need treatment referrals for both. Misdiagnosis can also have longer-term treatment consequences: unnecessary treatment with an antipsychotic medication can cause a significant side-effect burden, including movement disorders, diabetes, and cardiovascular disease.

While the presenting symptoms of SIP and primary psychotic illness may be clinically indistinguishable, there are some factors that can be helpful in differentiating the two disorders. Eliciting a careful history is invaluable in determining the etiology of the psychosis. Establishing a temporal relationship between the onset of psychotic symptoms and substance use can help clinicians determine the likely cause of psychosis. If a patient is a poor historian due to acute intoxication or psychosis, collateral information from family, friends, outpatient clinicians, and medical records will be critical to aid in diagnosis. It is also important to determine past history of SIP: those individuals who have prior history of SIP have increased risk of repeated episodes compared to those individuals who have not. Similarly, those individuals who have a history of a primary psychotic illness, such as schizophrenia, and no history of substance use are likely to be presenting with an acute primary psychotic illness exacerbation. Patients with SIP tend to have a later age of onset of psychosis, poor family support, more frequent comorbid antisocial personality disorder diagnosis, longer periods of substance use, and history of multiple illicit drugs used compared to those with a primary psychotic illness [30]. With regard to family history, parental substance abuse increases the likelihood of SIP, while parental history of other mental illness increases the likelihood of a primary psychotic illness [31]. Clinically, patients with SIP have a significantly shorter duration of untreated psychosis and more positive psychotic symptoms [32]. By contrast, patients with a primary psychotic illness are more likely to experience greater general psychopathology, have more severe psychotic symptoms (when accounting for both positive and negative symptoms), and have less insight [30]. While both groups have similar rates of auditory hallucinations, visual hallucinations are more common in those with SIP (see Table 7.2). While these clinical and demographic characteristics may help in differentiating a primary psychotic disorder from a SIP, many presentations to the ED will be complex and unclear, particularly for patients who have both a primary psychotic disorder and a co-occurring substance use disorder.

The Psychiatric Research Interview for Substance and Mental Disorders (PRISM) is a semi-structured interview developed to differentiate between substance-induced and primary psychiatric illnesses based on DSM-IV diagnostic criteria and can be used in clinical settings [33]. While a complete semi-structured interview is typically not feasible in the acute setting given the duration and training required to administer, aspects of the PRISM may be useful in an emergency department evaluation. Specifically, the PRISM interview begins with obtaining a detailed history of substance use so that when psychiatric symptoms are explored later in the interview, they can be placed within the timeline of known substance use. This approach may be helpful if the clinician has a high suspicion of a SIP.

Table 7.2 Differentiating clinical characteristics of SIP and primary psychotic illness

Substance-induced psychosis	Primary psychotic illness
Psychotic symptoms only with intoxication or withdrawal	Psychotic symptoms independent of substance use
Later age at onset of psychosis	Greater general psychopathology
Poor family support	More severe psychotic symptoms (both positive and negative)
Comorbid antisocial personality disorder diagnosis	Less insight into psychotic illness
Prolonged periods of substance use	
Multiple substance use disorders	
Visual hallucinations	
Family history of substance use disorder	
Shorter duration of untreated psychosis	

Objective findings can also be helpful in determining an accurate diagnosis or, at the very least, suggesting the presence of substance use and a possible SIP. For example, acute cocaine, amphetamine, or other stimulant intoxication may present with tachycardia, elevated blood pressure, chest pain, shortness of breath, pupillary dilation, formication, perspiration, and stereotyped behaviors. Most standard urine toxicology screens can reveal the presence of drugs of abuse including cannabis, amphetamines, benzodiazepines, opioids, and cocaine. Cannabinoids can remain in the urine up to 10 days after use and even up to a month in chronic users. While not frequently done in the emergency setting, measuring an inactive metabolite of tetrahydrocannabinol (THC), 9-carboxy THC, in the urine can help to quantify the amount of cannabis used. A high level of 9-carboxy THC (e.g., >500 ng/mL) may suggest regular, frequent use, or a large recent ingestion, suggesting cannabis-induced psychosis. Depending on the testing methods and amount used, amphetamines may be detected in the urine up to 7 days after use, and cocaine metabolites can be detected in urine up to 4 days after use. It is important to note that the presence of a positive urine toxicology screen does not definitively confirm a SIP but can help the clinician make a more informed diagnosis. The converse is true as well – a negative urine drug screen does not rule out the diagnosis of SIP. Substances such as synthetic cannabinoids ("spice" or "K2") are often not detected in standard urine toxicology assays; newer, more sensitive, and specific assays have been developed in order to detect synthetic cannabinoids [34], but are not consistently available in most general hospital EDs.

Acute Management in the ED

While the underlying cause of acute psychotic symptoms may differ, the acute management of SIP or an exacerbation of a primary psychotic disorder, with or without co-occurring substance use, can be similar. Vital signs must be monitored for instability in heart rate, blood pressure, and oxygenation. An electrocardiogram (EKG) may also be indicated in certain situations, such as acute amphetamine or cocaine intoxication. Acute amphetamine intoxication and acute cocaine intoxication can produce a hyperadrenergic state, resulting in elevated heart rate and blood pressure (both systolic and diastolic), elevated respiratory rate, and elevated body temperature, with potentially lethal outcomes including stroke, acute coronary syndrome, or pulmonary hypertension. Synthetic cannabinoids can also cause cardiovascular instability and seizures. One case report describes rhabdomyolysis and hyperthermia requiring an intensive care unit stay after synthetic cannabis (K2) use [35]. Other hallucinogens, such as LSD and N,N-dimethyltryptamine (DMT), can cause rhabdomyolysis [36]. Cannabis intoxication can cause cardiovascular side effects, including elevated heart rate and blood pressure (through increasing sympathetic tone). These physical symptoms are discussed further in the corresponding individual substance use disorder chapters.

Depending on the substance and the chronicity and intensity of use, both patients with SIP and patients with a primary psychotic disorder with co-occurring substance use are at risk for withdrawal syndromes. Even patients who initially present to the ED while acutely intoxicated may develop withdrawal symptoms over the course of their ED stay. Psychotic symptoms may be present in alcohol, benzodiazepine, and barbiturate withdrawal, with or without delirium, as discussed above. These withdrawal syndromes can be managed by using oral or parenteral benzodiazepines or barbiturates, titrated to normalize vital signs (and subsequently tapered over days, ideally on an inpatient unit), in addition to giving thiamine and folate for prevention of Wernicke's syndrome associated with poor nutrition in those at risk for alcohol withdrawal. Severe alcohol withdrawal can lead to alcohol withdrawal delirium as discussed above: this entity is a medical emergency, and the mortality rate can be as high as 5–10%. Immediate medical care with parenteral benzodiazepines, antipsychotics, fluids, and thiamine is required.

Patients with psychotic symptoms due to either a primary psychotic disorder, with or without co-occurring substance use, or a SIP will benefit from acute treatment with antipsychotic medication while in the ED. Regardless of etiology, patients with psychotic symptoms are often suffering: they are frequently frightened, confused, overwhelmed, and distressed. Acute treatment with antipsychotic medication can alleviate their suffering and improve psychotic symptoms. Patients with an exacerbation of a known psychotic disorder for which they have received treatment may benefit from an additional dose of an antipsychotic medication they are already taking or have taken and tolerated in the past. Patients who are antipsychotic naïve can be offered an antipsychotic medication, ideally one with more sedating properties, such as risperidone or olanzapine or quetiapine, in order to prevent or treat agitation. Antipsychotic medication should also be used to treat the acute psychotic symptoms associated with SIP. For amphetamine-induced psychosis, two randomized clinical trials, each comparing haloperidol to a second-generation antipsychotic medication (olanzapine and quetiapine), found all of the agents to be equally effective, with haloperidol causing more extrapyramidal side effects [37, 38]. Another small randomized double-blind 6-week trial showed significant rates of reduction of positive psychotic symptoms after treatment with risperidone compared to aripiprazole among patients with amphetamine-induced psychosis [39]. It is important to note that amphetamine intoxication can be associated with hyperthermia, cardiac arrhythmias, dystonias, and seizures; antipsychotic medications may exacerbate these symptoms, and benzodiazepines should be the initial treatment in this population. For the treatment of cannabis-induced psychosis, olanzapine and haloperidol have been found to be equally effective, although haloperidol was again associated with more extrapyramidal symptoms [40].

Substance intoxication and withdrawal and psychosis with co-occurring substance use may result in varying degrees of agitation. An agitated patient must be urgently treated to ensure the safety of the patient and those around the patient. Patients must also be in behavioral control in order to participate meaningfully in the psychiatric assessment and treatment planning. Clinicians may use non-pharmacologic methods to decrease agitation. These methods include verbal de-escalation, which involves empathic listening, validation, respectfully stating expectations for behavior, and offering choices when possible. The physical environment should also be modified to decrease external stimuli. When possible, the patient can be moved to a quiet, private room. The room should provide ample space for the patient and staff, including security staff, as psychotic patients may be particularly sensitive to personal space. The environment should be safe and free of potential weapons. Offering comforting measures (such as food or drink, a warm blanket) may also help de-escalate a patient. If a patient remains agitated despite the aforementioned interventions, physical restraints may be used to keep both the patient and those around the patient, including hospital workers and other patients, safe. Medication to help calm the patient should always be given in conjunction with the restraints, and restraints should be removed as soon as safely possible.

In the setting of agitation and psychosis, treatment with antipsychotic medication is indicated. The Best practices in Evaluation and Treatment of Agitation (BETA) psychopharmacology work group was convened by the American Association for Emergency Psychiatry and consists primarily of emergency psychiatrists and emergency medicine physicians. The BETA Project work group recommends offering oral medications prior to intramuscular injections, if safe for the patient's clinical and medical situation [41]. The BETA work group advises treating agitation occurring in the setting of psychosis due to a primary psychotic disorder with oral risperidone (2 mg), olanzapine (5–10 mg), or haloperidol (5 mg) and a benzodiazepine (lorazepam 2 mg). There may be a slight preference for choosing a second-generation antipsychotic in the acute setting, given the lower rates of extrapyramidal side effects. Further, the onset of action differs between these oral antipsychotic preparations: risperidone reaches maximum concentration after 1 hour, olanzapine after 4 hours, and haloperidol between 2 and 6 hours. If the patient is unable to take oral medication, then a parenteral antipsychotic medication should be given – olanzapine (10 mg) alone or haloperidol (5 mg) plus a parenteral benzodiazepine lorazepam (2 mg) [41]. Intramuscular olanzapine and lorazepam should not be given together given the potential risk of hypotension and respiratory suppression [42].

Specific recommendations for the management of agitation in SIP are lacking, although some research does exist. Overall, antipsychotic medication remains the mainstay of treatment of both agitation and psychotic symptoms in SIP. The management of agitation in alcohol intoxication, with or without psychosis, should include the use of haloperidol (given that haloperidol has the most data to support safety and efficacy in this population), but optimally without additional benzodiazepines (given the risks of respiratory suppression) [41]. In contrast, the management of agitation in alcohol or benzodiazepine withdrawal should always include administration of a benzodiazepine. Benzodiazepines may also be helpful in treating agitation associated with amphetamine or other stimulant intoxication [41], and beta-blockers and alpha-2 agonists may be used to treat hyperadrenergic symptoms. Both second-generation antipsychotic medications and benzodiazepines are recommended for cannabis-associated psychosis and agitation [40].

Disposition

A thorough medical workup will help determine the patient's ultimate disposition from the ED. Individuals needing acute medical intervention (e.g., those with unstable vital signs, complicated withdrawal, and delirium) must remain in the ED for stabilization and may require admission to a medical unit. These patients may benefit from ongoing psychiatric consultation during this medical treatment for further assessment and assistance in managing psychotic symptoms, substance withdrawal, and potential agitation.

Once medically stable, patients can be referred for further psychiatric treatment including substance use treatment. A thorough risk assessment, which can only be completed when the patient is clinically sober, is one important factor in determining disposition. This risk assessment should elucidate whether a patient is (1) at imminent risk of harm to self, (2) at imminent risk of harm to others, or (3) gravely disabled due to psychiatric illness such that the individual cannot adequately care for him or herself in the community. In the USA, individual states vary on their legal criteria for involuntary psychiatric hospitalization, but, in general, if any of these three aforementioned criteria are met, the patient warrants admission to an inpatient psychiatric unit for further care, even involuntarily. Some states, such as Massachusetts, specify that the risk of harm must be due to a mental illness, excluding substance use. However, in the case of a SIP presenting acutely to the ED, it is often difficult to completely exclude an underlying psychiatric illness, and the primary objective must be to protect the patient's safety. A parallel process for primary substance use disorders is civil commitment to mandate an individual to undergo substance abuse treatment. Thirty-seven states in the USA allow civil commitment for substance abuse treatment, and most laws include language that the individual must pose a significant risk of harm to self or others because of the substance use. Commitments range from less than a month to a year or more [43].

As previously mentioned, distinguishing between primary psychosis and SIP is important for determining disposition. Patients with a primary psychotic disorder without significant comorbid substance use will benefit from psychiatric treatment with antipsychotic medication and additional psychosocial treatments, either on an inpatient or outpatient basis, depending on safety factors, level of disorganization, and available social supports. Patients with a primary psychotic disorder with co-occurring substance use, or patients with SIP with ongoing psychotic symptoms, may benefit from "dual diagnosis" treatment: treatment of both psychosis and comorbid substance use. Patients with SIP whose psychotic symptoms resolve quickly in the ED with sobriety may benefit from treatment more focused on substance use, including detoxification programs. Other patients, for example, those who have presented after only their first use, may not be referred for further substance use treatment and instead follow-up with their primary care physician. When achieving diagnostic clarity is not possible, disposition determination should be guided by the best possible assessment of the patient's current symptoms and the type of treatment that is most suited to addressing those symptoms.

Both dual diagnosis and substance use disorder programs exist in several levels of intensity. Patients who pose a risk of harm to themselves or others, cannot safely care for themselves in the community, require ongoing monitoring for substance withdrawal, or have severe symptoms will likely require inpatient hospitalization. Patients without these safety concerns and who do not require inpatient detoxification may be appropriate for referral to outpatient treatment. Outpatient treatment options include partial hospitalization programs, intensive outpatient programs, outpatient care under a psychiatrist (including possible medication-assisted treatment) and/or therapist, and peer support groups in the community.

Conclusions

Distinguishing a primary psychotic disorder from SIP presents a challenge to the ED clinician. Assuming medical causes have been ruled out, the clinician's responsibility is to ensure the safety of the patient and those around him or her and to treat the patient's symptoms, regardless of the underlying cause. Acute psychotic symptoms should be treated with an antipsychotic medication; in most cases there is little evidence suggesting benefit of one antipsychotic medication over another. Agitation associated with acute intoxication or underlying psychotic illness can be treated with an antipsychotic medication plus or minus a benzodiazepine. A thorough clinical history should be obtained to help determine diagnosis; some clinical features such as the nature of the psychotic symptoms, level of insight, and comorbid personality traits may help guide the diagnosis. Ongoing medical evaluation and risk assessment, in addition to the clinical assessment, will guide the ultimate disposition for this challenging population.

References

1. Larkin GL, Claassen CA, Emond JA, Pelletier AJ, Camargo CA. Trends in U.S. emergency department visits for mental health conditions, 1992 to 2001. Psychiatr Serv. 2005;56(6):671–7.
2. Sara GE, Burgess PM, Malhi GS, Whiteford HA, Hall WC. Stimulant and other substance use disorders in schizophrenia: prevalence, correlates and impacts in a population sample. Aust N Z J Psychiatry. 2014;48(11):1036–47.
3. Kessler RC, Birnbaum H, Demler O, Falloon IR, Gagnon E, Guyer M, et al. The prevalence and correlates of nonaffective psychosis in the National Comorbidity Survey Replication (NCS-R). Biol Psychiatry. 2005;58(8):668–76.
4. Larsen TK, Melle I, Auestad B, Friis S, Haahr U, Johannessen JO, et al. Substance abuse in first-episode non-affective psychosis. Schizophr Res. 2006;88(1–3):55–62.
5. American Psychiatric Association. Diagnostic and statistical manual of mental disorders. 5th ed. Arlington: American Psychiatric Association; 2013.
6. Niemi-Pynttari JA, Sund R, Putkonen H, Vorma H, Wahlbeck K, Pirkola SP. Substance-induced psychoses converting into schizophrenia: a register-based study of 18,478 Finnish inpatient cases. J Clin Psychiatry. 2013;74(1):e94–9.
7. Ross JD, Gastfriend DR, Renner JA. Massachusetts General Hospital handbook of general hospital psychiatry. 6th ed. Philadelphia: Saunders/Elselvier; 2010.
8. Mirijello A, D'Angelo C, Ferrulli A, Vassallo G, Antonelli M, Caputo F, et al. Identification and management of alcohol withdrawal syndrome. Drugs. 2015;75(4):353 65.
9. Perala J, Kuoppasalmi K, Pirkola S, Harkanen T, Saarni S, Tuulio-Henriksson A, et al. Alcohol-induced psychotic disorder and delirium in the general population. Br J Psychiatry. 2010;197(3):200–6.
10. Schuckit MA. Recognition and management of withdrawal delirium (delirium tremens). N Engl J Med. 2014;371(22):2109–13.
11. Perry EC. Inpatient management of acute alcohol withdrawal syndrome. CNS Drugs. 2014;28(5):401–10.
12. Petursson H. The benzodiazepine withdrawal syndrome. Addiction. 1994;89(11):1455–9.
13. Sato M, Numachi Y, Hamamura T. Relapse of paranoid psychotic state in methamphetamine model of schizophrenia. Schizophr Bull. 1992;18(1):115–22.
14. Zweben JE, Cohen JB, Christian D, Galloway GP, Salinardi M, Parent D, et al. Psychiatric symptoms in methamphetamine users. Am J Addict. 2004;13(2):181–90.
15. Grant KM, LeVan TD, Wells SM, Li M, Stoltenberg SF, Gendelman HE, et al. Methamphetamine-associated psychosis. J Neuroimmune Pharmacol. 2012;7(1):113–39.
16. Thirthalli J, Benegal V. Psychosis among substance users. Curr Opin Psychiatry. 2006;19(3):239–45.
17. Glasner-Edwards S, Mooney LJ. Methamphetamine psychosis: epidemiology and management. CNS Drugs. 2014;28(12):1115–26.
18. Roncero C, Daigre C, Grau-Lopez L, Barral C, Perez-Pazos J, Martinez-Luna N, et al. An international perspective and review of cocaine-induced psychosis: a call to action. Subst Abus. 2014;35(3):321–7.
19. Manschreck TC, Laughery JA, Weisstein CC, Allen D, Humblestone B, Neville M, et al. Characteristics of freebase cocaine psychosis. Yale J Biol Med. 1988;61(2):115–22.
20. SAMHSA. Treatment for stimulant use disorders. Rawson RA, editor. Rockville; 1999.
21. Chen CK, Lin SK, Sham PC, Ball D, Loh EW, Hsiao CC, et al. Pre-morbid characteristics and co-morbidity of methamphetamine users with and without psychosis. Psychol Med. 2003;33(8):1407–14.

22. Thomas H. A community survey of adverse effects of cannabis use. Drug Alcohol Depend. 1996;42(3):201–7.
23. Sewell RA, Ranganathan M, D'Souza DC. Cannabinoids and psychosis. Int Rev Psychiatry. 2009;21(2):152–62.
24. Nunez LA, Gurpegui M. Cannabis-induced psychosis: a cross-sectional comparison with acute schizophrenia. Acta Psychiatr Scand. 2002;105(3):173–8.
25. Kuepper R, van Os J, Lieb R, Wittchen HU, Hofler M, Henquet C. Continued cannabis use and risk of incidence and persistence of psychotic symptoms: 10 year follow-up cohort study. Br Med J. 2011;342:d738.
26. Hall W, Degenhardt L. Cannabis use and psychosis: a review of clinical and epidemiological evidence. Aust N Z J Psychiatry. 2000;34(1):26–34.
27. Moore TH, Zammit S, Lingford-Hughes A, Barnes TR, Jones PB, Burke M, et al. Cannabis use and risk of psychotic or affective mental health outcomes: a systematic review. Lancet. 2007;370(9584):319–28.
28. Schanzer BM, First MB, Dominguez B, Hasin DS, Caton CL. Diagnosing psychotic disorders in the emergency department in the context of substance use. Psychiatr Serv. 2006;57(10):1468–73.
29. Drake RE, Caton CL, Xie H, Hsu E, Gorroochurn P, Samet S, et al. A prospective 2-year study of emergency department patients with early-phase primary psychosis or substance-induced psychosis. Am J Psychiatry. 2011;168(7):742–8.
30. Caton CL, Drake RE, Hasin DS, Dominguez B, Shrout PE, Samet S, et al. Differences between early-phase primary psychotic disorders with concurrent substance use and substance-induced psychoses. Arch Gen Psychiatry. 2005;62(2):137–45.
31. Caton CL, Hasin DS, Shrout PE, Drake RE, Dominguez B, First MB, et al. Stability of early-phase primary psychotic disorders with concurrent substance use and substance-induced psychosis. Br J Psychiatry. 2007;190:105–11.
32. Weibell MA, Joa I, Bramness J, Johannessen JO, McGorry PD, Ten Velden Hegelstad W, et al. Treated incidence and baseline characteristics of substance induced psychosis in a Norwegian catchment area. BMC Psychiatry. 2013;13:319.
33. Hasin DS, Trautman KD, Miele GM, Samet S, Smith M, Endicott J. Psychiatric Research Interview for Substance and Mental Disorders (PRISM): reliability for substance abusers. Am J Psychiatry. 1996;153(9):1195–201.
34. Spinelli E, Barnes AJ, Young S, Castaneto MS, Martin TM, Klette KL, et al. Performance characteristics of an ELISA screening assay for urinary synthetic cannabinoids. Drug Test Anal. 2015;7(6):467–74.
35. Sweeney B, Talebi S, Toro D, Gonzalez K, Menoscal JP, Shaw R, et al. Hyperthermia and severe rhabdomyolysis from synthetic cannabinoids. Am J Emerg Med. 2016;34(1):121 e1–2.
36. Paterson NE, Darby WC, Sandhu PS. N,N-dimethyltryptamine-induced psychosis. Clin Neuropharmacol. 2015;38(4):141–3.
37. Leelahanaj T, Kongsakon R, Netrakom P. A 4-week, double-blind comparison of olanzapine with haloperidol in the treatment of amphetamine psychosis. J Med Assoc Thai. 2005; 88(Suppl 3):S43–52. PubMed: 16858942.
38. Verachai V, Rukngan W, Chawanakrasaesin K, Nilaban S, Suwanmajo S, Thanateerabunjong R, et al. Treatment of methamphetamine-induced psychosis: a double-blind randomized controlled trial comparing haloperidol and quetiapine. Psychopharmacology (Berl). 2014;231(16):3099–108.
39. Farnia V, Shakeri J, Tatari F, Juibari TA, Yazdchi K, Bajoghli H, et al. Randomized controlled trial of aripiprazole versus risperidone for the treatment of amphetamine-induced psychosis. Am J Drug Alcohol Abuse. 2014;40(1):10–5.

40. Bui QM, Simpson S, Nordstrom K. Psychiatric and medical management of marijuana intoxication in the emergency department. West J Emer Med. 2015;16(3):414–7.
41. Wilson MP, Pepper D, Currier GW, Holloman GH Jr, Feifel D. The psychopharmacology of agitation: consensus statement of the american association for emergency psychiatry project Beta psychopharmacology workgroup. West J Emerg Med. 2012;13(1):26–34.
42. Zacher JL, Roche-Desilets J. Hypotension secondary to the combination of intramuscular olanzapine and intramuscular lorazepam. J Clin Psychiatry. 2005;66(12):1614–5.
43. Christopher PP, Pinals DA, Stayton T, Sanders K, Blumberg L. Nature and utilization of civil commitment for substance abuse in the United States. J Am Acad Psychiatry Law. 2015;43(3):313–20.

Chapter 8
Substance-Induced Anxiety and Co-occurring Anxiety Disorders

Daryl Blaney Jr., Annise K. Jackson, Ozan Toy, Anna Fitzgerald[†], and Joanna Piechniczek-Buczek

Introduction

Anxiety is an unpleasant emotional state with psychological and physiological symptoms, typically experienced as a normal response to stress, but also occurring pathologically in anxiety disorders, and as a symptom of medical or other psychiatric conditions, including substance use disorders (SUDs). Anxiety disorders are relatively common in the general population, with a 12-month prevalence of 11% and lifetime prevalence of 16.6% [1, 2]. Data from the National Epidemiologic Survey on Alcohol and Related Conditions (NESARC) suggest the prevalence of substance-induced anxiety (SIA) disorders is around 1% of all anxiety disorders [1]. While some studies suggest a higher prevalence of SIA versus independent anxiety disorders among substance users, these are limited by diagnostic methods that do not conform to DSM criteria [1]. Though the prevalence of SIA in those using substances is relatively low, co-occurring anxiety disorders and SUDs are common, with one study suggesting nearly 15% of those with a known anxiety disorder had at least one independent co-occurring SUD and 17% of those with a known SUD had at least one independent co-occurring anxiety disorder over a single 12-month period [1]. These findings may explain why anxiety is a frequent clinical complaint in substance-using ED patients.

[†](Deceased)

D. Blaney Jr. · A. K. Jackson · O. Toy
Boston University Medical Center, Department of Psychiatry, Boston, MA, USA

J. Piechniczek-Buczek (✉)
Boston Medical Center/Boston University School of Medicine, Department of Psychiatry, Boston, MA, USA
e-mail: Joanna.buczek@bmc.org

A. L. Donovan, S. A. Bird (eds.), *Substance Use and the Acute Psychiatric Patient*, Current Clinical Psychiatry, https://doi.org/10.1007/978-3-319-23961-3_8

The Diagnostic and Statistical Manual of Mental Disorders (DSM-5) identifies SIA as the induction of clinically predominant fear, worry, or panic after ingestion, intoxication, or withdrawal from a substance or medication [3]. Per DSM-5, the prevalence of SIA is thought to be rare in the general population, with an estimated 12-month prevalence of 0.002%, though the prevalence in clinical populations is thought to be higher. SIA is known to occur in the context of acute substance intoxication or withdrawal and can persist for weeks after the cessation of use [1, 3]. With the increasing numbers of individuals using illicit drugs, many are likely to develop SIA. This phenomenon should prompt the inclusion of SIA on the differential for patients presenting to the ED with a variety of anxiety-related chief complaints.

Making a diagnosis of SIA can be difficult, as independent mood and anxiety disorders co-occur frequently with SUDs. When substance use and anxiety are comorbid, they frequently reinforce each other [4] and comorbidity tends to be the rule, rather than the exception. Often, those with anxiety disorders will attempt to alleviate their symptoms through substance use, colloquially referred to as "self-medicating." One systematic review and meta-analysis found that nearly 50% of those with lifetime illicit drug dependence had a comorbid anxiety disorder [5]. This finding is clinically important because the presence of comorbid substance use and anxiety disorders is linked to poorer treatment outcomes [6]. With an estimated 27.1 million Americans currently using illicit substances, and the number of first-time illicit substance users increasing yearly [7], the comorbidity of substance use and anxiety cannot be ignored.

Although often challenging to tease out, it is important to attempt to distinguish SIA from comorbid anxiety and SUDs because treatment approaches may be different. A thorough history with a focus on establishing an accurate time course of symptoms and substance use is critical to making an accurate diagnosis. Accurate diagnosis, combined with other clinical information, then informs appropriate treatment planning, which can decrease the risk of adverse patient outcomes, including reckless behavior while intoxicated, high-risk withdrawal syndromes, and potentially lethal overdoses.

Substances Causing Anxiety

The number of substances that induce or exacerbate anxiety is substantial and includes consumer products, prescription medications, and illicit substances (See Table 8.1). Eight of the nine substance classes in DSM-5 are recognized to cause SIA disorders during intoxication, withdrawal, or both [3]. Conspicuously absent from this DSM-5 list is nicotine, though clinical experience and research suggest that nicotine is indeed capable of inducing significant anxiety, specifically during withdrawal.

Individuals who present to an ED with SIA may be under the influence of a single substance or many. Currently, there is little published data on SIA in the psychiatric emergency setting, particularly during substance withdrawal. The substances

Table 8.1 Common substances that induce anxiety [3]

Substance	Anxiety with intoxication	Anxiety in withdrawal
Alcohol	+	+
Caffeine	+	+
Cannabis	+	+
Stimulants	+	+
Sedatives, hypnotics, anxiolytics		+
Opioids		+
Hallucinogens (PCP, other)	+	
Inhalants	+	

discussed in this section do not represent a comprehensive list of anxiety-inducing substances. Rather, they reflect those most frequently seen and implicated in the development of anxiety in the clinical setting.

Alcohol

51.7% of Americans report current alcohol use, making it one of the most used substances in the United States [7]. Exact mechanisms remain unclear, but alcohol has been shown to have both anxiolytic and anxiogenic effects, which are correlated with the time course of use. Short-term use of alcohol is thought to be anxiolytic and affects multiple neurotransmitter systems in the brain, including catecholaminergic, GABAergic, glutaminergic, and serotonergic systems [8]. Its initial action at ligand-gated ion channel receptors of GABA, the primary inhibitory neurotransmitter in the brain, contributes to the anxiolytic effects [8]. Intoxication typically results in initial mood elevation and relaxation, then behavioral disinhibition, impulsivity, and gait instability, but may also result in depression, rage, and gross cognitive deficits in memory, executive planning, and motor control. Severe neurologic changes, including stupor, coma, brain damage, and death, may also occur at high levels of intoxication [8, 9]. Alcohol can also be anxiogenic. Individuals with vulnerability to experiencing anxiety may experience transient anxiety after alcohol intoxication [10]. In addition, those who are alcohol dependent may experience anxiety, in addition to autonomic hyperarousal, during withdrawal and then develop anticipatory anxiety during periods of waning intoxication [11].

Not all individuals that present with anxiety will report alcohol use, but it is critical to take an alcohol use history regardless. Prevalence rates for anxiety disorders range from 15% to 26% among patients with alcohol use disorders [6]. The severity of anxiety has been demonstrated to be higher when comorbid with alcohol use disorder, and some studies demonstrate decreased relapse rates when anxiety is treated [4]. It is important to rule out alcohol-induced anxiety before diagnosing an independent anxiety disorder, since the former is likely to be transient and will resolve without further treatment, if alcohol use is stopped. Alcohol withdrawal can initially present as anxiety. Diagnosing and treating the withdrawal is critical, as withdrawal can be severe in some patients, leading to complications such as seizures, delirium tremens, and even death [9, 12].

Caffeine

Caffeine is the most widely consumed stimulant worldwide [13]. It is estimated that nearly 90% of the US population consumes caffeinated products (including coffee and soft drinks) regularly [14], and recent FDA estimates indicate that the average adult in the United States over 22 years old consumes 300 mg of caffeine daily [15]. While up to 97% of this intake is from coffee and tea [15], caffeine is often added to other beverages, food items, medications, and is even sold as a supplement.

Caffeine is a methylxanthine that exerts most of its effects through blocking multiple adenosine receptors throughout the body [13]. This blockade results in the stimulation of the central nervous system [13]. At low doses, this stimulation provides a boost in energy and alertness [9]. High doses result in a condition called caffeinism, the signs and symptoms of which closely resemble natural anxiety [16]. Caffeinism is characterized by restlessness, agitation, excitement, rambling thoughts and speech, insomnia, and may precipitate sinus tachycardia [16]. These symptoms may explain why individuals with a known anxiety disorder often avoid caffeine. Though caffeine withdrawal characteristically consists of fatigue, depressed mood, headache, and difficulty concentrating, some studies demonstrate that withdrawal can also cause increased anxiety, insomnia, and restlessness [3, 17].

Cannabis

Marijuana is the most commonly used illicit substance in the United States, with 8.3% of the population 12 years and older reporting current use [7]. Expectedly, marijuana use disorder is also the most common illicit SUD [7]. The impact of growing social acceptance and legalization of marijuana on usage patterns and health issues remains a debated topic, though reports suggest these changes have led to increased marijuana use overall [7]. Cannabis use disorder is highly comorbid with other SUDs and primary psychiatric disorders, with a 24% rate of comorbidity with anxiety disorders [3].

The individual response to marijuana is multifactorial and likely depends on the strain of marijuana, absorbed dose, setting, personality, and expectations of the user [9]. The effects of marijuana are modulated by delta-9-tetrahydrocannabinol's (THC) interaction with cannabinoid receptors within the central nervous system [9]. Cannabis intoxication is typically characterized by euphoria and relaxation [9], but it can also cause anxiety, paranoia, and dysphoria [18]. Anxiety and dysphoria are the most common presentations to the emergency department following marijuana use [9]. Cannabis withdrawal is marked by anxiety, irritability, sleep disturbance, and decreased appetite [3]. Withdrawal symptoms, including anxiety, appear within 1–3 days after cessation of use and peak within the first week [3]. Anxiety may persist for several weeks in dependent users [19].

Synthetic Cannabinoids

Synthetic cannabinoids, commonly known by the street names of K2 and spice, are often sold under the guise of being "herbal incense" [9]. The synthetic cannabinoids are generally more potent than THC, likely due to their stronger affinity for cannabinoid receptors [9]. Whereas THC is a partial agonist, the synthetic cannabinoids are full agonists and demonstrate 4–10 times greater affinity for the cannabinoid receptor [9].

Symptoms of intoxication parallel those of cannabis. Anxiety is prominent [20] and intoxicated individuals frequently experience palpitations. Users are also at risk for seizures and psychosis [9, 21]. Multiple case reports indicate a link between new onset encephalopathy and recent synthetic cannabinoid use, which may help to explain the onset of seizures and psychotic symptoms [21]. Case reports also highlight the potential for a withdrawal syndrome in chronic users characterized by anxiety, drug cravings, and dysautonomia [9].

Stimulants

Peaking in the mid-1980s with 7.1 million users [9], cocaine and crack use in the United States continue to decline, with recent estimates suggesting 1.9 million current users [7]. There is nearly the same estimated number of current users of other stimulants (excluding cocaine and methamphetamine) at 1.7 million people [7]. Though legally available by prescription, beginning in 2015, the National Survey on Drug Use and Health began including specific questions regarding illicit methamphetamine use, due to its production and use being overwhelmingly illicit in the United States. Data from the survey indicate an estimated 0.9 million current users of methamphetamine in the United States, though it is the second most popular illicit substance worldwide, behind marijuana [7, 9].

The intoxication phase of cocaine and other stimulants frequently includes increased alertness and elevated mood but can also include paranoid delusions, tactile hallucinations, agitation, and anxiety due to sympathomimetic effects and modulation of neurotransmitters, including dopamine, norepinephrine, and serotonin [9, 22]. This phase typically lasts longer with amphetamines than with cocaine [9]. "Bath salts," the synthetic cathinones (e.g., mephedrone, methylone), have demonstrated psychiatric side effects with acute intoxication, including anxiety and agitation [9]. Anxiety is common in patients with stimulant use disorders; samples suggest 15–40% of patients with stimulant use disorders have a co-occurring anxiety disorder [22], including panic attacks, social phobia, and generalized anxiety. Comorbidity with sedative SUDs is common, as these substances are frequently taken to reduce the unpleasant side effects associated with stimulant use [3].

Sedatives, Hypnotics, Anxiolytics

Nearly two million Americans report current misuse of prescription sedatives and tranquilizers, including benzodiazepines and barbiturates [7]. Benzodiazepines are a class of drugs that have widespread medicinal use for treatment of anxiety, seizure disorders, sleeping disorders, and as muscle relaxants [23, 24]. They exert their effect by binding to sites on $GABA_A$ receptors which increases the receptors' affinity for the inhibitory neurotransmitter GABA, potentiating GABA's effect on the central nervous system (CNS), resulting in mental and physical relaxation [25]. Barbiturates modulate GABA and have similar CNS depressant effects [9].

Benzodiazepine and barbiturate intoxication are marked by somnolence, ataxia, and reduced concentration [9, 26]. Clinical appearance mimics that of alcohol intoxication. Withdrawal from these medications may be severe and is typically marked by anxiety, insomnia, panic attacks, tremors, sweating, autonomic hyperarousal, and mood lability [9, 26]. If the duration and intensity of use is substantial, dysautonomia, visual hallucinations, seizures, and delirium may also occur, especially in the setting of abrupt withdrawal [9]. It can be difficult for clinicians to distinguish between the acute symptoms of an anxiety disorder and recurrent or worsening anxiety associated with withdrawal in a patient being tapered off a prescribed anxiolytic medication. Especially after protracted use, withdrawal symptoms, including anxiety and sleep disruption, can linger for weeks [9].

Opioids

The primary medical uses of opioids include the treatment of pain, anesthesia, cough suppression, and medication-assisted treatment (MAT) for those with opioid use disorders [9, 27]. Increasing rates of illicit use [7] have prompted new focus on treating opioid use disorders and preventing opioid-related overdose deaths.

Opioid-induced anxiety during acute intoxication is uncommon, though thought to be mediated by the effect of opioids and corticotropin-releasing factor (CRF) on the locus coeruleus, the major norepinephrine (NE)-containing nucleus in the brain [28]. It has been hypothesized that chronic opioid use results in tolerance at the level of the locus coeruleus, which decreases the ability of opioids to hyperpolarize and inhibit locus coeruleus neurons [29–31]. The development of opioid tolerance causes an imbalance in the locus coeruleus-NE system in favor of CRF-induced activation, which predisposes individuals to anxiety disorders [28].

Opioid intoxication is characterized by a state of euphoria and sedation [27]. Opioid withdrawal onset and severity of symptoms is influenced by the type of opioid used, duration of use, and degree of dependence [32]. Individuals abusing short-acting opioids, like fentanyl or heroin, typically begin to experience withdrawal symptoms within 6–12 hours after use, whereas those using methadone or buprenorphine may only begin to experience symptoms more than 24 hours after their last dose. Signs and symptoms of withdrawal most commonly include tachycardia, hypertension, diaphoresis, tremor, joint pain, diarrhea, nausea, vomiting, anxiety, and agitation [9]. Some patients develop an abstinence phobia, defined as anxiety in the context of fear of withdrawing from a substance [11], and will often present to the emergency department seeking a medication-assisted detoxification or the initiation of substitution therapy. Anxiety symptoms outside withdrawal states are uncommon.

Hallucinogens

Lysergic acid diethylamide (LSD), phencyclidine (PCP), peyote, mescaline, psilocybin mushrooms, "ecstasy" (MDMA or "Molly"), ketamine, N,N-dimethyltryptamine (DMT)/α-methyltryptamine (AMT)/"foxy," and *Salvia divinorum* are categorized as hallucinogens, which are currently used by 1.2 million people in the United States [7]. This heterogeneous category of substances has substantial interindividual variability in response to intoxication and withdrawal [9]. These substances exert their effects by modulation of different neurotransmitters. PCP primarily antagonizes NMDA receptors, modulating glutamate [9]. LSD is a mixed serotonin receptor partial agonist [9]. Ketamine also modulates glutamate through antagonism of NMDA receptors, though it additionally impacts other receptors, such as opioid, noradrenaline, serotonin, and cholinergic receptors [9]. The most common effects experienced with hallucinogen intoxication are altered perceptions and behavior, with variable sympathomimetic activity [9]. Adverse effects include paranoia, panic, and anxiety [9]. The hallucinations or aberrant behaviors are typically the impetus for seeking medical assistance, but both need not be present simultaneously [9]. Significant agitation and destructive behavior may also occur in the absence of altered sensorium due to significant disinhibition [9].

Inhalants

Glue, shoe polish, toluene, spray paints, gasoline, and lighter fluid are among the inhalants most commonly abused, though the number of consumer products that may produce intoxication when inhaled is innumerable [33]. Despite more than 22 million Americans reporting historical inhalant use, this form of substance abuse remains relatively unstudied [33]. Users are often male adolescents (12–17-year-old peak age range), disproportionately socioeconomically disadvantaged, or involved in the criminal justice system [9, 33]. Efforts to identify individuals at risk for inhalant use have found elevated use rates among youth who use inhalants to "self-medicate" anxiety [33].

Though not well understood, many inhalants are thought to exert their effects through modulation of GABA and NMDA receptors [9]. Typically, 10–15 inhalations are all that is required to achieve euphoria and drowsiness, which occur within seconds to minutes [9]. High doses may result in severely distressing hallucinations [9]. Chronic use can lead to significant behavioral changes, including hostility and paranoia [9]. The existence of a withdrawal syndrome is not universally accepted, but some reports suggest that it could include symptoms of intense craving for the substance, increased irritability, anxiety, headaches, nausea, vomiting, hallucinations, tachycardia, rhinorrhea, and epiphora [33, 34]. Presumably due to the low prevalence rates of inhalant use disorders, disproportionately affected subpopulations, and rapid and short-lived intoxication, inhalant-associated symptoms are an uncommon presentation to most emergency settings.

Emergency Assessment

Emergency evaluations of anxious patients with either SIA disorders or comorbid anxiety and SUDs involve the same principles of thorough assessment that apply to other medical and psychiatric illness presentations. Potentially serious and reversible medical causes for anxiety (Table 8.2) should first be ruled out. Emergent psychiatric evaluations should always include a safety assessment for evidence of acute dangerousness toward self or others, including ED staff.

Substances have complex physiological and psychological effects on patients, and it can be difficult to differentiate between a SIA disorder and comorbid substance use and anxiety disorders. The key to differentiation is to determine whether anxiety is present when an individual is not intoxicated or withdrawing from substances [3]. DSM-5 criteria for a SIA disorder also require that the severity of anxiety exceeds the expected anxiety during intoxication or withdrawal and warrants separate clinical attention [3]. A thorough history of present illness, including a detailed timeline of symptom evolution, medication history, social history, and substance use history are important in this determination. Patients with both anxiety disorders and SUDs will frequently need prolonged observation in the early stages of treatment, beyond the initial ED assessment, to clarify the diagnosis with confidence [35].

Table 8.2 Medical causes of anxiety

Cardiovascular	Myocardial ischemia and infarction, valvular disease, dysrhythmias, heart failure
Pulmonary	Asthma, COPD exacerbation, pulmonary embolus
Endocrine	Pheochromocytoma, hyperthyroidism, hypoglycemia, hypercalcemia
Neurologic	Delirium

Time Course

Delineating the time course of anxiety symptoms is diagnostically important, as the anxiety or panic symptoms must have started during or soon after the substance intoxication or withdrawal to be considered SIA [3]. If the onset of anxiety symptoms preceded substance intoxication or withdrawal, other etiologies should be considered. Substance-induced anxiety symptoms are, by definition, time-limited and will generally resolve within hours to one month from the time of use or withdrawal, depending on the half-life of the substance used [3]. In contrast, patients with comorbid anxiety and SUDs will have significant anxiety symptoms, even during periods of sobriety.

Identifying time of last use can be helpful for establishing a prospective time frame for expected symptom resolution. In addition, a history of brief substance use with substances known to cause anxiety only in withdrawal (e.g., opioids, sedatives, hypnotics) may suggest a diagnosis other than SIA because brief use is unlikely to cause a withdrawal syndrome. Symptoms that persist longer than typically associated with discontinuation should raise the question of an underlying primary anxiety disorder.

Severity

The intoxication and withdrawal syndromes of many substances produce physical and psychological signs and symptoms also commonly seen in primary anxiety disorders, such as tachycardia, sweating, trembling, fearfulness, and sleep disturbance [3, 9]. DSM-5 differentiates SIA from substance intoxication or withdrawal by symptom severity. In SIA disorders, the severity of symptoms must exceed that usually associated with intoxication or withdrawal, dominate the clinical presentation, or warrant independent clinical attention [3]. In comorbid anxiety and SUDs, symptom severity for both disorders must meet DSM-5 diagnostic thresholds. Therefore, one must make a (subjective) assessment of symptom severity and its relationship to expected and/or diagnostic thresholds.

Physical exam, vital signs, and lab work, including toxicology, can provide much needed objective information to help inform the diagnosis. Due to the overlapping signs and symptoms of independent anxiety and SIA, it can be challenging to differentiate between the two. The presence of nystagmus, slurred speech, gait disturbance, hyperpyrexia, or hyperthermia should prompt consideration of acute intoxication and may therefore better support a diagnosis of SIA. Toxicology tests may be helpful in determining substance use, though these are limited in their ability to detect many potential substances of abuse. Synthetic cannabinoids may cross-react, or not react at all, with a THC screen. Often, screens for benzodiazepines are not all-inclusive, and common drug screens only check for some opioids, such as morphine, heroin, and codeine, and exclude oxycodone and fentanyl. It is helpful to know the specific substances detectable by the screening assay in use so that more specific tests may be ordered if needed, such as tests for specific benzodiazepines and metabolites, or an expanded opioid panel to assess for the presence of synthetic opioids. However, it is important to remember that SIA may also present during a withdrawal syndrome, during which drug screens may be negative but substance use still etiologically implicated.

Collateral information from medical records, family members, and medical providers can also contribute to diagnostic clarity. A documented history of substance use in the absence of a known anxiety disorder suggests a substance-induced etiology, whereas a historical anxiety disorder in the absence of substance use would support an independent anxiety disorder. Family members can frequently provide information on the differences in the individual's mood and behavior while intoxicated and sober. Medical providers, particularly established outpatient providers, can be a wealth of information and often provide substantial history of substance use and anxiety.

Emergency Management

Standard pharmacologic treatment regimens for primary and comorbid anxiety disorders include selective serotonin reuptake inhibitors (SSRIs), selective norepinephrine reuptake inhibitors (SNRIs), buspirone, and benzodiazepines. Treatment with SSRIs, SNRIs, or buspirone is not typically initiated in the emergency setting due to the time to onset of effect (typically weeks), though these medications may be initiated, if a plan for outpatient follow-up and management can be determined.

Substance-induced anxiety dissipates once the effects of the substance have resolved [3], so emergent treatment is largely supportive, but may warrant pharmacologic intervention for patients in significant distress [9]. Acute intoxication or withdrawal may require active management prior to establishing a clear diagnosis and initiating longer-term definitive treatment.

Management of Anxiety Occurring with Specific Substances

Alcohol

Anxiety associated with alcohol use is most common during withdrawal. Benzodiazepines are the first-line treatment of both alcohol and benzodiazepine withdrawal and should be initiated immediately to avoid progression to potentially life-threatening withdrawal. Symptom-triggered therapy is preferred, as it has been shown to result in reduced duration and cumulative dose of benzodiazepines [36]. Prior to obtaining evidence of intact liver function, agents that are metabolized outside the liver, including lorazepam and oxazepam, are recommended.

Anxiety in the alcohol-withdrawing ED patient will typically resolve with appropriate medication administration. Blood alcohol level (BAL) may be helpful if the patient is profoundly intoxicated or unable to provide coherent history. Clinical presentation should guide treatment, as heavy users will start experiencing withdrawal symptoms even when BALs remain elevated. Alcohol detoxification may take multiple days, so admission to an inpatient detox facility or referral to a provider or program capable of managing outpatient detox may be considered after the patient has been acutely stabilized.

While acute treatment in the emergency setting typically consists of benzodiazepines regardless of the etiology of the anxiety, long-term treatments differ considerably. Long-term use of benzodiazepines in outpatients with alcohol or benzodiazepine use disorders is controversial due to the abuse potential and safety concerns of these medications, given that benzodiazepines can be lethal in combination with alcohol. Thus, it is common for outpatient providers to avoid using benzodiazepines to treat comorbid anxiety disorders in patients with alcohol use disorders. Comorbid anxiety and alcohol use disorders increase the prospective risk for relapse on alcohol, though conflicting reports exist on the benefits of specific anxiety treatment on the outcomes of alcohol use disorder treatment [4, 22]. Outpatient treatment for these patients generally consists of naltrexone for alcohol cravings, referral to community substance use support groups, and SSRIs/SNRIs for treatment of comorbid anxiety disorder. Treatment for patients with alcohol-induced anxiety should focus primarily on the SUD, as the anxiety will resolve with cessation of alcohol use.

Caffeine

Caffeine-induced anxiety is often unrecognized because medical providers frequently fail to ask about consumption [16]. Anxiety secondary to caffeine intake often resolves with the discontinuation of caffeine-containing products [9]. Patients can be managed conservatively by being placed in a quiet, non-stimulating environment. Severe anxiety may be managed with short-acting benzodiazepines. Symptoms of withdrawal generally begin within 24 hours of cessation, peak by 48 hours, and resolve typically within 1 week, if abstinence is maintained [9].

Cannabis

Psychotropic effects of cannabis begin up to 90 minutes after ingestion or inhalation, peak within 3 hours, and usually resolve within 12 hours [9]. Withdrawal symptoms may occur in chronic users and typically begin 1–3 days after last use, peak within 6 days, and resolve within 2 weeks [9]. Anxiety associated with acute intoxication may be managed with rest, reassurance, and reduction of environmental stimuli [9]. A urine drug screen for THC may serve to confirm the suspected diagnosis. Low-dose, short-acting benzodiazepines may be helpful in the ED for those acutely anxious patients who do not respond to conservative treatment. Temporary use of mirtazapine for 2 weeks following cessation may help with cannabis withdrawal-associated insomnia [37]. High-dose gabapentin (1200 mg/day) has also been shown to improve cannabis withdrawal symptoms [37]. While THC analogs may improve symptoms, these are not typically prescribed [37]. Though not extensively researched, one study suggested treatment of anxiety disorders in cannabis users and replacement cannabinoid use to treat anxiety did not promote long-term reductions in cannabis use but did have a positive therapeutic benefit on anxiety [38, 39]. Treatment of cannabis use disorder has been modeled after treatment for alcohol use disorder. Specifically, 12-step programs and CBT modalities have been developed to treat cannabis use disorder [40], and patients should be provided with information on local addiction treatment programs.

Synthetic Cannabinoids

Synthetic cannabinoids usually cannot be detected by standard urine toxicology tests, though some formulations which include THC may screen positive. Clinical judgment and patient history are important in determining if an individual has used a synthetic cannabinoid compound. Due to inconsistent purity and potent cannabinoid receptor agonism, medical management in the ED is important, as individuals who have used synthetic cannabinoids can develop seizures and tachycardia [41]. There is limited research on treatment of synthetic cannabinoid intoxication and withdrawal, but discontinuation of the substance has been shown to improve symptoms [9]. Evidence-based treatment is lacking, but supportive care, including placing the patient in a non-stimulating, quiet environment, may be beneficial [9] (see Chap. 4 for additional information).

Stimulants

The clinical effects of cocaine intoxication, including anxiety, typically develop within an hour of use and will resolve within 3 hours, in the absence of secondary sequelae [9]. The effects of amphetamines develop in a similar time frame and generally resolve within 4–6 hours [9].

Currently, there are no Food and Drug Administration (FDA)-approved pharmacologic treatments for stimulant use disorders [42]. Patients presenting during acute intoxication can usually be managed conservatively with a quiet and non-stimulating environment, but should be monitored and observed, specifically for cardiovascular complications. Significant anxiety and agitation may require pharmacologic treatment with short-acting benzodiazepines. Severe agitation and psychotic symptoms nonresponsive to benzodiazepines alone may require treatment with antipsychotics.

Although physiological withdrawal from cocaine and other stimulants is not life-threatening, the resulting dysphoria can be [9], and patients should be monitored for suicidal ideation and self-injurious behaviors. Withdrawal symptoms peak within

2–4 days but may persist for many weeks [9]. In some cases, acute cocaine withdrawal may reach the threshold of a panic attack and evolve into a seemingly autonomous and independent anxiety disorder [22]. Long-term pharmacologic treatments for both cocaine-induced anxiety and cocaine use disorder are experimental, with research suggesting a possible role for various agents, including mood stabilizers, antidepressants, disulfiram, and dopamine agonists [9].

Sedatives, Hypnotics, and Anxiolytics

Anxiety is a symptom of sedative, hypnotic, and anxiolytic withdrawal and will usually develop within 36 hours of last use, depending on the chronicity of use and the pharmacokinetics of the substance being used [9]. Patients with a significant history of chronic and heavy use will develop symptoms earlier in withdrawal, a phenomenon like what is seen in chronic heavy alcohol use. Symptom severity typically peaks within 48 hours of last dose, though seizures, psychosis, and delirium are possible for up to 5 days [9]. Withdrawal symptoms may persist for up to 2 weeks [9], and sleep disturbance may persist even longer.

There are no FDA-approved treatments for anxiety secondary to the use of sedatives, hypnotics, and anxiolytics (SHA). As previously mentioned, treatment for benzodiazepine withdrawal is like that for alcohol withdrawal and includes administration of benzodiazepines based on presenting signs and symptoms, followed by subsequent taper. A symptomatic approach in dealing with SHA-induced anxiety may be most helpful. It is important to know why patients are using SHA to better inform treatment approaches. If an individual uses SHAs for their sedative properties, a discussion may be had in the ED about sleep hygiene or the use of other medications, such as trazodone or mirtazapine, which have sleep-promoting properties [43]. If SHAs are being used for anxiety, it may be helpful to discuss the use of other agents to treat anxiety, such as SSRIs, SNRIs, or propranolol [44]. Being familiar with other substances of potential abuse can be invaluable, as patients may request less common agents which also have abuse potential, such as gabapentin and quetiapine. While psychoeducation can be provided in the ED, the longer-term prescribing of these psychopharmacologic agents should be managed by an outpatient treater, either a primary care physician or a psychiatrist.

Hallucinogens

Effects from LSD typically begin within 90 minutes of ingestion, peak within 3 hours, and resolve within 6–12 hours, though this timing may be influenced by dose and frequency of use [9]. PCP effect onset is usually within 30 minutes and may last for 4–6 hours [9]. MDMA effects typically begin within 1 hour and resolve within 4–6 hours [9]. The effects of psilocybin are like LSD and generally resolve within 6 hours [9]. Nystagmus is a common finding in PCP intoxication, and its presence or absence on physical exam can help differentiate PCP intoxication from

LSD intoxication [9]. Serotonin syndrome is a known complication of MDMA use and should be considered in patients with consistent signs and symptoms [9], such as hyperthermia, hyperreflexia, mydriasis, arrhythmias, tremor, hyperhidrosis, hypertension, and diarrhea.

Treatment for hallucinogen-induced anxiety is primarily supportive, and most patients respond well to reassurance, rest, and reduction of stimuli [9]. Severe anxiety may warrant pharmacologic intervention in the ED with short-acting benzodiazepines. Patients should be monitored for psychiatric and medical complications until sensorium clears and behavior returns to baseline. It may be beneficial to assess for suicidal ideation following resolution of intoxication, as severe depression is known to develop [9]. Though there is little data to support a characteristic withdrawal syndrome, individuals may experience cravings and dysphoric mood for up to one month following last use [9]. Residual perceptual disturbances after 1 month from last use should prompt consideration and assessment for hallucinogen persisting perception disorder.

Inhalants

Inhalant-induced anxiety is primarily associated with acute intoxication, which rapidly resolves with removal of the inhalant, frequently in less than an hour [9]. Symptoms persisting longer than a few hours should prompt consideration of alternative diagnoses, including a comorbid anxiety disorder. Long-term treatment is structured around cognitive behavioral therapy, 12-step programs, and motivational enhancement [9].

Opioids

There is little research on the treatment of opioid-induced anxiety. Diagnosing comorbid anxiety disorders in patients who present with acute heroin or other opioid use is challenging, as withdrawal symptoms may mimic an anxiety disorder. Treatment of the withdrawal and continuous reassessment of the anxiety will help to clarify diagnoses and inform treatment decisions and referrals. Detoxification from opioids may be useful in helping to relieve anxiety, and ED providers should consider referring the opioid-dependent patient to a detox facility if more efficacious treatments, such as medication-assisted treatment (MAT), are unavailable.

Clonidine, an alpha 2-adrenergic agonist, may be used as an anxiolytic in acute opioid withdrawal [45]. Short-term buprenorphine tapers have been demonstrated to be more effective in maintaining engagement in long-term treatment than clonidine (80% vs 30% retention) and appear to be a viable alternative treatment [46], especially in the context of withdrawal and anticipatory anxiety. Evidence and support for initiating buprenorphine maintenance in the ED [47] is growing. One such study examined treatment retention for those started on buprenorphine in the ED versus screening, brief intervention, and referral to treatment. The results of the study indicated that, 30 days post intervention, those that initiated buprenorphine in the ED were substantially more likely to be engaged in substance use treatment after 30 days than those receiving brief interventions or referrals (78% vs 45% and 37%, respectively) [47]. Methadone may also be helpful in the treatment of acute opioid withdrawal-related symptoms, particularly if aftercare planning involves referral to facilities which utilize methadone for detox or maintenance treatment. Evidence routinely supports the safety and superior efficacy of medication-assisted treatment versus detoxification and abstinence-only approaches, though significant barriers to widespread adoption persist and may be particularly challenging in the ED setting. For MAT induction in the ED to be successful, a network of community-based treatment services for follow-up care must also be available, and providing MAT without outpatient follow-up for continued management is strongly discouraged. Should anxiety persist despite adequate management of withdrawal symptoms, a comorbid anxiety disorder is likely and treatment addressing both the substance use disorder and suspected anxiety disorder should be sought.

General Treatment Approaches

The mainstays of treatment for SIA and comorbid anxiety and SUDs include detoxification, medication to assist with management of substance use and anxiety, motivational therapies, contingency management, and cognitive behavioral therapy [9, 48]. Treating comorbid anxiety and substance use poses unique challenges given the limited research. There has been some disagreement about whether comorbid anxiety and substance use should be treated simultaneously or separately [49]. Specifically, in comorbid anxiety and alcohol use disorder, conflicting evidence both suggests and refutes a role for the treatment of anxiety in patients with alcohol use disorder [4, 49]. Despite the conflicting research, current clinical practice recommends treatment of comorbid anxiety, and it is reassuring that some studies suggest this approach may prevent worsening of the alcohol use disorder [22]. The health benefits of the reduction, or cessation, of alcohol, tobacco, and illicit substance use cannot be understated, and treatment of SUDs should always be a clinical priority.

The clinician's role in the ED is to make appropriate diagnoses, assess safety, identify treatment recommendations, and motivate and educate the patient about what treatment entails for both the anxiety and any coexisting SUD. Brief intervention in the ED can be useful for patients who appear to have mild symptoms of SIA and for those who return to a stable mental state once sober from an uneventful intoxication. The purpose of brief intervention is to provide psychoeducation about, and coping strategies for, SIA and comorbid anxiety and SUDs [50]. A medical professional can provide patients and their families with reassurance, education on substance use and its role in modulating anxiety, as well as motivational interviewing for recovery. Educating the patient on the interconnectedness of their substance use and their anxiety is imperative. Patients with SIA should have a clear understanding that abstinence is critical for remission of their anxiety. Those with comorbid disorders should understand that their substance use, despite potentially being used to "self-medicate," is very likely making their anxiety symptoms worse. The ED visit is also an opportune time to provide the patient with information regarding local community support groups for substance use and mental health treatment resources for persistent anxiety.

All patients should be counseled about potential interactions associated with substances of abuse, whether illicit, legal, or prescribed. For example, patients abusing alcohol, sedatives, hypnotics, anxiolytics, or opioids should be counseled on the increased risk of respiratory depression and death by combining any of these substances with other CNS depressants. Those using MDMA should be cautioned against combining it with cocaine, serotonin reuptake inhibitors, and monoamine oxidase inhibitors, due to increased risk of precipitating serotonin syndrome [9].

Disposition

There are several options to consider in the disposition of individuals with SIA and comorbid disorders. Following medical assessment and stabilization, and assuming no active safety concerns persist, patients should be stratified according to the severity of their substance use and comorbid disorders. Once patients are stratified, the clinician can begin to evaluate appropriate treatment options based on the working diagnosis. Patients with lower severity disorders may do well with only outpatient clinic treatment. Those with moderate severity disorders generally require the higher level of care provided by intensive outpatient programs or partial hospitalization programs. Individuals with high severity disorders may benefit from inpatient services. Patients with SIA should have dispositions focused on treatment of substance use, whereas those with comorbid anxiety disorders and SUDs will benefit most from treatment that addresses both disorders.

Engagement with an outpatient provider with expertise in managing SUDs and anxiety is an instrumental part of treatment. These providers offer a source of stable support and provide longitudinal management of medications that may be indicated. The outpatient clinic setting allows for a more in-depth interview, discussion of the motivations for using, and barriers to stopping use of substances. Additionally, evaluation by an outpatient provider may reveal previously undisclosed factors suggesting the need for more intensive psychiatric treatment (e.g., safety concerns). Cognitive behavioral therapy (CBT) is a therapeutic tool that promotes behavioral modification through evaluation of emotional state and reasoning involved in decision-making and can be offered through outpatient behavioral health follow-up [48]. Outpatient clinics routinely have available resources regarding on-site and local area recovery groups that can be of tremendous benefit for those in treatment for substance use or anxiety.

If a patient is amenable to further outpatient treatment, partial hospitalization programs (PHPs) and intensive outpatient programs (IOPs) provide significant daily structure and additional treatment for patients with significant treatment needs but who do not require inpatient level of care. PHPs are typically 5 days a week and require transportation to the program location daily for the duration. Treatment duration varies from one to several weeks and usually consists of multiple daily group and individual therapy sessions, evaluation by a psychiatrist for medication management, and consultation with current outpatient treatment providers. IOPs are similar but generally less intense, meeting less frequently and for fewer hours of treatment.

For dependent patients at risk for physiologic withdrawal from alcohol, benzodiazepines, or opioids, detoxification may be warranted prior to initiation of treatment for any comorbid anxiety symptoms. Evidence unequivocally supports initiation of MAT for opioid-dependent patients over detox, and MAT should be sought for all interested opioid-dependent patients. However, some patients are uncomfortable with maintenance treatment and prefer detox. Detox may take place in an inpatient or outpatient setting, depending on medical and psychiatric risk stratification. Following completion of a detox program, an individual should pursue additional outpatient mental health follow-up treatment, including therapy and psychopharmacology, as needed. Residential programs are available and often require the patient to complete detox prior to admission, which may include detox from substances used for MAT. Policies regarding the continued use of MAT while in residential treatment vary and should be a consideration for final disposition.

Admission to an inpatient dual diagnosis program can be beneficial for those with severe SIA or SUDs comorbid with conditions such as psychosis, mood disorders, or posttraumatic stress disorder. There should be significant concern about the ability of the patient to function safely in the community, due to risk of suicide, homicide, or inability to care for self, to prompt referral to an inpatient dual diagnosis unit. The dual diagnosis program will treat the substance-induced symptoms, as well as the underlying psychiatric disorder. Upon discharge from a dual diagnosis program, an individual can then pursue outpatient mental health treatment for further assistance with maintaining stability and sobriety.

Conclusion

Individuals who present with substance use and anxiety must be evaluated comprehensively to establish a correct diagnosis. A thorough interview and collection of collateral information with specific focus on time course of illness can help differentiate between comorbid substance use and anxiety disorders and SIA disorders. Urine or serum toxicology can provide necessary objective information for patients who are under the influence of substances with known behavioral effects. Though most SIA will resolve with conservative measures, substance withdrawal can be life-threatening and should be managed aggressively to prevent poor outcomes. While there are standard practices for treating generalized anxiety, social phobias, and specific phobias, more research is needed on the treatment of those people with SIA. Multiple disposition options exist, and referral should be based on the specific needs of the patient.

References

1. Grant B, Stinson F, Dawson D, Chou S, Dufour MC, Compton W, et al. Prevalence and co-occurrence of substance use disorders and independent mood and anxiety disorders – results from the national epidemiologic survey on alcohol and related conditions. Arch Gen Psychiatry. 2004;61(8):807–16.
2. Somers JM, Goldner EM, Waraich P, Hsu L. Prevalence and incidence studies of anxiety disorders: a systematic review of the literature. Can J Psychiatr [Internet]. 2006;51(2):100–13. Available from:. https://doi.org/10.1177/070674370605100206.
3. American Psychiatric Association. Diagnostic and statistical manual of mental disorders. 5th ed. Washington, D.C.: American Psychiatric Association; 2013.
4. Kushner MG, Krueger R, Frye B, Peterson J. Epidemiological perspectives on co-occurring anxiety disorder and substance use disorder. In: Stewart SH, Conrod PJ, editors. Anxiety and substance use disorders: the vicious cycle of comorbidity. New York: Springer; 2008. p. 3–17.
5. Lai HMX, Cleary M, Sitharthan T, Hunt GE. Prevalence of comorbid substance use, anxiety and mood disorders in epidemiological surveys, 1990–2014: a systematic review and meta-analysis. Drug Alcohol Depend. 2015;154:1–13.
6. Moss HB, Chen CM, Yi H. Prospective follow-up of empirically derived alcohol dependence subtypes in wave 2 of the National Epidemiologic Survey on Alcohol and Related Conditions (NESARC): recovery status, alcohol use disorders and diagnostic criteria, alcohol consumption behavior, health status, and treatment seeking. Alcohol Clin Exp Res. 2010;34(6):1073–83.
7. Center for Behavioral Health Statistics and Quality. Key substance use and mental health indicators in the United States: results from the 2015 National Survey on Drug Use and Health (HHS Publication No. SMA 16-4984, NSDUH Series H-51). 2016. Retrieved from http://www.samhsa.gov/data/.
8. Goudriaan AE, Sher KJ. Alcohol. In: Verster JC, Brady K, Galanter M, Conrod P, editors. Drug abuse and addiction in medical illness: causes, consequences and treatment [internet]. New York: Springer; 2012. p. 123–36. Available from:. https://doi.org/10.1007/978-1-4614-3375-0_9.
9. Barceloux DG. Medical toxicology of drugs abuse: synthesized chemicals and psychoactive plants [Internet]. New York: Wiley; 2012. [cited 2017 Sept 25]. Available from: ProQuest Ebook Central.
10. Matt G, Kenneth J, Bernard D. The relation between alcohol problems and the anxiety disorders. Am J Psychiatry. 1990;147(6):685–95.
11. Robinson J, Sareen J, Cox BJ, Bolton JM. Role of self-medication in the development of comorbid anxiety and substance use disorders: a longitudinal investigation. Arch Gen Psychiatry. 2011;68(8):800.
12. Mayo-Smith MF, Beecher LH, Fischer TL, Gorelick DA, Guillaume JL, Hill A, et al. Management of alcohol withdrawal delirium. An evidence-based practice guideline. Arch Intern Med. 2004;164(13):1405–12.
13. Benowitz NL. Clinical pharmacology of caffeine. Annu Rev Med. 1990;41:277–88.
14. Frary CD, Johnson RK, Wang MQ. Food sources and intakes of caffeine in the diets of persons in the United States. J Am Diet Assoc. 2005;105(1):110–3.
15. Somogyi L. Caffeine intake by the U.S. population: Food and Drug Administration. Oakridge National Laboratory; 2010. [2015 27 July]. Available from: http://www.fda.gov/downloads/AboutFDA/CentersOffices/OfficeofFoods/CFSAN/CFSANFOIAElectronicReadingRoom/UCM333191.pdf.
16. Winston AP, Hardwick E, Jaberi N. Neuropsychiatric effects of caffeine. Adv Psychiatr Treat [Internet]. The Royal College of Psychiatrists. 2005;11(6):432–9. Available from: http://apt.rcpsych.org/content/11/6/432.
17. Bernstein GA, Carroll ME, Thuras PD, Cosgrove KP, Roth ME. Caffeine dependence in teenagers. Drug Alcohol Depend. 2002;66(1):1–6.

18. Thomas H. Psychiatric symptoms in cannabis users. Br J Psychiatry. 1993;163:141–9.
19. Budney AJ, Hughes JR, Moore BA, Vandrey R. Review of the validity and significance of cannabis withdrawal syndrome. Am J Psychiatry. 2004;161:1967–77.
20. Schneir AB, Cullen J, Ly BT. "Spice" girls: synthetic cannabinoid intoxication. J Emerg Med. 2011;40(3):296–9.
21. Louh IK, Freeman WD. A "spicy" encephalopathy: synthetic cannabinoids as cause of encephalopathy and seizure. Crit Care. 2014;18:553.
22. Vorspan F, Mehtelli W, Dupuy G, Bloch V, Lepine J-P. Anxiety and substance use disorders: co-occurrence and clinical issues. Curr Psychiatry Rep. 2015;17(2):4.
23. Amato L, Minozzi S, Vecchi S, Davoli M. Benzodiazepines for alcohol withdrawal. Cochrane Database Syst Rev. 2010;(3):CD005063.
24. Baldwin DS, Aitchison K, Bateson A, Curran HV, Davies S, Leonard B, et al. Benzodiazepines: risks and benefits. A reconsideration. J Psychopharmacol. 2013;27(11):967–71.
25. Soyka M. Treatment of benzodiazepine dependence. N Engl J Med. 2017;376(12):1147–57.
26. Ashton H. Benzodiazepine abuse. In: Caan W, de Belleroche J, editors. Drink, drugs and dependence from science to clinical practice. London: Routledge; 2002. p. 197–212.
27. Schuckit MA. Treatment of opioid-use disorders. N Engl J Med. 2016;375:1596–7.
28. Van Bockstaele EJ, Reyes BAS, Valentino RJ. The locus coeruleus: a key nucleus where stress and opioids intersect to mediate vulnerability to opiate abuse. Brain Res. 2010;1314:162–74.
29. Aghajanian GK. Tolerance of locus coeruleus neurones to morphine and suppression of withdrawal response by clonidine. Nature. 1978;276(5684):186–8.
30. Christie MJ, Williams JT, North RA. Mechanisms of tolerance to opiates in locus coeruleus neurons. NIDA Res Monogr. 1987;78:158–68.
31. Rasmussen K, Beitner-Johnson DB, Krystal JH, Aghajanian GK, Nestler EJ. Opiate withdrawal and the rat locus coeruleus: behavioral, electrophysiological, and biochemical correlates. J Neurosci. 1990;10(7):2308–17.
32. Farrell M. Opiate withdrawal. Addiction. 1994;89(11):1471.
33. Howard MO, Bowen SE, Garland EL, Perron BE, Vaughn MG. Inhalant use and inhalant use disorders in the United States. Addict Sci Clin Pract. 2011;6(1):18–31.
34. Perron BE, Howard MO, Vaughn MG, Jarman CN. Inhalant withdrawal as a clinically significant feature of inhalant dependence disorder. Med Hypotheses. 2009;73(6):935–7.
35. McHugh RK. Treatment of co-occurring anxiety disorders and substance use disorders. Harv Rev Psychiatry. 2015;23(2):99–111.
36. Taheri A, Dahri K, Chan P, Shaw M, Aulakh A, Tashakkor A. Evaluation of a symptom-triggered protocol approach to the management of alcohol withdrawal syndrome in older adults. J Am Geriatr Soc. 2014;62(8):1551–5.
37. Bonnet U, Preuss UW. The cannabis withdrawal syndrome: current insights. Subst Abuse Rehabil. 2017;8:9–37.
38. Hoch E, Bonnetn U, Thomasius R, Ganzer F, Havemann-Reinecke U, Preuss UW. Risks associated with the non-medicinal use of cannabis. Dtsch Arztebl Int. 2015;112(16):271–8.
39. Allsop DJ, Copeland J, Lintzeris N, Dunlop AJ, Montebello M, Sadler C, et al. Nabiximols as an agonist replacement therapy during cannabis withdrawal: a randomized clinical trial. JAMA Psychiat. 2014;71(3):281–91.
40. Copeland J, Swift W, Roffman R, Stephens R. A randomized controlled trial of brief cognitive-behavioral interventions for cannabis use disorder. J Subst Abuse Treat. 2001;21(2):55–6.
41. Lapoint J, James LP, Moran CL, Nelson LS, Hoffman RS, Moran JH. Severe toxicity following synthetic cannabinoid ingestion. Clin Toxicol (Phila). 2011;49(8):760–4.
42. Douaihy A, et al. Medications for substance use disorders. Soc Work Public Health. 2013;28(3–4):264–78.
43. Nissen C, Frase L, Hajak G, Wetter TC. Hypnotics – state of the science. Nervenarzt. 2014;85(1):67–76.

44. Mariani JJ, Malcolm RJ, Mamczur AK, Choi JC, Brady R, Nunes E, et al. Pilot trial of gabapentin for the treatment of benzodiazepine abuse or dependence in methadone maintenance patients. Am J Drug Alcohol Abuse. 2016;42(3):333–40.
45. Gowing L, Farrell MF, Ali R, White JM. Alpha2-adrenergic agonists for the management of opioid withdrawal. Cochrane Database Syst Rev. 2014;(3):CD002024.
46. Brigham GS, Amass L, Winhusen T, Harrer JM, Pelt A. Using buprenorphine short-term taper to facilitate early treatment engagement. J Subst Abuse Treat. 2007;32(4):349–56.
47. D'Onofrio G, O'Connor PG, Pantalon MV, Chawarski MC, Busch SH, Owens PH, et al. Emergency department-initiated buprenorphine/naloxone treatment for opioid dependence: a randomized clinical trial. JAMA. 2015;313(16):1636.
48. Hofmann SG, Smits JAJ. Cognitive-behavioral therapy for adult anxiety disorders: a meta-analysis of randomized placebo-controlled trials. J Clin Psychiatry. 2008;69(4):621–32.
49. Stewart SH, Conrod PJ. Anxiety and substance use disorders: the vicious cycle of comorbidity [Internet]. 2008. Available from: http://uwo.summon.serialssolutions.com/2.0.0/link/0/eLvHCXMwlV3dS8MwED9kA5kIOj9qdULBJx9amn4mjzIVQR-d-FaSNdXhrB-roP71Xtpmade91TSpCXkLr_c5XK_APie49pLmCA4SXmc-SqRMaPSRYRQ2hVLN0WFSkSZ5I338nIXxwdoCxxW6e-LYhh0bdT2dCIwiopWF19ORrNd1mUt4FOWB2mxaaUkZp2R5c9Hetc9dd.
50. Center for Substance Abuse Treatment. Brief interventions and brief therapies for substance abuse. Rockville: Substance Abuse and Mental Health Services Administration (US); 1999. (Treatment Improvement Protocol (TIP) Series, No. 34.) Available from: https://www.ncbi.nlm.nih.gov/books/NBK64947/.

Chapter 9
Patients with Co-occurring Substance Use and Personality Disorders

Daniel P. Johnson and Karsten Kueppenbender

Introduction

Individuals who are struggling with a substance use disorder (SUD) and comorbid personality disorder (PD) are often challenging patients in the ED. They present frequently to the ED, require intensive care, and evoke strong and often negative emotions among healthcare providers. Individuals with SUDs and individuals with PDs are also among the most stigmatized patients by the public, healthcare providers, and the patients themselves. In this chapter, we aim to present an understanding of PDs and comorbid SUDs in the ED, using a phenomenological and behavioral perspective. We will include a brief review of the literature on these comorbidities, highlight how stigma interferes with optimal care and impacts provider burnout, and make recommendations for assessment, management, treatment planning, and disposition consideration. We will also suggest clinical techniques that promote effective "in the room" interactions with patients during stressful, often emotionally charged, and frequently high-risk clinical encounters.

D. P. Johnson
Department of Psychiatry, Massachusetts General Hospital, Boston, MA, USA

K. Kueppenbender (✉)
Pavilion Center, McLean Hospital, Belmont, MA, USA
e-mail: kkueppenbender@partners.org

A. L. Donovan, S. A. Bird (eds.), *Substance Use and the Acute Psychiatric Patient*, Current Clinical Psychiatry, https://doi.org/10.1007/978-3-319-23961-3_9

Prevalence of Substance Use Disorders and Comorbid Personality Disorders

Studies indicate substantial comorbidity rates between SUDs and PDs. In the National Epidemiologic Survey on Alcohol and Related Conditions (NESARC; collected 2001–2002), a representative sample including over 40,000 respondents, 29% of individuals with alcohol use disorder (AUD) and 48% of individuals with other SUDs also met criteria for at least one of the PDs assessed in Wave 1 (avoidant, dependent, obsessive-compulsive, paranoid, schizoid, histrionic, and antisocial). In Wave 2 of the study, collected 2004–2005, 25.5% of individuals meeting criteria for an SUD also met criteria for borderline personality disorder (BPD). Similarly high rates of comorbidity between SUDs and PDs have been found in outpatient treatment samples [1] and institutionalized samples [2].

Of the ten personality disorder diagnoses, BPD and antisocial personality disorder (ASPD), both part of "cluster B" PDs according to past DSM categorizations, are most likely to overlap with SUDs [1, 3, 4]. Furthermore, studies have also shown that individuals with BPD, ASPD, or significant characteristics of these disorders have high rates of presentation to the ED [5, 6]. For these reasons, we will focus our attention and examples on BPD and ASPD; however, many of the recommendations and much of the discussion can be useful when applied to other PD presentations as well.

Stigma and Burnout

High rates of functional impairment, distress, service utilization, and recurrence rates make SUDs and PDs some of the most difficult disorders to treat [7, 8], particularly within the time and resource constraints of the ED setting. These factors all represent potential barriers for patients to effectively seek, engage in, and receive care. A barrier worthy of particular attention is stigma. Stigma, as it relates to health, describes the process by which certain groups, based on a socially discredited health condition, are devalued, rejected, and excluded [9]. SUDs and PDs have been shown to be highly stigmatized mental health conditions [10, 11] in the population at large ("social stigma"), among health professionals ("structural stigma"), and among patients themselves ("self-stigma") [9]. For example, individuals with alcohol use disorders are less likely to be seen as having an illness, more likely to be held responsible for their condition, and provoke more social rejection and structural discrimination than individuals with other mental health problems [12]. Health providers endorse less empathy and hold antagonistic views toward individuals with BPD [10, 13, 14] and more frequently report feeling mistreated and overwhelmed by patients with BPD [15].

Stigma can influence health and healthcare in myriad ways, and importantly, it may influence treatment decisions and the quality of care provided to patients.

Providers state they prefer to avoid BPD patients when possible [13] and view inpatient hospitalization as less justified for a patient with BPD, compared to a patient with major depressive disorder [16]. Similarly, health providers hold more negative views and feel less empathy for patients with SUDs and feel a diminished sense of impact on patient outcomes. These beliefs and emotional experiences contribute to a more task-oriented approach in treating patients with SUDs, with less personal engagement by providers, compared to treating other patients [11].

Of course, it makes sense that healthcare providers could form negative attitudes, experience reduced empathy, and have painful emotional reactions to patients with SUDs and PDs. Patients with SUDs and PDs are very likely to present to the ED repeatedly in crisis situations, to display emotional dysregulation, engage in ineffective and harmful interpersonal behaviors during clinical encounters, and often have significant personal histories with medical and psychiatric care institutions that influence their presentation (e.g., lack of follow-through with treatment recommendations, court-ordered treatment, involvement with the legal system). Burnout rates are significant among providers who work with these patients on a regular basis and special attention must be paid to self-care, receiving support, and developing robust coping skills among providers. Increasingly, research suggests there are effective interventions – on individual and organizational levels – for reducing burnout (for a review of the burnout literature and interventions, see [17]). Thus, we must consider the potential impact of stigma on patients and the impact of provider burnout when discussing clinical strategies for the ED setting.

A phenomenological and behaviorally based approach to clinical interactions in the ED is a first step to addressing these barriers to care. This approach focuses on observed behaviors, contextual factors contributing to the occurrence of behaviors, and the consequences (positive and negative) of behaviors. This approach can serve to reduce the use of labels and the tendencies (intentional or unintentional) to overpathologize, to speculate about intentions behind observed behaviors, and to judge the behaviors of patients. In conjunction with support from colleagues and self-care skills, such as mindfulness, behavioral approaches may also serve to reduce burnout among providers [18, 19]. With an eye toward the impact of stigma on patients and burnout on providers, we take this phenomenological perspective in our discussion of assessment and treatment considerations when interacting with patients with SUDs and comorbid PDs.

Clinical Assessment

When patients present to the ED with an acutely altered mental status or unusual behavior, it is critical to assess for intoxication, intentional or unintentional drug overdose, or toxic ingestion. A waxing and waning mental status suggests delirium and requires assessment of potential organic or medical etiology. Patients who are intoxicated or delirious are typically unable to provide the detailed history necessary to make a diagnosis of a personality disorder.

According to the DSM-5, personality disorders are characterized by an enduring pattern of inner experience and behavior that deviates markedly from the individual's culture. The pattern is manifested in two (or more) of the following areas: cognition, affectivity, interpersonal function, and impulse control [20].

Patients with BPD are often able and willing to describe a history of symptoms and experiences that allow a diagnosis of personality disorder to be made, even in the emergency room setting, unless there is acute impairment of mental status. Medical records, outpatient providers, family members, or friends may provide valuable collateral information. It is helpful to take the time necessary to make an accurate diagnosis of BPD and discuss the implications with the patient, when possible. The conversation with a skilled clinician is often a relief to the patient: an understanding of the BPD diagnosis offers an integrating framework to the patient, which puts a chaotic and distressing inner experience into perspective [21].

BPD is characterized by a pervasive pattern of instability of interpersonal relationships, self-image, and affects and marked impulsivity beginning by early adulthood and present in a variety of contexts. These patients often report feeling "empty" and can be described as having an unstable sense of self. Patients with BPD tend to form intense personal relationships, in which the other person (a partner, friend, clinician) is perceived and responded to through a lens of emotional extremes (i.e., "idealization" and "devaluation"), sometimes in succession. Patients tend to act impulsively, often with little regard for their own safety, sometimes in efforts to avoid real or perceived abandonment. The emotional experience of the patient is intense, often characterized by dysphoria, intense anger, or feelings of emptiness, which are difficult to bear – both for the patient and for his/her close social relations and clinicians.

Patients with BPD are prone to feeling rejected, and these feelings are magnified at times of stress, when frank paranoid ideation can occur. In contrast to a psychotic disorder, however, the underlying cognitive distortions are short-lived, and typically remit within hours, even minutes, depending on how quickly the patient calms down emotionally. States of intense anxiety and dysphoria or their opposite, a less common experience of elation, tend to be short-lived, on the order of hours, which differentiates BPD from typical bipolar disorder, where mood states persist with undiminished intensity for five or more days. Patients with BPD often have a history of non-suicidal self-injury (NSSI) and suicide attempts and are at risk for future self-harm. While the functions of self-harming behavior vary depending on the patient and context, patients often describe a desire to use self-injury as a means of achieving temporary emotional relief. When a patient presents to the ED after self-injurious behavior, regardless of the intent, a thorough medical clearance is indicated.

Patients with ASPD, especially when their mental status is not impaired, are typically less forthcoming about inner experiences and behaviors associated with their personality disorder than patients with BPD. ASPD is characterized by failure to conform to social norms with respect to lawful behaviors, as indicated by repeatedly performing acts that are grounds for arrest; deception, as indicated by repeatedly lying, or conning others for the purpose of personal profit or pleasure; impulsiveness or failure to plan ahead; irritability and aggressiveness, as indicated by repeated physical fights or assaults; reckless disregard for safety of self or others; consistent irresponsibility, as indicated by repeated failure to sustain consistent work behavior or honor financial obligations; and lack of remorse, as indicated by being indifferent to or rationalizing having hurt, mistreated, or stolen from another. For a formal diagnosis, there must be evidence of conduct disorder with onset before age 15 years [20]. Intelligent persons with ASPD may successfully subvert social norms, prevail in civil and sometimes criminal litigation, and paradoxically increase their social status, flagrant violations of social norms notwithstanding.

Disordered substance use may be associated with inner experiences and behaviors which overlap with diagnostic criteria for BPD or ASPD [22]. Therefore, for an accurate diagnosis and prognostic assessment, it is critical to determine if the disordered inner experience and behavioral pattern preceded the onset of disordered substance use or if they are secondary manifestations. If most symptoms manifested after the onset of a substance use disorder, then a complete rehabilitation of personality functioning is likely with remission of the substance use disorder. Patients will be "back to their old selves" and recover premorbid capacities for self-regulation and interpersonal functioning. Better yet, the learning, which occurs during the recovery process, often strengthens adaptive traits of character, including good humor, humility, altruism, and wisdom.

ED Management: Managing Patients' Skill Deficits to Promote Effective Care

Individuals with SUDs are likely to have functional deficits in their ability to regulate emotions, communicate with others, and tolerate distress, the impacts of which can be increased by acute intoxication and/or withdrawal states. These deficits are also the core deficits found in personality disorders according to the DSM-5 (e.g., intimacy, empathy, and identity impairments) and are primary treatment targets in evidence-based interventions for PDs [14, 19, 23]. Such impairments can manifest in myriad behaviors, including aggression, impulsive attempts to seek relief from emotional or physical pain (e.g., urges for self-harm, requests for hospitalization or medication), and inappropriate and ineffective forms of communication. Chapters 10 and 11 thoroughly cover the issues of SUDs and aggressive behavior and requests for medication in the ED, and thus we will not cover those topics in depth. Instead, we will focus on how SUDs and comorbid PDs can contribute to highly emotionally charged and ineffective communications with the ED team. The negative impact of these behaviors can be significantly mitigated by effective communication among ED team members, validation techniques, and functional analysis of the patient's behaviors.

Promote and Model Effective Communication

In the ED, interpersonal skill deficits in patients with SUDs and PDs may be evident in behaviors labeled as "idealization" or "devaluation" of certain providers (e.g., expressing disproportionate positive/negative affect or opinions, such as telling one provider she is a genius, while refusing to work with another provider, saying she is incompetent) or "splitting" among providers (e.g., providing different information to different providers or expressing opinions about one provider to another).

"Idealization," "devaluation," and "splitting" are labels used to describe sets of patient behaviors, and these behaviors can be reinforced or extinguished by providers' responses. The following recommendations are likely to reduce ineffective interpersonal behaviors by extinguishing them. *Have a team leader that is clearly identified to the treatment team and to the patient.* This may seem intuitive but is critically important to reduce reinforcement of ineffective strategies employed by the patient to get his/her needs met. If a patient makes differing requests to team members, or his/her requests change throughout the phases of the ED visit, team members can refer the patient to the team leader or offer to relay the patient's message to the team leader. This process can serve to extinguish ineffective communication, as it provides a delay between request and response; it reinforces a collaborative approach to treatment ("that's a good question, let's check in with Dr. X about that") and models thoughtful responding rather than impulsive reacting. If nothing else, deferring to a team leader models *clear, consistent communication between the team and the patient.* Moment-to-moment changes in treatment decisions, providers, disposition considerations, and even the clinical environment (e.g., room changes) are standard course for ED team providers. However, to the SUD/PD patient, these changes can feel abrupt, invalidating, and surprising and can leave a patient feeling "out of the loop," all experiences that can trigger the interpersonal/affective skill deficits described above. Updating the patient as often as is clinically relevant, ideally by the same staff member (or fewest staff possible), can promote stability in clinical interactions. Additionally, as early as possible during treatment, *set mutually understood boundaries and expectations with the patient that are reinforced by all team members.* For example, if a patient engages in abusive language toward team members, clearly stating to the patient what language is acceptable and unacceptable and informing the patient, respectfully but firmly, of the consequences of using this language: "I understand that you are frustrated *and* insulting our staff is not acceptable behavior. If you continue to speak like that, we will not address your requests until you are willing to communicate respectfully." Importantly, hold this limit! If the patient uses abusive language, team members should respond consistently with agreed-upon limit (e.g., not respond and leave the room). Finally, make efforts to *minimize judgment, criticism, and labeling of the patient in communications among team members (and in those with the patient).* This recommendation is related to the discussion of stigma and burnout earlier in this chapter. It is more likely than not that patients with SUDs/PDs have experienced explicit and implicit stigmatization in past treatment settings, and thus patients have good reason to be vigilant for signs of it in the ED interaction. Labeling a patient as "defensive" will do little to facilitate effective care. Instead, removing stigmatizing language, as much as possible, from the treatment context can serve to extinguish the patient's vigilance, increase the patient's receptivity to treatment decisions and recommendations, and reinforce collaboration. Additionally, judgmental language and labeling of patients among staff members is likely to reinforce negative attitudes and feelings toward patients and thereby *increase* provider burnout, rather than reduce it. Conversely, clinicians may choose to manage proactively their own negative arousal before an encounter with a "dreaded" patient, which helps prevent burnout. Stepping away from the patient to take a couple of minutes for an awareness exercise (e.g., RAIN; see Box 9.1) may help to engage with a challenging patient more effectively.

Validation Strategies

Patients with SUDs/PDs are likely to have experienced trauma, intense painful emotions, damaging interpersonal relationships, and stigma. These experiences, and responses to them, often lead to individuals feeling that their emotions, thoughts, or perceptions of events are "wrong" or "bad." Marsha Linehan, developer of dialectical behavior therapy (DBT), identified the profound impact of such invalidation on individuals with BPD and the importance of using validation in communicating with patients [19]. Research suggests validation strategies are also effective for individuals with other PDs, as well as those with SUDs and comorbid PDs and SUDs [23, 24]. Linehan [25] and her colleagues [18] suggest there are six levels of validation that can serve to improve communication, increase compassion, and reduce emotional distress among patients and healthcare providers alike. Table 9.1 describes the six levels of validation, what behaviors they may entail, and a clinical example of the strategy in the room.

Levels of Validation

- Level 1: Be present
- Level 2: Accurate reflection
- Level 3: Guessing about unstated feelings
- Level 4: Validate in terms of past history
- Level 5: Validate in terms of present events and the way most people would react
- Level 6: Radical genuineness

Table 9.1 Six levels of validation

Levels of validation	What does it look like?	Example
1. Be present	Focus on the patient; do not multitask; make eye contact; listen and nod; use facial expressions effectively	As often as possible, look away from the computer screen, stop typing, lean toward the patient, make eye contact, and listen without comment, judgment, or trying to problem-solve, even just for a few moments
2. Accurate reflection	Say back what you heard/saw as accurately as you can to confirm you got it right. Be open to the patient correcting you, and refrain from using a judgmental tone of voice	After a patient describes a fight with her partner as the reason for her suicidal ideation, you can say, "So you got in the fight with him and then started thinking suicide was the only way out of the relationship. Do I have that right?"
3. Guess unstated feelings	Notice and attend to what is *not* being said. Notice body language and facial expressions and consider what you know about the patient. Be receptive to correction!	Patient: "You're not admitting me? Typical! You guys just see me as another addict!" Provider: "You're really frustrated that doctors seem to treat you differently because of your substance use. It might even feel like you will never get your needs met when you ask for help."
4. Validate in the context of past history	Look for how the patient's thoughts/feelings make sense given his/her history. You don't have to agree with the patient or approve of the behavior to validate him/her	Patient: "I'm so pathetic. I have one argument at work and I blow two solid weeks of sobriety." Provider: "Look, you've spent the last 20 years in and out of jail, and the rest of that time using heroin to cope with life. When would you have learned another way to handle stress like this? It makes sense that you would turn to what you know."
5. Validate in the context of present events and how "most people" would react	Acknowledge what is valid in the patient's thoughts, feelings, and behaviors. Act as if their behavior is valid	Provider: "It makes sense that you are feeling frustrated. Your partner just walked out on you, you're coming down from a high, you've been in the ED for several hours and now I'm asking you the same questions three other people have already asked you…I think most people in your spot would be giving me some attitude!"
6. Be radically genuine/show your equality	Be human! Show respect and validation through honesty. Admit mistakes when appropriate; give honest feedback in a gentle manner. Don't fragilize the patient	Patient: "Thanks for your help doctor. I'm glad you're taking care of me now. That intake person was such an a------! So I let him know it!" Provider: "I can understand that you're in a tough spot and need help. From where I sit, calling my colleague an a------ is not going to get you what you want. Can we agree to focus on what we need to do and be respectful along the way?"

Functional Analysis and Nonjudgmental Assessment

Functional analysis can prove to be hugely beneficial in promoting effective interactions and treatment engagement, because it may reveal the causes and conditions of patient behavior in precise detail. Diagnosing BPD or ASPD, or a specific SUD, in the ED provides a helpful general direction for the treatment. Confusion arises, however, because an acute presentation of dysfunctional behavior is typically determined by concrete individual, relational and social factors that are not captured in the diagnosis. A functional approach classifies and intervenes with behaviors according to the processes (i.e., antecedents and consequences) that produce and maintain those behaviors. (For example, a patient may ask for pain pills because she has received pain pills after making requests in the ED before, and when she takes pain pills she feels relief from persistent trauma flashbacks and a sense of control over her physiological symptoms of anxiety.) There is considerable evidence that interventions focused on functional assessment and behavioral strategies are effective for PDs [26] and SUDs [27, 28] and may reduce the impact of stigma and burnout in the treatment context. For these reasons, we recommend bringing functional analytic strategies into the ED interaction.

The basic elements of a functional and contextual assessment [29] are:

1. Assessment of problem behaviors, including frequency, duration, and variability.
2. Assessment of relevant antecedents of the problem behavior, which can be external (contexts, people, events) and internal (thoughts, feelings, sensations). These are often referred to as "triggers" or "risk factors."
3. Assessment of consequences, including "positive" consequences that reinforce the problem behavior, and "negative" consequences that punish the behavior.
4. Assess treatment options by intervening on identified antecedents or consequences.

A full functional analysis of a patient's SUD or PD is unlikely to be completed in the ED; however, this tool can be used even in a time-limited interaction, making it invaluable in the ED context. We suggest a functional analysis of specific patient behaviors in the clinical interaction, such as requests for medication, for hospitalization, or for specific treatment options that may not be first-line or optimal. To illustrate this technique, we provide an example based on a recent clinical encounter experienced by one of the authors.

Terry, a patient with BPD and severe alcohol use disorder, presents to the ED for suicidal ideation. He provides a vague plan to drive off the road and reports his intent to die inconsistently, stating to some providers that he is "ready to do it" and others "it's just thoughts, I wouldn't actually kill myself." After assessment, Terry agrees to voluntary inpatient hospitalization, but states "I better be going to Hospital X for inpatient treatment. If you aren't sending me there, I am going to leave. You can't keep me here." Hospital X does not have a bed available and is not a realistic option at this time. A functional analysis of the Terry's demand for Hospital X follows. Notice, also, how validation can be integrated into the assessment. Validation of the patient's feelings, thoughts, and perspectives is critical to maintain an empathic connection with the patient, increasing the potential for a therapeutic interaction and behavioral change.

Provider: "Hospital Y has a bed and Hospital X doesn't. I can't change that unfortunately. It sounds like you and I are both worried about your safety and that being in the hospital is the best option right now. Hospital Y is a great hospital."

Terry: "I want Hospital X. They know how to take care of me. It's Hospital X, or I'm out of here. You can't stop me. I'm not sectionable."

Provider (assessing the problem behavior): "Ok. I want to understand more about this. Can you tell me more about why Hospital X seems like the right place for you?"

Terry: "They know me, they are safe, all the nurses like me there."

Provider (further assessing problem behavior): "Have you always asked to go to Hospital X? Are there other hospitals that you like?"

Terry: "The last three times I was in this ED I told them to send me to Hospital X and they did. Other hospitals aren't as good. Hospital X knows how to take care of me. So why can't you make that happen?"

Provider (assessing antecedents): "Ah ok, so you've made this request at this ED before and it's been granted. It makes sense you'd ask again. You've had positive experiences at Hospital X. Have you had other inpatient hospital experiences?"

Terry: "Yes! I went to Hospital A in the late 90s, it was a horror show! They treated me like a crazy person and just pumped me full of drugs. I'm pretty sure I have PTSD from that."

Provider (assessing antecedents and consequences): "That sounds awful! I'm pretty sure no one would want to be treated that way, especially when they are trying to get help! No wonder you are anxious about the idea of a different hospital. So, since Hospital A in the late 90s, you've come to this ED 3 times, asked for Hospital X in the same way you are right now and you got to go to Hospital X. And Hospital X worked out well for you. Do I have that right?"

Terry: "Yeah. Exactly. So you see what I mean now. I don't know if I can handle another hospital. Hospital X would be such a relief. Please help me."

Provider (assessing consequences): "So the fear of another 'horror show' like Hospital A goes away when you learn that you can stay at Hospital X."

Terry: "Yes! I can't add more bad memories. I have so many already."

From this brief exchange, we can extract some information about the problem behavior (demanding Hospital X) and its antecedents and consequences. The patient's behavior is preceded by feelings of anxiety related to past negative experience with Hospital A and past experiences of the behavior being reinforced (receiving Hospital X admission) and emotional relief associated with positive Hospital X experience and feeling cared for. The anticipated consequences of demanding Hospital X appear to be (1) increased likelihood of receiving Hospital X admission,

(2) anticipated relief from the anxiety associated with past Hospital A experience, and (3) anticipated positive experience of feeling cared for at Hospital X.

The provider, now with valuable information from this brief exchange, can choose which behaviors to reinforce, which behaviors to extinguish, and, working collaboratively and flexibly with the patient, identify alternative ways that he or she may receive anticipated consequences without engaging in the problematic behavior. See below, noticing validation techniques:

Provider: "That makes so much sense Terry. I don't want you to be creating more bad memories either. You've been through so much already. So I'm in a bind. On one hand, I really want to provide you what you need to feel safe and get better and on the other, you are saying you can only feel safe and get better at a Hospital that simply cannot be an option right now. How about we work together to come up with some way to solve this problem?"

Terry: "Ok. Yeah, I mean I don't think Hospital X is the ONLY safe hospital in the world, I'm just scared....Tell me about Hospital Y. What do you like about it? How is it different than Hospital A?"

Box 9.1 Maintaining Professionalism in the Heat of the Moment with RAIN

***R**ecognize what is happening in this moment.* Frustration, disgust, contempt, avoidance, and outright hatred, along with urges to punish an argumentative patient, stand less of a chance to take over your decision-making when you allow awareness of these dispositions within yourself and recognize the resultant feelings soon after they arise.

***A**ccept.* Acknowledge negative emotions when they are present and accept them. This is a balancing act. Neither indulge your emotions by becoming fused with them nor deny, avoid, or distract yourself from the experience. Stay curious and open to your experience.

***I**nvestigate with interest and care.* While the situation is medically urgent, you are here because this is a psychiatric emergency. The well-being of the patient in front of you depends critically on your ability to help contain a disturbed and disturbing mind and body. Tolerating distressing emotions requires care. Take a moment to slow down and investigate your inner state. After all, you do take time to look up information and check with colleagues, why not check in with yourself? If the patient is agitated, remain beyond the physical reach of the patient while you do this. For a moment, turn your attention inward. Direct awareness to your breath, without actively influencing your breathing. Is your breath short or long? Do you feel the expansion of your diaphragm into your abdomen with each in-breath, or are you more aware of the extension of your rib cage or movement in your shoulders? If your mind is racing, or when emotions are strong, support your awareness with silent self-talk, "Breathing in, I know I am breathing in. Breathing out, I know I am breathing out," or shorter, "In, Out" [30]. Extend your awareness toward tension and other sensations in your body and urges that may have arisen. There is information about you and the quality of your relationship to the patient in front of you, in your felt experience. If you feel overwhelmed, angry, or a sense of dissociation, you will be less able to assess the situation and the patient accurately, and you will be prone to misjudgments. If so, redirect your attention to your breathing, perhaps gently focusing on the movements of your diaphragm and abdomen, and use gentle self-talk or another strategy to ground yourself. If you feel defensive or angry, consider taking a posture that promotes and signals openness: uncross your arms and position yourself at eye level with your patient. Stand or sit up straight and pull back your shoulders slightly, opening your chest. Check in with a trusted member of your team, if frustration, anger, fear, or other negative emotions persist. Appreciate your own vulnerability and don't worry alone!

Nourish goodwill and respect. Focus your mind on an attribute of your patient that evokes your warmth and goodwill [33] – perhaps a vulnerability that you noticed in your patient – or that you respect, e.g., her or his persistent or shrewd self-advocacy. Set limits on verbal abuse and allow agitated patients time and space to calm down, potentially with the aid of medication. Nourish your capacity for re-spect (Latin: *re* (back) and *specere* (to look at)), i.e., the ability to look back at yourself, as you anticipate and consider the impact of your actions on others from their respective points of view. This process may include taking the perspective of your patient and his or her loved ones, your colleagues and members of your team, the other patients in the ED, and the community outside the hospital to whom your patient is going to return. Sooner or later, these groups are going to be affected, more or less, by your decision-making and behavior in this moment. Nourishing goodwill and respect are antidotes to alienation, cynicism, and compassion fatigue.

Adapted from a mindfulness practice described by several contemporary meditation teachers [31, 32].

See writings by Thanissaro Bhikkhu for an elaboration on the meaning and importance of goodwill [33].

Risk Assessment

The increased risk of violence toward others in patients with ASPD [34] and violence toward self through NSSI and suicide attempts in BPD [35] are well-documented. Reported histories of self-harm and suicide attempts are strongly associated with completed suicides and the presence of a SUD diagnosis is also associated with completed suicide [36]. As described in Chap. 10, the systematic assessment of risk for suicide and homicide weighs risk factors and protective factors. The purpose of the emergency evaluation is the identification of both modifiable and static risk factors and the determination of the need for hospitalization to protect the patient or third parties from imminent harm. When possible, collateral sources, including the medical record and treaters, family, friends, and others who know the patient well, are contacted to corroborate information. An insightful patient, perhaps in collaboration with a skilled outpatient therapist, may be able to develop a narrative with the emergency consultant, about why, and why now, a suicidal crisis occurred. This narrative, and its implications, facilitates a formulation of risk that goes beyond a mere weighing of risk and protective factors [34]. If the patient refuses contact with sources of collateral information, it is important to understand what motivates the patient's refusal (i.e., the function of the refusal). For example, shame, fear of abandonment, or other repercussions, or a desire to maintain control of the situation, could precede such a refusal. As in most difficult negotiations, effectively conveying an empathic understanding of the position of the patient and acknowledging underlying fears and misgivings are skillful means of swaying the negotiation partner toward one's own agenda [37], in this case, toward consent to contact collaterals. There are times when it may be critical to contact a family member or friend to obtain information needed for a safety risk assessment. In such critical situations, the benefit of receiving the information may well outweigh the cost of violating the patient's wishes or right to privacy, and in those cases, it is permissible to contact the collateral. It is important to focus those collateral conversations on only the information needed for the risk assessment and to limit the release of information about the patient to only what is necessary to facilitate that process.

Dialectical behavior therapy (DBT) and other structured treatments for BPD [19, 35] encourage formal safety planning that enables patients to use the least restrictive interventions to contain the risk of imminent self-harm or suicide. It is important to ask the patient about a safety or crisis plan. Healthcare organizations that deliver integrated mental healthcare may maintain individualized mental health crisis plans in the electronic medical record and flag the crisis plan for easy access by emergency room clinicians. If the patient is engaged in outpatient psychiatric treatment, contact with the treatment team to clarify the context of the acute crisis can help gauge the risk of imminent harm and may facilitate referral to the least restrictive treatment setting. Perhaps the temporary containment of the emergency ward suffices, the acute crisis wanes, and the patient may return to the care of the outpatient team, without accessing a higher level of care.

As discussed in Chap. 10, acute suicidality may be compounded by alcohol or drug intoxication and symptoms of withdrawal. The patient must be assessed and treated for symptoms of dangerous intoxication (including intentional overdose) or substance withdrawal. Acute intoxication with alcohol, sedative-hypnotics, or opioids, especially when the patient ingested a combination of these substances, may require emergency medical intervention to prevent death or irreversible injury, as is discussed in other chapters. Intoxicated patients must be observed until their mental status clears and they must be monitored for symptoms of withdrawal. A thorough risk assessment cannot be completed until the patient has been assessed when clinically sober.

Substance intoxication and withdrawal can also influence the capacity to make medical decisions, even more so when comorbid with a personality disorder. A patient who acutely overdosed on opioids and exhibited respiratory depression may have received the opioid antagonist naloxone prior to arrival in the ED from emergency medical services (EMS), other first responders, or, in states where naloxone is widely available, from peers. The experience of acute withdrawal precipitated by the naloxone rescue is distressing. Patients with BPD are vulnerable to paranoia, cognitive dysfunction, and emotional/behavior dysregulation during times of stress. In addition, patients struggling with BPD and ASPD often lack distress tolerance skills. As a result, when experiencing withdrawal, these patients may display agitated and disturbing behavior and demand to leave the ED against medical advice. A patient with BPD traits whose cognitive function is sufficient at baseline may have cognitive impairment under stress and, thus, lack capacity to decide to leave the ED. A formal assessment of capacity prior to discharge may be indicated and could result in the involuntary commitment of the patient, until discharge is medically safe. Likewise, the acute withdrawal from alcohol, benzodiazepines, and other sedative-hypnotics is potentially lethal (see Chap. 2), and a patient with BPD traits (or any patient with potentially impaired decision-making), who demands to leave against medical advice, deserves an assessment of capacity to make this decision.

The impact of comorbid PD and SUD on a patient's relationships can be profound and may be of great importance to the treatment process in the ED. Patients with ASPD and BPD are at increased risk of involvement in domestic abuse (as perpetrators and victims) and intimate partner violence [34]. Screening and referral to appropriate agencies as needed is important. It is also necessary to assess if children or elderly parents are currently at imminent risk of abuse or neglect. The notification of protective services may be mandated by state law. Additionally, family members of patients with personality disorders, even if they are not abused or abusive, are often burdened and overwhelmed [38]. They may benefit from referral to advocacy organizations, such as the New England Personality Disorder Association (http://www.nepda.org/) and the National Education Alliance for Borderline Personality Disorder (www.neabpd.org).

Disposition and Treatment Planning

The assessment of imminent risk to the patient and third parties is a major determinant of disposition and treatment planning. Acute intoxication with alcohol, sedative-hypnotics, and/or opioids requires careful monitoring and medical management, as described above and in Chaps. 1 and 2. Intoxication with other common substances, while usually not life-threatening, may require observation and containment until the mental status of the patient has normalized and he/she has capacity to engage in aftercare planning. Patients in withdrawal from alcohol or sedative-hypnotics often require inpatient admission for medical detoxification and referral to outpatient care. Medical detoxification without subsequent inpatient or outpatient care leads to higher rates of relapse and poorer outcomes [39].

As described in Chap. 1, opioid withdrawal may be treated in the ED symptomatically with comfort medications, with full opioid agonists (e.g., methadone), or with the partial opioid receptor agonist buprenorphine, in conjunction with referral to follow-up outpatient care. D'Onofrio and colleagues [40, 41] compared addiction treatment referral, a brief intervention combined with treatment referral, and initiation of buprenorphine-naloxone treatment in the ED, and found that the latter resulted in higher treatment engagement at 2 months and no difference in outcome at 6 and 12 months follow-up. There are multiple ways to organize buprenorphine-naloxone maintenance treatment in primary care successfully [42] but treatment retention remains a challenge. Retention is worse when there is psychiatric comorbidity, including personality disorders [43]. Thus, patients with SUDs and co-occurring PDs may benefit from referral to an addiction psychiatry clinic, when this option is available, wherein the treatment for SUD and co-occurring disorders can occur simultaneously.

Patients with ASPD or antisocial traits may be pursuing secondary gain, e.g., asserting suicidality when psychiatric inpatient hospitalization is advantageous for one reason or another or to receive a prescription for a controlled substance. A record review of previous ED visits, perhaps including encounters at other institutions, which are increasingly available through shared electronic medical records, as well as checking with available prescription drug databases, helps to put the current presentation in perspective and formulate risk, as described above. Often, these patients may engage in behaviors that evoke strong negative emotions and thus may require extra effort by the clinical team to maintain professional excellence (see Box 9.1). If the patient's threats of suicide are incongruent with the overall presentation and history, then the risk of reinforcing maladaptive behavior by gratifying the demand of inpatient care is greater than the benefit of hospitalization, if any. An urgent referral to addiction psychiatric outpatient treatment or partial hospital program, instead, is the appropriate disposition. If the same patient returns frequently with a similar presentation, the ED evaluation and disposition may be accelerated by an individualized protocol, ideally developed in collaboration with the outpatient treatment team, if any, saved in the patient record and flagged upon the patient's arrival in the ED. This type of individualized plan can be implemented to reinforce adaptive behaviors and extinguish ineffective behaviors in the treatment context.

Conclusion

There are many individuals who suffer from SUDs and co-occurring PDs and these individuals often seek treatment in ED settings. The complexity and severity of this clinical presentation can leave ED providers facing difficult decisions in the diagnostic, intervention, and disposition phases of ED encounters, often in the context of disruptive behavior, emotion dysregulation, and ineffective interpersonal behaviors on the part of the patient. We have reviewed how these individuals are also among the most stigmatized patients and how this stigma contributes to difficult ED encounters and treatment engagement and how ED providers have a unique opportunity to engage these patients through "in the room" behavioral interventions, such as validation techniques and functional analysis. Finally, we stress the importance of self-care of the treatment team, acknowledging the intense emotional and interpersonal reactions patients may display and elicit and providing skills, such as mindfulness, self-compassion, and team support, to promote provider well-being and prevent burnout. In acknowledging the many factors that contribute to ED encounters with SUD/PD patients, we hope this chapter provides clinicians with a fresh perspective on these individuals, as well as a set of practical tools to promote effective clinical care and ED interactions.

References

1. Casadio P, Olivoni D, Ferrari B, Pintori C, Speranza E, Bosi M, et al. Personality disorders in addiction outpatients: prevalence and effects on psychosocial functioning. Subst Abuse Res Treat. 2014;8:17–24.
2. Regier DA, Farmer ME, Rae DS, Locke BZ, Keith SJ, Judd LL, et al. Comorbidity of mental disorders with alcohol and other drug abuse. JAMA. 1990;264(19):2511–8.
3. Grant BF, Chou SP, Goldstein RB, Huang B, Stinson FS, Saha TD, et al. Prevalence, correlates, disability, and comorbidity of DSM-IV borderline personality disorder: results from the Wave 2 National Epidemiologic Survey on Alcohol and Related Conditions. J Clin Psychiatry. 2008;69(4):533–45.
4. Grant BF, Stinson FS, Dawson DA, Chou SP, Ruan WJ, Pickering RP. Co-occurrence of 12-month alcohol and drug use disorders and personality disorders in the United States: results from the National Epidemiologic Survey on Alcohol and Related Conditions. Arch Gen Psychiatry. 2004;61(4):361–8.
5. Pasic J, Russo J, Roy-Byrne P. High utilizers of psychiatric emergency services. Psychiatr Serv. 2005;56:687–4.
6. Zaheer J, Links PS, Liu E. Assessment and emergency management of suicidality in personality disorders. Psychiatr Clin. 2008;31(3):527–43.
7. McLellan AT, Lewis DC, O'Brien CP, Kleber HD. Drug dependence, a chronic medical illness: implications for treatment, insurance, and outcomes evaluation. JAMA. 2000;284(13):1689–95.
8. White WL. Recovery-remission from substance use disorders: an analysis of reported outcomes in 415 scientific reports. Chicago: Great Lakes Addiction Technology Transfer Center; 2012.
9. Livingston JD, Milne T, Fang ML, Amari E. The effectiveness of interventions for reducing stigma related to substance use disorders: a systematic review. Addiction. 2012;107(1):39–50.
10. Aviram RB, Brodsky BS, Stanley B. Borderline personality disorder, stigma, and treatment implications. Harv Rev Psychiatry. 2006;14(5):249–56.
11. Van Boekel LC, Brouwers EP, Van Weeghel J, Garretsen HF. Stigma among health professionals towards patients with substance use disorders and its consequences for healthcare delivery: systematic review. Drug Alcohol Depend. 2013;131(1):23–35.

12. Schomerus G, Lucht M, Holzinger A, Matschinger H, Carta MG, Angermeyer MC. The stigma of alcohol dependence compared with other mental disorders: a review of population studies. Alcohol Alcohol. 2010;46(2):105–12.
13. Black DW, Pfohl B, Blum N, McCormick B, Allen J, North CS, et al. Attitudes toward borderline personality disorder: a survey of 706 mental health clinicians. CNS Spectr. 2011;16(3):67–74.
14. Bateman A, Bolton R, Fonagy P. Antisocial personality disorder: a mentalizing framework. Focus. 2013;11(2):178–86.
15. Betan E, Heim AK, Zittel Conklin C, Westen D. Countertransference phenomena and personality pathology in clinical practice: an empirical investigation. Am J Psychiatry. 2005;162(5):890–8.
16. Bodner E, Cohen-Fridel S, Mashiah M, Segal M, Grinshpoon A, Fischel T, et al. The attitudes of psychiatric hospital staff toward hospitalization and treatment of patients with borderline personality disorder. BMC Psychiatry. 2015;15(1):2.
17. Morse G, Salyers MP, Rollins AL, Monroe-DeVita M, Pfahler C. Burnout in mental health services: a review of the problem and its remediation. Adm Policy Ment Health Ment Health Serv Res. 2012;39:341–52.
18. Koerner K, Linehan MM. Doing dialectical behavior therapy: a practical guide. New York: The Guilford Press; 2011.
19. Linehan M. Cognitive-behavioral treatment of borderline personality disorder. New York: Guilford Press; 1993. 584 p.
20. American Psychiatric Association. Diagnostic and statistical manual of mental disorders. 5th ed. Washington, D.C.: APA; 2013.
21. Gunderson JG. Making the diagnosis. In: The handbook of good psychiatric management for borderline; 2014. p. 21–6.
22. Center for Substance Abuse Treatment. Substance abuse treatment for persons with co-occurring disorders. 2005. [Internet]. Rockville: Substance Abuse and Mental Health Services Administration; 2005. (Treatment Improvement Protocol (TIP) Series; vol. 42). Available from: https://www.ncbi.nlm.nih.gov/books/NBK64203/.
23. Linehan MM, Dimeff LA, Reynolds SK, Comtois KA, Welch SS, Heagerty P, et al. Dialectical behavior therapy versus comprehensive validation therapy plus 12-step for the treatment of opioid dependent women meeting criteria for borderline personality disorder. Drug Alcohol Depend. 2002;67(1):13–26.
24. van den Bosch LMC, Verheul R, Schippers GM, van den Brink W. Dialectical Behavior Therapy of borderline patients with and without substance use problems: implementation and long-term effects. Addict Behav. 2002;27(6):911–23.
25. Linehan MM. Validation and psychotherapy. In: Empathy reconsidered: new directions in psychotherapy. Washington, D.C.: American Psychological Association; 1997. p. 353–92.
26. Linehan MM, Comtois KA, Murray AM, Brown MZ, Gallop RJ, Heard HL, et al. Two-year randomized controlled trial and follow-up of dialectical behavior therapy vs therapy by experts for suicidal behaviors and borderline personality disorder. Arch Gen Psychiatry. 2006;63(7):757–66.
27. Dimeff LA, Linehan MM. Dialectical behavior therapy for substance abusers. Addict Sci Clin Pract. 2008;4(2):39–47.
28. Dutra L, Stathopoulou G, Basden SL, Leyro TM, Powers MB, Otto MW. A meta-analytic review of psychosocial interventions for substance use disorders. Am J Psychiatry. 2008;165(2):179–87.
29. Wilson KG, Murrell AR. Functional analysis of behavior. In: Encyclopedia of psychology. New York: Academic. p. 833–9.
30. Hanh TN. Breathe, you are alive! The sutra on the full awareness of breathing. Berkeley: Parallax Press; 2008.
31. Brach T. The RAIN of self-compassion [Internet]. 2013. Available from: https://www.tarabrach.com/wp-content/uploads/pdf/RAIN-of-Self-Compassion2.pdf.

32. McDonald M. RAIN: the nourishing art of mindful inquiry. Tricycle Online Course [Internet]. 2018. Available from: https://learn.tricycle.org/courses/rain.
33. Bhikkhu, Thanissaro. Metta means goodwill [Internet]. Available from: https://www.accesstoinsight.org/lib/authors/thanissaro/metta_means_goodwill.html.
34. Logan C, Johnstone L. Personality disorder and violence: making the link through risk formulation. J Pers Disord. 2010;24(5):610–33.
35. Gunderson JG. Managing suicidality and non-suicidal self-harm. In: Handbook of good psychiatric management for borderline personality disorder. Washington, D.C.: American Psychiatric Publishing; 2014. p. 37–46.
36. Yoshimasu K, Kiyohara C, Miyashita K. Suicidal risk factors and completed suicide: Meta-analyses based on psychological autopsy studies. Environ Health Prev Med. 2008;13:243–56.
37. Fisher R, Ury W, Patton B. Getting to yes: negotiating agreement without giving in. 2nd ed. Houghton Mifflin: New York; 1991.
38. Bauer R, Döring A, Schmidt T, Spießl H. "Mad or bad?": burden on caregivers of patients with personality disorders. J Pers Disord. 2012;26(6):956–71.
39. Ivers J-H, Zgaga L, Sweeney B, Keenan E, Darker C, Smyth BP, et al. A naturalistic longitudinal analysis of post-detoxification outcomes in opioid-dependent patients. Drug Alcohol Rev [Internet]. 2017.; Available from:;37:S339. https://doi.org/10.1111/dar.12597.
40. D'Onofrio G, Chawarski MC, O'Connor PG, Pantalon MV, Busch SH, Owens PH, et al. Emergency department-initiated buprenorphine for opioid dependence with continuation in primary care: outcomes during and after intervention. J Gen Intern Med. 2017;32(6):660–6.
41. D'Onofrio G, O'Connor PG, Pantalon MV, Chawarski MC, Busch SH, Owens PH, et al. Emergency department-initiated buprenorphine/naloxone treatment for opioid dependence: a randomized clinical trial. JAMA. 2015;313(16):1636–44.
42. Chou R, Korthuis PT, Weimer M, Bougatsos C, Blazina I, Zakher B, et al. Medication-assisted treatment models of care for opioid use disorder in primary care settings. [Internet]. Rockville: Agency for Healthcare Research and Quality; 2016. Available from: http://www.ncbi.nlm.nih.gov/books/NBK402352/.
43. Litz M, Leslie D. The impact of mental health comorbidities on adherence to buprenorphine: a claims based analysis. Am J Addict. 2017;26(8):859–63.

Chapter 10
Preventing and Managing Risk of Violence and Suicide in Substance-Abusing Patients in the Emergency Department

Michael Murphy and Suzanne A. Bird

Introduction

There is a well-established association between violent behavior and substance use—especially when combined with comorbid psychiatric disorders [1, 2]. This association contributes to violent and self-destructive behaviors in the community and is demonstrated on a regular basis in hospital EDs where clinicians interact directly with people with violent histories, those who may be acutely violent, or those whose lives have been recently impacted by violence [3, 4]. Patients using substances, with and without other mental health conditions, may come to the ED to receive treatment for a variety of clinical presentations. These presentations include medical and psychiatric disorders in association or comorbid with substance use, as well as accidental or intentional injuries. Such injuries may include the physical sequelae of self-destructive or overtly suicidal behavior, or trauma experienced as a result of reckless or aggressive behavior during periods of intoxication and impaired judgment. Other patients may be brought to the hospital specifically for assessment and containment of violent or agitated behavior—most frequently while intoxicated—and this behavior may persist or even worsen during the process of ED evaluation and stabilization [5, 6]. Patients in any of these groups, even when initially presenting without obviously concerning behavior, are considered to be potentially at risk for agitation and aggression while receiving treatment in the ED. Violence and the threat of violence compromise the quality of emergency care delivered to all patients. Violent behavior also jeopardizes the safety of

M. Murphy (✉)
McLean Hospital, Belmont, MA, USA
e-mail: mmurphy56@partners.org

S. A. Bird
Acute Psychiatry Service, Massachusetts General Hospital, Department of Psychiatry, Boston, MA, USA

A. L. Donovan, S. A. Bird (eds.), *Substance Use and the Acute Psychiatric Patient*, Current Clinical Psychiatry, https://doi.org/10.1007/978-3-319-23961-3_10

ED personnel. Thus, ED staff must learn to anticipate, identify, and manage the associated risks in these common clinical scenarios with the overarching goal of maintaining safety for all involved.

Emergency departments are commonly cited as particularly high-risk environments, and multiple surveys have suggested that threatening or aggressive behavior toward medical personnel is a common occurrence [7, 8]. Workplace violence in the medical occupations represents 10% of all workplace violence reported in the United States, and healthcare workers have a significantly higher than the average rate of being injured at work, even though there is considerable evidence that such incidents tend to be vastly underreported [9]. Although there is a lack of high-quality and current research, EDs and inpatient psychiatric units have been found to have the highest rates of workplace violence experienced by hospital staff [9]. One study found that more than 75% of emergency physicians reported having experienced at least one violent incident while at work in the past year [10]. Another study of ED nurses found that over 70% had experienced physical or verbal assault by ED patients or visitors [11]. The latter study reported that violence against nurses occurred most often during triage, the performance of invasive procedures, or during the process of restraining patients. Diagnoses causing alterations in brain functioning are the most commonly implicated among perpetrators of violent behavior against staff in healthcare settings [9]. Such diagnoses include a wide variety of traumatic and medical illnesses, neurocognitive disorders, acute intoxication or withdrawal from substances, and acute psychiatric presentations.

In addition to increasing patients' risk for violent behavior toward others, substance use disorders have been shown to be significantly associated with an increased risk of suicide and suicide attempts [12]. Suicide is a leading cause of death among individuals with SUDs, and any patient presenting to an emergency department with active substance use should be considered potentially at risk for suicide and screened accordingly [13]. Alcohol has been the most widely studied substance in relation to suicide, with 22% of US suicide deaths and 30–40% of suicide attempts involving acute alcohol intoxication (BAL at or above the legal limit/CDC) [14]. Opioids, including both heroin and prescription narcotics, are present in 20% of US suicide cases. Surveillance data demonstrate that a diagnosis of alcohol use disorder or a history of intravenous drug use are associated with suicide risks 10 and 14 times greater, respectively, than in the general population [13, 15]. From 2005 to 2011, there was more than a 50% increase in ED visits for drug-related suicide attempts among patients aged 12 or older, and, although data are very limited regarding statistical risks of suicide associated with use of more than one substance, there is some consensus that the number, rather than the specific types of substances used, is more predictive of risk [16].

Protecting patients at risk of suicide from self-harm while in the hospital is one of the Joint Commission's National Patient Safety Goals, and alcohol and drug abuse were included by the Joint Commission as suicide risk factors in their 2016 Sentinel Event Alert [17]. Although data is scant regarding suicides and suicide attempts occurring in hospitals, the Joint Commission has reported that ~8% of all reported inpatient suicides occurred in EDs. Similarly, a VA study found that the ED had the second highest number of reported suicide attempts and completions in their healthcare system, second only to inpatient psychiatric units [18]. Thus, emergency clinicians working with substance-using and potentially suicidal patients must be vigilant about the risk of self-directed violence in the ED setting, assessing patients carefully and monitoring them closely until they have been determined to be either safe for discharge or stable for transfer. Preventing violence toward self and others is a primary clinical goal in the emergency management of patients with substance use disorders and associated psychological and behavioral sequelae.

Alcohol

While there are regional differences in the distribution of substance use, for most hospitals, alcohol is the most significant driver of substance-related violence in the ED setting. Alcohol use disorder has multiple comorbidities, both medical and psychiatric, and establishing a clear causal relationship can be difficult. However, chronic alcohol use, acute intoxication, and withdrawal have all been clearly and repeatedly linked to aggression, violence, self-injury, and suicide [2, 14, 19, 20].

Acute alcohol intoxication is hypothesized to increase the risk of violence toward self or others by direct pharmacological inhibition of frontal cortex functioning with resultant disinhibition, increased impulsivity, and impaired problem-solving [21]. Alcohol intoxication may also interfere with the appropriate processing of sensory and autonomic stimuli in a way that increases the likelihood of aggressive behavior by increasing the emotional and physiological response to potential threat signals [22]. Several studies have shown a dose-dependent relationship between blood alcohol levels (BALs) and aggression [23]. However, a BAL alone is an unreliable predictor of both clinical intoxication and risk. The same BAL may induce toxic delirium in an inexperienced drinker while being associated with active withdrawal in an individual who has been drinking heavily over time. The pharmacological effects of alcohol intoxication alone are not sufficient to produce aggression or violent behavior; most people who use alcohol, even to excess, do not become violent or self-destructive. The relationship between alcohol use and violence, therefore, relies on the presence of multiple mediating factors, only some of which are understood [24].

Several epidemiological studies have shown that alcohol use and dependence strongly increase the risk of violence in individuals with comorbid psychiatric diagnoses, such as psychotic disorders and bipolar disorder [4, 25]. People with antisocial personality disorder are more likely to be violent while intoxicated than alcohol users who do not have a personality disorder [26]. In addition, both acute alcohol intoxication and a history of chronic alcohol abuse are strongly linked to suicidality [27]. People who attempt suicide while acutely intoxicated with alcohol are more likely to use more lethal methods with a higher likelihood of success [14]. Individuals with a diagnosis of depression and alcohol use disorder have a much higher risk of suicide than those with depression alone [28].

Nicotine

Nicotine is one of the most widely used substances in the world, and up to 20% of adults in the United States use nicotine daily [29]. Nicotine can have either stimulating or relaxing effects depending on the dose, method of delivery, and individual [30]. Nicotine withdrawal is characterized by intense cravings and irritability. There is no evidence linking nicotine use or nicotine withdrawal with violence in community or general hospital settings [2]. However, nicotine use is highly comorbid with psychiatric illness, especially with psychotic disorders and substance use disorders [31]. It has been proposed that nicotine withdrawal, with its associated irritability, may exacerbate the risk of violent behavior in individuals with comorbid substance and/or psychiatric disorders [32]. Nicotine-dependent patients in the ED often struggle with long waiting times and no smoking policies, and routine orders for nicotine replacement patches, gums, lozenges, or inhalers tend to be underutilized.

Marijuana (Cannabis)

There are few studies looking at the effect of marijuana use on the risk of violence in the ED. Increasingly, marijuana is considered to be a largely benign drug by the lay public, as well as by some healthcare providers. However, marijuana use has been associated with interpersonal violence in epidemiological studies [33, 34]. This relationship exists even after effects of alcohol and other illicit substances are accounted for. Clinical observation suggests that marijuana intoxication can produce symptoms of anxiety and psychosis, particularly in patients with a history of psychiatric illness, but observed administration of marijuana or cannabis has not been reliably associated with increases in violent behavior or aggression [35, 36]. Therefore, it remains unclear whether marijuana intoxication is causally linked to violence or whether people who are more likely to be violent are also more likely to use marijuana.

Daily users of cannabis are susceptible to developing a withdrawal syndrome upon discontinuation. This cannabis withdrawal syndrome can be characterized by agitation and irritability [37]. Multiple studies have shown increases in self-reported scores for aggression and violent behavior in people experiencing cannabis withdrawal [36, 38]. This effect is strongest in individuals with a pre-existing history of violence [38]. However, no epidemiological studies have demonstrated an increase in violence toward self or others during cannabis withdrawal.

Hallucinogens

Phencyclidine (PCP) is a dissociative hallucinogen that first rose to prominence in the 1970s. Use of PCP declined after the 1980s; however, it has seen a resurgence in use since 2005 [39]. PCP has properties of both a stimulant and a depressant. The PCP toxidrome is characterized by autonomic instability, analgesia, nystagmus, and waxing and waning periods of agitation and sedation [40]. PCP intoxication can also induce psychotic symptoms, such as paranoia and thought disorganization, especially in patients with a history of a psychotic disorder [41]. Therefore, it is not surprising that individuals intoxicated with PCP are often violent and aggressive toward others [40]. There is no evidence for an increased risk of suicide during acute PCP intoxication. Most patients who presented to the ED with PCP intoxication will experience complete, or nearly complete, resolution of psychiatric symptoms occurring secondary to the drug within 24 hours of use; however, some patients will take up to several weeks before full symptom resolution [40].

Patients intoxicated with other hallucinogens, such as psilocybin, lysergic acid diethylamide (LSD), N,N-Dimethyltryptamine (DMT) and mescaline, may present to the ED with altered mental status and bizarre behavior. While there is a popular conception that hallucinogens are associated with violence, there is little evidence to support this idea for hallucinogens other than PCP [1, 2]. While use of these substances can precipitate the development of a psychotic disorder, particularly in prodromal individuals, most users do not develop long-lasting psychosis. Intoxication with LSD or psilocybin mushrooms is rarely associated with violence or suicidality [2]. With these patients, the greater risk is from accidental injuries to self or others due to impaired reality testing and disorganization [42]. Less commonly encountered agents include salvinorins (Salvia), dextromethorphan, and research chemicals (several of which are not regulated and can be legally purchased). There are scattered case reports of violence associated with intoxication with these agents [43–45].

Opioids

Opioid abuse and dependence is a growing public health concern in the United States. Intoxication with opioids generally produces sedation and, in the absence of other substance use, it is not associated with violence or aggression. Opioid-dependent individuals may also use other substances, such as cocaine [46]. In such cases, patients may become impulsive, violent, or aggressive [47]. Opioid withdrawal is extremely uncomfortable and is characterized by muscle aches, cramps, anxiety, irritability, dysphoria, insomnia, and intense cravings [48]. Patients who are actively withdrawing from opioids are at risk for agitation. This presentation is most likely to be encountered in the ED when a patient has been waiting for treatment and then begins to enter withdrawal [2]. Irritability and risk for agitation may be compounded by difficulty in providing opioid replacement therapy in the ED. This presentation may also be encountered when patients receive naloxone for suspected opioid overdose. These patients often undergo an intense, acutely uncomfortable opioid withdrawal syndrome potentially associated with agitation and combativeness [49, 50]. In patients with polysubstance use, naloxone may eliminate the sedating effect of the opioid and unmask the psychogenic effects of other drugs. A history of opioid use disorder is strongly associated with suicidality [51]. In addition, many individuals with opioid use disorder present to the ED following overdoses which may or may not have been intentional acts of self-harm [52]. Careful assessment for depression and suicide risk is particularly important in post-overdose patients, once clinically sober.

Stimulants

The most commonly encountered stimulants in the ED setting are cocaine and various amphetamine derivatives. Cocaine intoxication induces psychomotor agitation which usually lasts for 1–2 hours and may be followed by a period of intense dysphoria and irritability ("crash"). Patients are at elevated risk for violence during the rush of intoxication and are at risk for both violence and suicide during the dysphoric period. While the literature is clear that cocaine use is linked to violence, it is not clear that this link is causal [1, 2]. The presence of a personality disorder, and, in particular, antisocial personality disorder, may strengthen the link between the use of cocaine and violent behavior [53]. Additionally, the effects of cocaine intoxication may be increased by concomitant alcohol use, which alters the metabolism of cocaine to produce cocaethylene—a longer-acting, psychoactive metabolite associated with increased impulsive aggression [54]. Overall, both the scientific literature and our own clinical experience suggest that known or suspected cocaine intoxication is accompanied by a higher likelihood of violence or aggression.

Acute amphetamine intoxication produces similar psychological effects as cocaine intoxication, although some data suggests that the "high" from amphetamine-like compounds may be associated with higher levels of irritability, impulsivity, and hypersexuality than other stimulants. Methamphetamine has a much longer half-life than cocaine and, therefore, the effects of this drug can persist for days [55]. Acute intoxication with methamphetamine is more likely than cocaine to produce psychotic symptoms in users and, therefore, greatly increases the risk of violence and self-harm [2]. Furthermore, chronic use of methamphetamines can be associated with the development of a paranoid psychosis in which patients are frequently fearful, violent, impulsive, and aggressive [56]. Amphetamine is neurotoxic, and prolonged use has been associated with degeneration of brain structures involved in emotional regulation, which may also increase the risk of violence [57]. Chronic users of methamphetamine experience a withdrawal syndrome following discontinuation of the drug. This withdrawal syndrome, like post-cocaine dysphoria, is characterized by depression, anxiety, and drug cravings [58]. While clinical experience suggests that these individuals are at an elevated risk of harm to self or others, further research is needed to clarify the relationship between amphetamine withdrawal and violence toward self or others.

"Toxicology-Negative" Substance Use

Many patients present to the ED with agitation and disorganization but have negative urine and/or serum toxicology screens. While toxicology screens are useful for ruling out a specific group of substances, a negative result does not mean that the patient is substance-free. Many substances associated with violence, such as synthetic cannabinoids and synthetic cathinones, are not routinely detected on toxicology screens. Testing for these substances may be too time-consuming or costly to be useful in the ED. In one study, patients who presented to an ED with agitation refractory to benzodiazepines had blood samples subsequently processed through extensive serum toxicology testing [59]. More than a quarter of these patients tested positive for chemical agents that are not typically included in routine screens.

Synthetic cannabinoid use has become increasingly common since 2000 [60]. Urban homeless patients, in particular, are overrepresented in those who use these drugs because they are inexpensive and easy to obtain on the street [61]. Such patients often have major mental illness and are especially vulnerable to the pro-psychotic effects of these drugs. Spikes of ED presentations of K2-related psychosis have been traced in some locales to a single homeless shelter [62]. Synthetic cannabinoids ("Spice" and "K2") have very different biochemical properties than naturally derived cannabinoids, and they produce sympathomimetic and hallucinogenic effects not typically seen with marijuana. Synthetic cannabinoid intoxication has been frequently associated with severe anxiety, paranoid delusions, and acute agitation requiring restraints, comprising a far more profound and disturbing alteration in mental status and behavior than that associated with marijuana alone [60]. In addition, both chronic synthetic cannabinoid use and acute intoxication are associated with suicidality and self-harm [60, 63].

Synthetic cathinones, commonly referred to as "bath salts," are another group of substances associated with acute agitation and potential violence during intoxication. The prevalence of synthetic cathinone use increased dramatically from 2010 to 2011, but this trend then appeared to plateau [64]. A recent large-scale survey of US high school students found that synthetic cathinone use remains rare, with only 1.1% of respondents reporting use within the past year [65]. The clinical presentation of cathinone intoxication is very similar to that of amphetamines—patients may be delirious, agitated, anxious, hallucinating, and aggressive [66–68]. These effects typically resolve within a few hours of use but may persist for up to a few days, particularly in patients with comorbid psychiatric disorders [69].

Many other substances are associated with violent or aggressive behavior. Healthcare providers may encounter patients who are intoxicated or withdrawing from inhalants; anabolic steroids; plant-derived intoxicants, such as jimson weed or kratom; as well as various research chemicals. This list is not exhaustive, and novel substances are continually being developed and ingested. In many cases, it will not be possible to definitively identify a substance of abuse, even when a patient appears grossly intoxicated. In these cases, it is often advisable to presume that the patient is intoxicated, carefully monitor for any evidence of medical instability, and follow a safe set of general principles to reduce the risk of harm to the patient or others.

Management Issues

Prevention

Preventing violence in the ED is far preferable to managing the sequelae after the fact. Various interventions may be helpful in reducing the risk of violence in the emergency department [70]. However, there is scant literature to support a direct effect from any specific intervention; therefore, determining reliable guidelines for clinical practice has been difficult [9]. Recognizing this need, the American Association for Emergency Psychiatry initiated Project BETA (Best practices in Evaluation and Treatment of Agitation) to attempt to identify and disseminate effective ways of reducing and managing violence and aggression in the ED setting [71]. Many of the suggestions in this chapter are derived from this project.

Screening for suicide risk is one aspect of preventing violence in the ED. In 2016, The Joint Commission released a sentinel event alert highlighting the importance of detecting and addressing suicide risk across all healthcare settings [17]. In this alert, as in virtually all suicide screening tools, substance use is identified as a key risk factor. Thus, all patients with substance use disorders should be considered to have an increased risk for suicide. The risk of violence toward others is often more obvious in patients presenting to EDs with substance-related complaints, but assessing risk of self-destructive behavior or suicide is equally important when these patients present to the ED.

Several hospital design elements have been suggested to create clinical environments in which the risk of violence or self-harm may be mitigated. In an effort to screen for weapons, some hospitals have installed metal detectors at the entrance to the ED, but the use of metal detectors remains controversial [72]. In one recent study examining the impact of metal detector use in an urban, teaching hospital ED, the authors reported that in a 26-month period, over 5800 weapons, including more than 280 firearms, were detected [73]. Despite such findings, other studies have shown no evidence that metal detectors actually decrease violent incidents in the ED, perhaps because the majority of hospital-based violence does not involve weapons [9, 74]. Less controversial is the recommendation that the entrance to the ED be restricted by requiring identification cards on all doors, thus decreasing the chance of a potentially violent patient or visitor having free access to the unit. Patients considered to be at high risk of harm to self or others may be asked to change into safe hospital clothing, with restricted access to personal belongings, or potentially undergo a search or "pat-down" in order to remove items that may be used to harm themselves or others. These practices also serve to minimize patients' access to potentially toxic substances that they may have brought with them to the hospital. Patient rooms can also be designed to decrease the risk of violence or self-harm. Furniture can be removed or attached to the walls or floor, and arranged in a way that allows staff an easy exit in an emergency. Smaller items, such as needles, medical instruments, tubing or IV poles, should be kept out of reach of patients who are at increased risk of harm to self or others, in order to minimize the risk of these items becoming weapons, projectiles, or means to self-injury. All clinical areas in the ED should be equipped with easily accessible panic buttons to allow immediate communication by staff of an emergency and the need for help. One-to-one observers and/or closed-circuit cameras are also useful for close monitoring of patients who are at risk of unsafe behavior to themselves and others. However, space and staffing constraints, as well as the need to provide medical care to potentially high-risk patients, often limit the ability of hospitals to provide optimally safe clinical environments. Furthermore, none of these interventions is able to fully eliminate the risk of violence, replace thorough risk assessment or the need for close monitoring.

Patients who are intoxicated and behaviorally labile will often do better in a more contained area of the ED, ideally while continuing to receive close clinical monitoring. Patients who present to the ED for issues involving substance use often wait for long periods of time to be evaluated, to achieve clinical sobriety, or to be admitted to a mental health or substance use treatment facility. These long waits can be frustrating for patients already disinhibited by intoxication or withdrawal states [11]. In order to minimize this frustration, withdrawal syndromes and physical complaints, such as hunger and pain, should be adequately addressed via supportive and specific treatments. Withdrawal status and physical comfort should be repeatedly monitored, as patients may present while intoxicated and then progress to withdrawal over the course of their ED encounter. Frequent verbal check-ins from staff can demonstrate to patients that their needs are being attended to and their treatment plans addressed. Increased staffing during high volume times, especially with clinicians with specialty training in addiction medicine and/or psychiatry, can help with providing appropriate, ongoing care to these frequently long-stay patients [9].

Properly trained staff are crucial to the prevention and management of violence and self-harm in the ED. Patients with substance use disorders frequently engender feelings of fear, helplessness, and anger in staff [75]. When desensitized or under-supported ED staff tolerate verbal threats and physical outbursts, there is the risk that opportunities to intervene in order to prevent more serious violent events have been missed. ED staff may also underestimate patients' risk of self-harm in the case of high-utilizing patients recurrently presenting with acute intoxication and suicidal ideation, and then recanting suicidality when sober. Having access to specialty consultation by clinicians trained in addiction medicine and/or psychiatry can assist all ED staff in maintaining an awareness of risk, as well as hope for all patients' recovery.

Screening

Rapid identification of patients who are acutely intoxicated or withdrawing is extremely important to optimize clinical assessments and management. The importance of history cannot be overstated, but it can be difficult to obtain from patients who might be unwilling or unable to provide accurate information. Identifying, pursuing, and reviewing past medical records and other collateral sources of information, while time-consuming, can be extremely valuable in the service of a thorough medical, psychiatric, and behavioral risk assessment.

Physical and mental status examinations should be done as early as possible upon arrival of the patient to the ED [76]. Even with patients who are combative or otherwise uncooperative, a cursory exam can be highly informative. Physical examinations should focus on signs of trauma, autonomic instability, and evidence of acute medical problems. Mental status examinations should focus on ruling out delirium and assessing for evidence of acute psychiatric illness. Even in the absence of history or toxicology reports, these examinations can often provide clues to the specific substances causing a patient's substance-related emergency (Table 10.1). For example, rotatory nystagmus is classically associated with phencyclidine intoxication. Lacrimation, yawning, and rhinorrhea, on the other hand, suggest opioid withdrawal. Tremulousness, tachycardia, confusion, and fruity-smelling breath indicate a possible diagnosis of alcoholic ketoacidosis.

Diagnostic laboratory testing can be helpful, depending on the history and examination findings. Toxicology screens, both serum and urine, should be obtained, if possible, but acute management should not be delayed pending these results [77]. These tests usually provide confirmation of clinically suspected substance intoxication, but they can also be helpful in identifying occult co-ingestions, as well as in ruling out suspected intoxication as the cause of an acute mental status change. Blood alcohol levels (BAL) can provide useful information regarding the severity of intoxication and the chronicity of use in patients with a known alcohol use disorder [78]. For example, a patient with a high BAL who appears clinically sober is likely to have a long history of heavy alcohol use and have developed tolerance. In fact, these patients may even experience alcohol withdrawal symptoms at BALs that would produce marked intoxication in a novice user. On the other hand, a negative BAL should be interpreted in light of a patient's known history of use and current presentation and may prompt consideration of other potential causes of agitation, including alcohol withdrawal, other substance use, and other medical or psychiatric conditions.

A vitally important component of screening is the assessment of potentially life-threatening medical issues which might be obscured by the patient's abnormal mental status [76]. Both acute intoxication and chronic substance use disorders can increase the risk of serious medical illness and trauma. Patients with substance use disorders, particularly those who recurrently present in an intoxicated and dysregulated state, may elicit dismissive responses from frustrated ED staff [79]. Often unable to give a reliable history, these patients are at risk of receiving perfunctory medical screening exams and then being placed in out-of-the-way corners of the ED

Table 10.1 Clinical features of intoxication and withdrawal for alcohol, sympathomimetics, opioids, and cannabis as well as risks of violence and suicide in the intoxicated and withdrawal states

Substance	Intoxication signs and symptoms	Risk of suicide	Risk of violence	Withdrawal signs and symptoms	Risk of suicide	Risk of violence
Alcohol and sedative hypnotics	Hypothermia, hypotension, decreased respiratory rate, slurred speech, ataxic gait, alcohol odor	+++	+++	Hyperthermia, hypertension or hypotension, tachycardia, increased respiratory rate, tremor, diaphoresis, nausea, irritability	++	+++
Sympathomimetics (cocaine, amphetamines, synthetic cannabinoids, cathinones, PCP)	Hyperthermia, hypertension, tachycardia, increased respiratory rate, diaphoresis, mydriasis, bruxism, nystagmus (PCP)	+	+++	Depression, irritability	+	+
Opioids	Hypothermia, bradycardia, hypotension, decreased respiratory rate, miosis, anhidrosis, constipation	++	–	Hypertension, yawning, lacrimation, mydriasis, rhinorrhea, piloerection, tremor, muscle cramps, diarrhea	+	+
Cannabis	Tachycardia, conjunctival injection, dry mouth, impaired motor coordination	–	–	Irritability, agitation	–	–/+

with little monitoring, in the hope that they will "sleep it off." This approach neglects the fact that such patients are at increased risk of acute trauma, cardiac abnormalities, rhabdomyolysis, and gross metabolic derangements, such as ketoacidosis [80–82]. Furthermore, many medical conditions may mimic the presentation of acutely intoxicated or violent patients, and even the presence of acute intoxication does not rule out the possibility of a co-existing medical issue or trauma [83]. Full consideration of a complete differential diagnosis is warranted at every encounter, even with patients who present frequently and have well-documented substance use and/or psychiatric disorders.

Management

Even in the presence of appropriate screening and prevention techniques, violent or self-destructive behavior related to substance use can still occur in ED patients. Maintaining safety for patients and others remains the primary clinical goal, and, when possible, verbal de-escalation with a respectful and empathetic approach should generally be attempted [19]. Verbal de-escalation can include listening to patient concerns, identifying shared goals, and even directly informing patients about the effect they are having on ED staff. Verbal de-escalation and transfer to a de-stimulating environment may be effective with some patients, but this supportive approach may not be possible with acutely agitated and combative patients, who require immediate containment for the purpose of safe assessment. Many patients presenting to the ED with acute intoxication or withdrawal states will require the use of emergency psychopharmacological and/or physical interventions, as well as the assistance of hospital security officers [5].

The choice of psychopharmacological agents for an agitated or violent patient with active substance use depends on the substance being used and the presence of intoxication or withdrawal. Voluntary medications are always preferred to involuntary medications for patients who are willing to accept appropriate agents [84]. Substance withdrawal should be treated with the most appropriate medication to provide medical stabilization, relieve subjective distress and maximize the ability of the patient to participate in their own care. For example, nicotine gum or patches can be given to patients who are experiencing or are at risk for nicotine withdrawal. Opioid withdrawal may require comfort medications, such as dicyclomine, if opioid replacement is not available in the ED.

For acutely agitated patients in alcohol or benzodiazepine withdrawal, benzodiazepines are the usual agents of choice to treat both the agitation and withdrawal, due to their direct treatment of the withdrawal process, as well as antiseizure efficacy. Acute agitation refractory to benzodiazepines is generally treated with high potency antipsychotics, such as haloperidol [85]. Antipsychotics should not be used in isolation for patients who are withdrawing from alcohol, as they will not treat the underlying withdrawal and they may also decrease the seizure threshold. Conversely, the use of benzodiazepines to treat agitation in a patient who is acutely intoxicated with alcohol, benzodiazepines, or other sedative drugs can worsen mental status and increase the risk of medical complications, such as respiratory suppression, ataxia, and falls [5]. Antipsychotics, either first or second generation, can be useful for treating agitation in patients who are delirious from alcohol intoxication [5]. Of note, intramuscular administration of the second-generation antipsychotic olanzapine has been associated with oxygen desaturations and cardiac events in patients who are intoxicated with alcohol and, therefore, should be avoided [86]. For this reason, if parental agents are required, haloperidol is generally the first-line choice. Close clinical monitoring is required for ongoing assessment of the patient's level of agitation, sedation, and neurologic and cardio-respiratory status. The Clinical Institute Withdrawal Assessment (CIWA) scale for alcohol is increasingly being used in emergency settings to monitor alcohol withdrawal, respond to observed signs and reported symptoms, and, thus, minimize the risk of alcohol withdrawal delirium [87, 88]. However, appropriate use of this scale requires close monitoring which may not be possible in a very busy ED.

In patients with acute cannabis intoxication presenting with psychosis, second-generation antipsychotics and benzodiazepines should be used to treat psychosis and minimize risk for agitation [5, 89]. Agitation related to stimulant intoxication is best treated with benzodiazepines, antipsychotics, and/or β-blockers [90]. Agitation secondary to PCP intoxication may be extremely severe and difficult to manage due to the combined presence of psychosis and decreased pain sensitivity. Antipsychotic medications and de-stimulation can be helpful for these patients, who are at increased risk for medical complications, including rhabdomyolysis, autonomic instability and cardiac arrhythmias, and, thus, require close medical monitoring, often including telemetry. When opioid intoxication is rapidly reversed with intranasal naloxone, patients may become acutely agitated [49]. Managing agitation in a patient who has recently used opioids can be challenging because the presence of opioids increases the risk of oversedation and respiratory suppression. Agitation in these patients should be treated with antipsychotic medications.

Some patients who are withdrawing from alcohol or intoxicated with stimulants may exhibit violent behavior that is refractory to the above agents. In these rare cases, sedation with alternative agents, such as phenobarbital or even dexmedetomidine, may be considered [91]. In the latter cases, the support of anesthesia staff may be necessary for patients who require intubation.

Often it is difficult to determine whether a patient's severely altered mental status is due to intoxication or withdrawal, or what substance-related state(s) may be contributing to the acute presentation. This challenge occurs commonly with patients who arrive at the ED in an acutely agitated state and require safety interventions before examination and labs can be performed, or in instances where the substances being used are undetected by available lab screening [59, 68]. In these cases, if emergency medication is required, antipsychotic medications with or without benzodiazepines may be tried first [5].

Physical restraint refers to any physical restriction of a patient's freedom to move. Types of physical restraint range from placing a patient in a locked seclusion room to using four-point leather restraints. The use of physical restraints should be undertaken carefully and selectively, and only as needed to protect the safety of the patient and others, including staff. In general, patients who are placed in physical restraints should also be offered, or, if necessary, given involuntarily, medication to treat agitation [5]. In practice, these medications are often a combination of antipsychotic, benzodiazepine, and anticholinergic medication delivered intramuscularly. These medications are used in combination because they are all sedating but act via different pharmacological pathways. In addition, benzodiazepines may reduce the risk of akathisia and anticholinergic medications reduce the risk of dystonia [92].

In addition to their potentially traumatic psychological effects, physical restraints expose patients to a variety of medical risks, and time spent in restraints should be minimized [93]. This guideline is especially true for patients intoxicated with phencyclidine or stimulants who are at increased risk for rhabdomyolysis, but it is also true for any patient whose mental status prevents communication about physical symptoms or distress [94]. Close monitoring, including frequent re-assessments of mental status and physical comfort, are clinical imperatives for the restrained patient, as well as an important area of regulatory requirement.

Risk Assessment

Risk assessment is extremely important for patients with substance use disorders presenting for emergency evaluation. As previously described, substance use increases the risk for both violence toward others and harm to self, but there is no specific calculus of risk vs. protective factors which can be applied to any individual patient with predictive accuracy. Furthermore, there is little evidence for how best to assess risk specific to patients in the ED setting. Risk assessments for patients with substance-related emergencies in the ED will thus depend on careful consideration of available clinical data to allow a determination of likely short-term risk, formulation of treatment recommendations, and an actionable safety plan. Historical domains of risk to be evaluated for both risk to self and others include patient demographics, medical, psychiatric and substance use diagnoses and symptoms, past history of high-risk behavior, and psychosocial status and stressors. In addition, findings must be synthesized from both the medical and psychiatric evaluation of the patient in the ED—evaluations which are often complicated by the presence of acute intoxication or withdrawal.

Risk factors for suicide or aggression may be divided into chronic or acute, and modifiable or non-modifiable factors. Chronic risk factors are not modifiable and may be useful in generally stratifying patients into higher and lower risk categories. Chronic, non-modifiable, risk factors for suicide include male sex, history of alcohol use disorder, family history of suicide, and personal history of previous suicide attempts [95]. Acute risk factors are often modifiable, and may be important targets of treatment. Acute risk factors for suicide include depressed mood, physical illness, pain, suicidal ideation, and the intensity and frequency of substance use [95]. Chronic risk factors for violent behavior include male sex and past history of having been a victim and/or a perpetrator of violence; acute risk factors include intoxication, homicidal ideation, untreated psychiatric illness, delirium, and impulsivity [1].

Serial examination and re-evaluation is often necessary for patients presenting to the ED with active substance use, especially for those who have been suicidal or violent while intoxicated. While many historical risk factors can be determined by way of the medical record or collateral sources, these patients should be evaluated when clinically sober before risk assessment can be considered complete. Decisions about disposition options for patients with substance use and violent or self-destructive behavior should take into account the mental status of the patient at the point when the patient became violent or expressed suicidal ideation. Depending on history and the presence of comorbid psychopathology, patients who were violent or suicidal while intoxicated but who regain behavioral control or recant their suicidality once sober, may be considered differently from patients who become or persist in being violent or suicidal after the effects of a substance subside [96, 97].

Many patients are brought to the ED having overdosed on a substance or substances of abuse. Initially, it may not be clear if the overdose was a suicide attempt or a reckless accident. When able to participate in an interview, these patients should be carefully screened for depression and suicidal thinking, and those who express suicidal thoughts should have a thorough psychiatric evaluation, including a risk assessment with referral for appropriate treatment. Even when acute suicide risk is determined to be low, any patient brought to the hospital having overdosed on a substance of abuse should be evaluated for the presence of a substance use disorder and offered a referral for treatment, if indicated [98].

After clinical stabilization in the ED, many initially high-risk patients may request discharge. Determining their safety for release vs. their need to be held against their will for further treatment can be challenging and often involves complex clinical, ethical, and medicolegal issues [99]. Resource availability, as well as regional differences in statutory allowances for involuntary treatment of substance use and psychiatric disorders, can add to clinical uncertainty about how best to manage the potential risk of patients refusing treatment, especially when they are likely to re-enter high risk mental states associated with ongoing substance use [100]. Such clinical scenarios necessitate a careful assessment of the patient's capacity to make a decision about discharge. Clinical sobriety and the ability to participate rationally in a verbal risk assessment can be reassuring, but many substance-using patients cannot resist the powerful cravings to resume using. Most states do not have clear statutes for holding people who want to leave the hospital but are intoxicated, or for those whose risk is a "state-dependent" phenomena, acutely increased when intoxicated [101]. While physicians often have the authority to involuntarily hospitalize high-risk patients with "mental illness," the determination of risk as a result of substance use is often excluded from such interventions. At the same time, patients who leave the hospital against medical advice (AMA) while intoxicated or after a high-risk presentation in the setting of intoxication have ongoing risk of bad outcomes [102]. As always, serial assessments, collateral history, and consultation with colleagues and specialists are important aspects contributing to safe treatment and optimal disposition planning.

Disposition

Disposition planning for patients with substance use disorders is often difficult, particularly for those whose ED course has included concerns about risk of violence or suicide [103, 104]. Disposition options are dictated by local resource availability and may include medical hospitalization, involuntary inpatient psychiatric, dual diagnosis, substance-abuse treatment, voluntary inpatient treatment, partial hospital or intensive outpatient programs, referral to outpatient treaters or community supports (e.g., self-help groups), or none of the above. Psychiatric consultation may be helpful in multiple domains, including determining the presence of a delirium, or any comorbid psychiatric illness, in addition to a possible substance use disorder.

In some cases, disposition may be influenced by previous history and contingency planning at a hospital level. For example, in many urban emergency departments, there is a cohort of individuals with substance use disorders, often chronically homeless, who are extremely high-utilizers of emergency department services. Despite frequent ED evaluations, stabilization, and treatment referrals, these patients repeatedly present to the ED acutely intoxicated, medically at risk, and either transiently suicidal or combative. There is an increasing recognition of the need for systems-based approaches for such patients, incorporating housing, substance-abuse treatment, and psychiatric care to target their refractory conditions and enormous healthcare utilization. "Acute Care Plans" can be useful additions to the medical records of such high-utilizing patients, flagging their charts upon entry to the ED and outlining suggested treatment approaches for both acute management and disposition, as well as contact information for outpatient treaters and involved community agencies [105].

Conclusion

Patients with acute substance use and violence toward self or others are frequently encountered in the ED. Intoxication and/or withdrawal can directly increase the risk of agitation or suicide. Therefore, patients with substance use disorders who present to the ED require careful evaluation and management to minimize the risk of harm to self or others. This evaluation may include a focused medical workup to identify other potential causes of altered mental status, as well as serial risk assessments. These patients may also require behavioral and psychopharmacological interventions to reduce the acute risk of violence. These interventions include verbal de-escalation, chemical and physical restraints, and aggressive treatment of withdrawal symptoms. Disposition options are often limited by local resources, and decisions about disposition should not be made until patients are clinically sober.

References

1. Tomlinson MF, Brown M, Hoaken PNS. Recreational drug use and human aggressive behavior: a comprehensive review since 2003. Aggress Violent Behav [Internet]. 2016;27:9–29. Elsevier Ltd. Available from: https://doi.org/10.1016/j.avb.2016.02.004.
2. Boles SM, Miotto K. Substance abuse and violence: a review of the literature. Aggress Violent Behav. 2003;8(2):155–74.
3. Behnam M, Tillotson RD, Davis SM, Hobbs GR. Violence in the emergency department: a national survey of emergency medicine residents and attending physicians. J Emerg Med [Internet]. 2011;40(5):565–79. Elsevier Inc. Available from: https://doi.org/10.1016/j.jemermed.2009.11.007.

4. Elbogen EB, Johnson SC. The intricate link between violence and mental disorder. JAMA Psychiat. 2009;66(2):152–61.
5. Wilson MP, Pepper D, Currier GW, Holloman GH, Feifel D. The psychopharmacology of agitation: consensus statement of the American Association for Emergency Psychiatry Project BETA Psychopharmacology Workgroup. West J Emerg Med. 2012;13(1):26–34.
6. Zun LS, Downey LVA. Level of agitation of psychiatric patients presenting to an emergency department. Prim Care Companion J Clin Psychiatry [Internet]. 2008;10(2):108–13. Available from: http://www.pubmedcentral.nih.gov/articlerender.fcgi?artid=2292436&tool=pmcentrez&rendertype=abstract.
7. James A, Madeley R, Dove A. Violence and aggression in the emergency department. Emerg Med J [Internet]. 2006;23(6):431–4. Available from: http://www.pubmedcentral.nih.gov/articlerender.fcgi?artid=2564335&tool=pmcentrez&rendertype=abstract.
8. Lavoie FW, Carter GL, Danzl DF, Berg RL. Emergency department violence in United States teaching hospitals. Ann Emerg Med. 1988;17(11):1227–33.
9. Phillips JP. Workplace violence against health care workers in the United States. N Engl J Med [Internet]. 2016;374(17):1661–9. Available from: http://www.nejm.org/doi/10.1056/NEJMra1501998.
10. Emergency Department Violence Fact Sheet [Internet]. American College of Emergency Physicians. Available from: http://newsroom.acep.org/fact_sheets?item=30010.
11. May DD, Grubbs LM. The extent, nature, and precipitating factors of nurse assault among three groups of registered nurses in a regional medical center. J Emerg Nurs. 2002;28(1):11–7.
12. U.S. Department of Health and Human Services Substance Abuse and Mental Health Services Administration. Substance abuse and suicide prevention: evidence & implications a white paper. 2008.
13. U.S. Department of Health and Human Services Substance Abuse and Mental Health Services Administration. Substance use and suicide: a nexus requiring a public health approach. 2016.
14. Kaplan MS, McFarland BH, Huguet N, Conner K, Caetano R, Giesbrecht N, et al. Acute alcohol intoxication and suicide: a gender-stratified analysis of the National Violent Death Reporting System. Inj Prev. 2012:38–43.
15. U.S. Surgeon General. 2012 National Strategy for Suicide Prevention. 2012.
16. U.S. Department of Health and Human Services Substance Abuse and Mental Health Services Administration. National Estimates of Drug-Related Emergency Department Visits. 2011.
17. Joint Commission. Detecting and treating suicide ideation in all settings. 2016. p. 1–7.
18. Mills PD, Watts BV, DeRosier JM, Tomolo AM, Bagian JP. Suicide attempts and completions in the emergency department in Veterans Affairs Hospitals. Emerg Med J. 2012;29(5):399–403.
19. Ferns T, Cork A. Managing alcohol related aggression in the emergency department (Part I). Int Emerg Nurs. 2008;16(1):43–7.
20. Macdonald S, Cherpitel CJ, DeSouza A, Stockwell T, Borges G, Giesbrecht N. Variations of alcohol impairment in different types, causes and contexts of injuries: results of emergency room studies from 16 countries. Accid Anal Prev. 2006;38(6):1107–12.
21. Peterson JB, Rothfleisch J, Zelazo PD, Pihl RO. Acute alcohol intoxication and cognitive functioning. J Stud Alcohol. 1990;51(2)
22. Pihl RO, Peterson J. Alcohol and aggression: three potential mechanisms of drug effect. In: Martin SE, editor. Alcohol and interpersonal violence: fostering multidisciplinary perspectives; 1993. p. 1–36.
23. Duke AA. Alcohol dose and aggression: another reason why drinking more is a bad idea. J Stud Alcohol Drugs. 2011;72(1):34–43.
24. Bègue L, Subra B, Arvers P, Muller D, Bricout V, Zorman M. A message in a bottle: extrapharmacological effects of alcohol on aggression. J Exp Soc Psychol. 2009;45(1):137–42.
25. Rasanen P, Tiihonen J, Isohanni M, Rantakauio P, Lehtonen J, Schizophrenia JM. Alcohol abuse, and violent behavior: a 26-year followup study of an unselected birth cohort. Schizophr Bull. 1996;24(3):437–42.
26. Moeller FG, Dougherty DM, Lane SD, Steinberg JL, Cherek DR. Antisocial personality disorder and alcohol-induced aggression. Alcohol Clin Exp Res. 1998;22(9):1898–902.

27. Mann JJ. A current perspective of suicide and attempted suicide. Ann Intern Med. 2002;136(4):302–11.
28. Koller G, Preuss UW, Bottlender M, Wenzel K, Soyka M. Impulsivity and aggression as predictors of suicide attempts in alcoholics. Eur Arch Psychiatry Clin Neurosci [Internet]. 2002;252(4):155–60. Available from: http://www.ncbi.nlm.nih.gov/pubmed/12242575.
29. Centers for Disease Control. Current cigarette smoking prevalence among working adults — United States, 2004–2010. 2016.
30. Gilbert D. Paradoxical tranquilizing and emotion-reducing effects of nicotine. Psychol Bull [Internet]. 1979;86(4):643–61. Available from: http://psycnet.apa.org/journals/bul/86/4/643/.
31. Grant BF, Hasin DS, Chou SP, Stinson FS, Dawson DA. Nicotine dependence and psychiatric disorders in the United States. Arch Gen Psychiatry. 2004;61:1107.
32. Lawn S, Pols R. Nicotine withdrawal: pathway to aggression and assault in the locked psychiatric ward? Australas Psychiatry. 2003;11(2):199–203.
33. Reingle JM, Staras AS, Jennings WG, Branchini J, Maldonado-Molina MM. The relationship between marijuana use and intimate partner violence in a nationally representative, longitudinal sample. J Interpers Violence [Internet]. 2012;27(8):1562–78. Available from: http://jiv.sagepub.com/cgi/doi/10.1177/0886260511425787.
34. Swartout KM, White JW. The relationship between drug use and sexual aggression in men across time. J Interpers Violence. 2010;25(9):1716–35.
35. Taylor SP, Vardaris RM, Rawtich AB, Gammon CB, Cranston JW, Lubetkin AI. The effects of alcohol and delta-9-tetrahydrocannabinol on human physical aggression. Aggress Behav [Internet]. 1976;2(2):153–61. Available from: http://doi.wiley.com/10.1002/1098-2337(1976)2:2%3C153::AID-AB2480020206%3E3.0.CO;2-9.
36. Moore TM, Stuart GL. A review of the literature on marijuana and interpersonal violence. Aggress Violent Behav. 2005;10(2):171–92.
37. Budney AJ, Hughes JR, Moore BA, Vandrey R. Review of the validity and significance of cannabis withdrawal syndrome. Am J Psychiatry. 2004;161(11):1967–77.
38. Smith PH, Homish GG, Leonard KE, Collins RL. Marijuana withdrawal and aggression among a representative sample of U.S. marijuana users. Drug Alcohol Depend [Internet]. 2013;132(1–2):63–8. Elsevier Ireland Ltd. Available from: https://doi.org/10.1016/j.drugalcdep.2013.01.002.
39. U.S. Department of Health and Human Services Substance Abuse and Mental Health Services Administration. The DAWN Report. 2013.
40. McCarron MM, Schulze BW, Thompson GA, Conder MC, Goetz WA. Acute phencyclidine intoxication: clinical patterns, complications, and treatment. Ann Emerg Med. 1981;10(6):290–7.
41. Roth JA. Psychoactive substances and violence: US Department of Justice, Office of Justice Programs, National Institute of Justice; 1994.
42. van Amsterdam J, Opperhuizen A, van den Brink W. Harm potential of magic mushroom use: a review. Regul Toxicol Pharmacol [Internet]. 2011;59(3):423–9. Elsevier Inc. Available from: https://doi.org/10.1016/j.yrtph.2011.01.006.
43. Tyler O, Matthew S, Melanie R, John H. A case of aggressive psychosis in the setting of regular dextromethorphan abuse. Psychosomatics [Internet]. Elsevier. 2016. Available from: http://linkinghub.elsevier.com/retrieve/pii/S0033318216300573.
44. Paulzen M, Grunder G. Toxic psychosis after intake of the hallucinogen Salvinorin A. J Clin Psychiatry. 2008;69(9):1501–2.
45. Chan WL, Wood DM, Hudson S, Dargan PI. Acute psychosis associated with recreational use of benzofuran 6-(2-aminopropyl)benzofuran (6-APB) and cannabis. J Med Toxicol. 2013;9(3):278–81.
46. Leri F, Bruneau J, Stewart J. Understanding polydrug use: review of heroin and cocaine co-use. Addiction. 2003;98:7–22.
47. Verdejo-garcía AJ, Perales JC, Pérez-garcía M. Cognitive impulsivity in cocaine and heroin polysubstance abusers. Addict Behav. 2007;32:950–66.
48. Wesson DR, Ling W. The clinical opiate withdrawal scale. J Psychoactive Drugs. 2003;35(2):253–9.

49. Buajordet I, Naess A-C, Jacobsen D, Brørs O. Adverse events after naloxone treatment of episodes of suspected acute opioid overdose. Eur J Emerg Med. 2004;11(1):19–23.
50. Eizadi-Mood N, Sabzghabaee A, Gheshlaghi F, Yaraghi A, Siadat S. The frequency of agitation due to inappropriate use of naltrexone in addicts. Adv Biomed Res [Internet]. 2014;3(1):249. Available from: http://www.advbiores.net/text.asp?2014/3/1/249/146373.
51. Bozkurt M, Evren C, Yilmaz A, Can Y, Cetingok S. Aggression and impulsivity in different groups of alcohol and heroin dependent inpatient men. Bull Clin Psychopharmacol. 2013;23(4):335–44.
52. Hasegawa K, Brown D, Tsugawa Y, Camargo CA. Epidemiology of emergency department visits. Mayo Clin Proc [Internet]. Elsevier Inc. 2014. Available from: https://doi.org/10.1016/j.mayocp.2013.12.008.
53. Fridell M, Hesse M, Meier M, Kühlhorn E. Antisocial personality disorder as a predictor of criminal behaviour in a longitudinal study of a cohort of abusers of several classes of drugs: relation to type of substance and type of crime. Addict Behav. 2008;33:799–811.
54. Pennings EJM, Leccese AP, de Wolff FA. Effect of concurrent use of alcohol and cocaine. Addiction [Internet]. 2002;97(7):773. Available from: http://search.ebscohost.com/login.aspx?direct=true&db=sih&AN=7157196&site=ehost-live.
55. Ciccarone D. Stimulant abuse: pharmacology, cocaine, methamphetamine, treatment, attempts at pharmacotherapy. Prim Care. 2011;38(1):41–58.
56. Meredith CW, Jaffe C, Ang-lee K, Saxon AJ. Implications of chronic methamphetamine use: a literature review. Harv Rev Psychiatry. 2005;13(3):141–54.
57. Sekine Y, Ouchi Y, Sugihara G, Takei N, Yoshikawa E, Nakamura K, et al. Methamphetamine causes microglial activation in the brains of human abusers. J Neurosci. 2008;28(22):5756–61.
58. Mcgregor C, Srisurapanont M, Jittiwutikarn J, Laobhripatr S, Wongtan T, White JM. The nature, time course and severity of methamphetamine withdrawal. Addiction. 2005;100(9):1320–9.
59. Lung D, Wilson N, Chatenet F-T, LaCroix C, Gerona R. Non-targeted screening for novel psychoactive substances among agitated emergency department patients. Clin Toxicol (Phila). 2016;3650(February):1–5. Available from: http://www.tandfonline.com/doi/full/10.3109/15563650.2016.1139714.
60. Huestis MA, Pirard S, Hartman RL, Desrosiers NA, Gorelick DA, Castaneto MS. Synthetic cannabinoids: epidemiology, pharmacodynamics, and clinical implications. Drug Alcohol Depend. 2015;1(0):12–41.
61. Joseph AM, Manseau MW, Lalane M, Rajparia A, Lewis CF. Characteristics associated with synthetic cannabinoid use among patients treated in a public psychiatric emergency setting. Am J Drug Alcohol Abuse. 2017;43(1):117–22.
62. Casey N. K2, a potent drug, casts a shadow over an East Harlem Block. The New York Times.
63. Thomas S, Bliss S, Malik M. Suicidal ideation and self-harm following K2 use. J Okla State Med Assoc. 2012;105(11):430–3.
64. Spiller HA, Ryan ML, Weston RG, Jansen J. Clinical experience with and analytical confirmation of "bath salts" and "legal highs" (synthetic cathinones) in the United States. Clin Toxicol (Phila) [Internet]. 2011;49(6):499–505. Available from: http://www.ncbi.nlm.nih.gov/pubmed/21824061.
65. Palamar JJ. "Bath salt" use among a nationally representative sample of high school seniors in the United States. Am J Addict. 2015;24(6):488–91.
66. Imam SF, Patel H, Mahmoud M, Prakash NA, King MS, Fremont RD. Bath salts intoxication: a case series. J Emerg Med [Internet]. 2013;45(3):361–5. Elsevier Ltd. Available from: https://doi.org/10.1016/j.jemermed.2013.04.017.
67. Khullar V, Jain A, Sattari M. Emergence of new classes of recreational drugs – synthetic cannabinoids and cathinones. J Gen Intern Med. 2014;29(8):1200–4.
68. Kadaria D, Sinclair SE. A case of acute agitation with a negative urine drug screen: a new wave of "legal" drugs of abuse. Tenn Med [Internet]. 2012;105(9):31–2. Available from: http://ovidsp.ovid.com/ovidweb.cgi?T=JS&PAGE=reference&D=emed11&NEWS=N&AN=23097956.
69. Caffery T, Musso M, Manause R, Everett J, Perret J. Riding High on Cloud 9. J Louisiana State Med Soc. 2012;164(4):186–9.

70. Henson B. Preventing interpersonal violence in emergency departments: practical applications of criminology theory. Violence Vict. 2010;25(4):553–65.
71. Holloman GH, Zeller SL. Overview of project BETA: best practices in evaluation and treatment of agitation. West J Emerg Med. 2012;13(1):1–2.
72. Gorman A. L.A. County removing metal detectors from some hospital facilities [Internet]. The Los Angeles Times. 2013 [cited 2016 Mar 8]. Available from: http://articles.latimes.com/2013/feb/03/local/la-me-metal-detectors-20130203.
73. Malka ST, Chisholm R, Doehring M, Chisholm C. Weapons retrieved after the implementation of emergency department metal detection. J Emerg Med [Internet]. 2015;49(3):355–8. Elsevier Ltd. Available from: https://doi.org/10.1016/j.jemermed.2015.04.020.
74. Rankins RC, Hendey GW. Effect of a security system on violent incidents and hidden weapons in the emergency department. Ann Emerg Med. 1999;33(6):676–9.
75. Van Boekel LC, Brouwers EPM, Van Weeghel J, Garretsen HFL. Stigma among health professionals towards patients with substance use disorders and its consequences for healthcare delivery: systematic review. Drug Alcohol Depend [Internet]. 2013;131:23–35. Elsevier Ireland Ltd. Available from: https://doi.org/10.1016/j.drugalcdep.2013.02.018.
76. Kanich W, Brady WJ, Huff JS, Perron AD, Holstege C, Lindbeck G, et al. Altered mental status: evaluation and etiology in the ED. Am J Emerg Med. 2002;20(7):613–7.
77. Meehan TJ, Bryant SM, Aks SE. Drugs of abuse: the highs and lows of altered mental states in the emergency department. Emerg Med Clin North Am. 2010;28:663–82.
78. Urso T, Galaver JS, Van Thiel DH. Blood ethanol levels in sober alcohol users seen in an emergency room. Life Sci. 1981;28:1053–6.
79. Svoboda T. Difficult behaviors in the emergency department: a cohort study of housed, homeless and alcohol dependent individuals. PLoS One [Internet]. 2015;10(4):e0124528. Available from: http://dx.plos.org/10.1371/journal.pone.0124528.
80. Wrenn KD, Slovis CM, Minion GE, Rutkowski R. The syndrome of alcoholic ketoacidosis. Am J Med. 1991;91:119–28.
81. Richards JR, Johnson EB, Stark RW, Derlet RW. Methamphetamine abuse and rhabdomyolysis in the ED: a 5-year study. Am J Emerg Med. 1999;17(7):681–5.
82. Biyik I, Ergene O. Alcohol and acute myocardial infarction. J Int Med Res. 2007;35(1):46–51.
83. Royl G, Katchanov J, Schultze J, Ploner CJ, Endres M. Diagnostic pitfall: wound botulism in an intoxicated intravenous drug abuser presenting with respiratory failure. Intensive Care Med. 2007;33:10117.
84. Gault TI, Gray SM, Vilke GM, Wilson MP. Are oral medications effective in the management of acute agitation? J Emerg Med [Internet]. 2012;43(5):854–9. Elsevier Ltd. Available from: https://doi.org/10.1016/j.jemermed.2012.01.028.
85. Mayo-Smith MF, Beecher LH, Fischer TL, Gorelick DA, Guillaume JL, Hill A, et al. Management of alcohol withdrawal delirium an evidence-based practice guideline. Arch Intern Med. 2004;164:1405–13.
86. Wilson MP, Chen N, Vilke GM, Castillo EM, Macdonald KS, Minassian A. Olanzapine in ED patients: differential effects on oxygenation in patients with alcohol intoxication. Am J Emerg Med [Internet]. 2012;30(7):1196–201. Elsevier Inc. Available from: https://doi.org/10.1016/j.ajem.2012.03.013.
87. Cassidy EM, Sullivan IO, Bradshaw P, Cassidy EM, Sullivan IO, Bradshaw P, et al. Symptom-triggered benzodiazepine therapy for alcohol withdrawal syndrome in the emergency department: a comparison with the standard fixed dose benzodiazepine regimen. Emerg Med Clin North Am. 2012;29:802–4.
88. Sullivan JT, Sykora K, Schneiderman J, Naranjo CA, Sellers EM. Assessment of Alcohol Withdrawal: the revised clinical institute withdrawal assessment for alcohol scale (CIWA???Ar). Br J Addict. 1989;84(11):1353–7.
89. Bui QM, Simpson S, Nordstrom K. Psychiatric and medical management of marijuana intoxication in the emergency department. West J Emerg Med [Internet]. 2015;16(3):414–7. Available from: http://www.scopus.com/inward/record.url?eid=2-s2.0-84929089046&partnerID=tZOtx3y1.

90. Richards JR, Albertson TE, Derlet RW, Lange RA, Olson KR, Horowitz BZ. Treatment of toxicity from amphetamines, related derivatives, and analogues: a systematic clinical review. Drug Alcohol Depend [Internet]. 2015;150:1–13. Elsevier Ireland Ltd. Available from: https://doi.org/10.1016/j.drugalcdep.2015.01.040.
91. Rovasalo A, Tohmo H, Aantaa R, Kettunen E, Palojoki R. Dexmedetomidine as an adjuvant in the treatment of alcohol withdrawal delirium: a case report. Gen Hosp Psychiatry. 2006;28:362–3.
92. Brown HE, Stoklosa J, Freudenreich O. How to stabilize an acutely psychotic patient. Curr Psychiatr. 2012;11(12):10–6.
93. Mohr WK, Petti TA, Mohr BD. Adverse effects associated with physical restraint. Can J Psychiatry. 2003;48(5):330–3.
94. Patel R, Connor G. A review of thirty cases of rhabdomyolysis-associated acute renal failure among phencyclidine users. J Toxicol Clin Toxicol. 1986;23(7):547–56.
95. Bohnert ASB, Roeder K, Ilgen MA. Unintentional overdose and suicide among substance users: a review of overlap and risk factors. Drug Alcohol Depend [Internet]. 2010;110(3):183–92. Elsevier Ireland Ltd. Available from: https://doi.org/10.1016/j.drugalcdep.2010.03.010.
96. McCaffery R, Lee A, Jauhar P, Scott J. A survey of opinions on the management of individuals who express suicidal ideation while intoxicated with alcohol. Psychiatr Bull. 2002;26:332–4.
97. Jones GN, Musso MW, Dodge V, Adams J, Lillich P, Woodward CJ. The role of alcohol intoxication in psychiatrists' recension of emergency physicians' involuntary admissions. Am J Emerg Med. 2013;34(11):2226.
98. Fenton JJ, Lee CI, Baldwin L, Elmore JG. Presentation of prescription and nonprescription opioid overdoses to US emergency departments. JAMA Intern Med. 2014;174(12):2035–7.
99. Goldberg JF, Ernst CL, Bird S. Predicting hospitalization versus discharge of suicidal patients presenting to a psychiatric emergency service. Psychiatr Serv. 2007;58(4):561–5.
100. Klag S, Callaghan FO, Creed P. The use of legal coercion in the treatment of substance abusers: an overview and critical analysis of thirty years of research. Subst Use Misuse. 2005;40:1777–95.
101. Brooks R. Psychiatrists' opinions about involuntary civil commitment: results of a national survey. J Am Acad Psychiatry Law. 2007;35:19–28.
102. Ding R, Jung JJ, Kirsch TD, Levy F, Mccarthy ML. Uncompleted emergency department care: patients who leave against medical advice. Acad Emerg Med. 2007;14:870–6.
103. Jayaram G, Triplett P. Quality improvement of psychiatric care: challenges of emergency psychiatry. Am J Psychiatry. 2008;165(10):1256–60.
104. Slade EP, Dixon LB, Semmel S. Trends in the duration of emergency department visits, 2001–2006. Psychiatr Serv. 2010;61(9):878–84.
105. Spillane LL, Lumb EW, Cobaugh DJ, Wilcox SR, Clark JS, Schneider SM. Frequent users of the emergency department: can we intervene? Acad Emerg Med. 1997;4(6):574–80.

Part III
Special Topics

Chapter 11
Responding to the Medication-Seeking Patient

Scott G. Weiner

Introduction

A 35-year-old male presents to the emergency department complaining of left shoulder pain. He is from out of town, visiting his mother. The patient has a distant history of injury to that shoulder and has had shoulder surgery. He is experiencing an exacerbation of pain (15 out of 10!), which he attributes to lifting his young child. He has tried ice packs, ibuprofen, acetaminophen, and a sling but they don't work. He specifically requests oxycodone. After an examination, you obtain radiographs that show evidence of prior surgery but no sign of acute bone injury. You counsel the patient that this is likely pain from a ligamentous injury and you recommend continuing anti-inflammatory medications and supportive care. The patient becomes angry and states: "I waited two hours to be seen, and all you are giving me is Motrin!" You stand your ground and counsel the patient on the risks of opioids and that they are not indicated for his condition. The patient becomes increasingly agitated and threatens you. Security is called and as he is escorted out, he yells, "You haven't heard the last from me. I'm going to sue!"

This dramatic case presentation is not an exaggeration but instead illustrative of a routine occurrence in the emergency department (ED). Taking care of medication-seeking patients is incredibly challenging in the ED setting. Whereas most patients are forthright with their clinicians about their signs and symptoms, medication-seeking patients may feign symptoms, falsify their histories and attempt other forms of deceit. These patients usually are not purposely malicious towards their clinicians. Instead, it is important to realize that they, too, are suffering from a legitimate medical problem (e.g., substance-use disorder) and that clinicians must be astute and vigilant in order to detect the problem and then effectively address it.

S. G. Weiner (✉)
Department of Emergency Medicine, Brigham and Women's Hospital, Boston, MA, USA
e-mail: sweiner@bwh.harvard.edu

A. L. Donovan, S. A. Bird (eds.), *Substance Use and the Acute Psychiatric Patient*, Current Clinical Psychiatry, https://doi.org/10.1007/978-3-319-23961-3_11

The scope of the problem is broad and patients with medication-seeking behavior have a profound effect on satisfaction and burnout of emergency physicians. One study estimated that an ED with 75,000 annual visits will likely have up to 262 annual visits from "fabricating drug-seeking patients" [1]. An informal survey revealed striking results: A sample of 135 emergency physicians was surveyed from two large online discussion groups in March, 2016. Physicians rated their experience, on a scale of 0–100 for (1) an elderly patient with pneumonia requiring intubation, (2) a young woman with pain and hypotension from an ectopic pregnancy, (3) a middle-aged man with an ST-elevation myocardial infarction, and (4) a 30-year-old patient with atraumatic back pain and a normal neurologic examination who was requesting an opioid pain reliever. When asked about the contribution of each case to "professional burnout," the average value for the first three cases was <20, but the value for the back pain patient was 79 out of 100. Likewise, the "satisfaction you have from taking care of the patients" was >80 for the first three cases but just 18 out of 100 for the patient with the back pain.

The goal of this chapter, therefore, is to provide definitions, evidence, and strategies that will help the prescribing clinician identify patients with medication-seeking behavior and provide strategies to treat these patients in an optimal fashion.

Definitions

The terminology surrounding medication-seeking is problematic because the definitions lack standardization. Common phrases found in the medical literature and vernacular are "drug-seeking," "doctor-shopping," or "malingering" [2, 3]. Although more inclusive of patients who visit the ED often, they are also sometimes referred to as "frequent fliers" [4]. These terms are vague and pejorative and should be eliminated from use in the clinical environment. The definitions are subjective; for example, the diagnoses of conditions like appendicitis and pneumonia are well defined and universally understood, and different practitioners may think of "drug-seekers" in different or often pejorative ways. For example, is a patient who is seeking a refill of their antihypertensive medicine a drug-seeker? Is another patient who presents requesting a second or third opinion for their skin condition a doctor-shopper?

Most clinicians understand that these terms imply some sort of behavior that deviates from the norm, which usually involves medications with addictive properties such as opioids and benzodiazepines. "Doctor-shopping" can be typically defined as obtaining medications for nonmedical use from multiple sources. We agree with Solis, who used the term "controlled medication seeker," which is defined as "intentionally feigning or exaggerating a medical condition, or otherwise using deception (e.g., prescription tampering) to obtain a controlled medication (medications that are classified as being schedule II-V of the U.S. "Controlled Substances Act") from the healthcare system for purposes not sanctioned by the medical profession and provider" [5].

Another acceptable term would be "aberrant drug-related (or medication-related) behavior," defined as any medication-related behavior that departs from strict adherence to the prescribed therapeutic plan of care [6]. This term is all-encompassing and includes behaviors that arise from abuse, misuse, addiction, diversion, physical dependence (e.g., pseudo-addiction), and tolerance. "Medication-seeking," as used in this chapter, indicates that the patient is purposely misrepresenting his/her condition by feigning, exaggerating, or otherwise attempting to deceive the clinician.

It is important to note that just as clinicians may have different ideas about the definitions of vernacular terms, so do patients. It is strongly advised not to use words such as "drug-seeker" or "doctor-shopper" in the clinical environment. Even an overheard conversation by the patient can be interpreted as derogatory and may trigger the perception of minimizing or discrediting the patient's concerns, instilling anger in the patient and leading to immediate degradation of the therapeutic relationship.

Although medication-seeking can happen with many different types of prescribed medications, including benzodiazepines, stimulants, gabapentin, and others, the remainder of the chapter will focus specifically on opioids. Given the current misuse, overdose, and death epidemic, clinicians must be specifically attuned to patients seeking opioids. Many of the principles will apply to other classes of medications, but the majority of research in this area focuses on opioids.

Identifying the Medication-Seeking Patient With Pain

There are several signs to look for when treating a patient with a painful condition. "Red flag" features for patients with medication-seeking behavior are described in Table 11.1 [7]. Unfortunately, several of these characteristics are not identifiable from a single ED visit. In addition, softer "yellow flag" symptoms should raise provider suspicion. These include the following: the patient is away from home or has passed closer health-care facilities, the patient gives an improbable story for running out of a medication, multiple allergies are reported to non-controlled medications, the patient has an unusual amount of knowledge about controlled substances, or has history of abuse of other substances, including alcohol or other recreational drugs. Clinicians should also have heightened awareness of patients presenting with common painful conditions that cannot be measured (e.g., headache, renal colic, abdominal pain) [8]. A patient who has multiple ED visits but no evidence of follow-up for routine longitudinal care for a chronic condition should also raise suspicion. Furthermore, patients who are more interested in the specific medicine itself, as opposed to the relief of pain, should prompt consideration [4].

Grover and colleagues examined characteristics of patients at high risk for medication-seeking behavior [9]. These patients were enrolled in a specialized addiction case management program due to a large number of ED visits, or nurse, physician, or state prescription drug-monitoring program (PDMP) concern for medication-seeking behavior. Thirteen characteristics of this population were

Table 11.1 Warning signs for medication-seeking behavior

"Red flags" (strong evidence) are present when the patient:
1. States that they have an addiction problem
2. Frequents multiple providers, institutions and pharmacies in a short period of time to obtain controlled medications.
3. Steals or diverts prescriptions from family members.
4. Obtains controlled medications from non-medical sources (diversion).
5. Steals medical goods, like prescription pads or syringes.
6. Forges or alters a prescription for a controlled medication.
7. Reports frequently losing their controlled medication by misplacing it, having it stolen, etc.
8. Has notification by another provider, institution, or a family member that the patient is addicted to controlled medications.
9. Has drug-related deterioration in work performance, family relationships, or other social dynamics.
10. Concurrently abuses illicit drugs, for example, positive urine drug screen for illicit drugs.
11. Asserts that they take a controlled medication regularly and recently for their condition, but the urine drug screen is negative; are they diverting the medication for resale?
12. Gives false or no identification information.

Adapted from Solis [5]

Table 11.2 Odds ratios for certain medication-seeking behaviors in a population enrolled in a care coordination program versus a control population

Characteristic	Odds ratio
Requesting parenteral pain medication	∞
>10 pain	∞
Three visits in 7 days	30.8
Over 3 pain complaints	29.3
Out of medication	26.9
Requests by name	26.3
Chief complaint of refill	19.2
Lost or stolen medication	14.1
10 out of 10 pain	13.9
Back pain	13.6
Headache	10.9
Dental pain	6.3
Non-narcotic allergy	3.4

Adapted from Grover [10]

identified, including reporting 10/10 pain, requesting parenteral medication, and requesting medication by name. See Table 11.2 for the complete list. While these characteristics should prompt clinicians to consider the presence of medication-seeking behavior, this list is neither exhaustive nor predictive. In a companion study [10], the investigators found that the most common feature, a complaint of 10/10 pain, was present in only 29.1% of the patients. Furthermore, the features most highly associated with medication-seeking behavior in the first study (requesting parenteral pain medication and having >10 pain) were present in only 4.3% and

1.8%, respectively, of these patients. These features are important clues to possible medication-seeking behavior, but are not sensitive and must be correlated with the overall clinical presentation.

Prescription Drug-Monitoring Programs

Perhaps the most important development in detecting medication-seeking behavior is the prescription drug-monitoring program (PDMP). Although primitive databases to monitor dispensing of controlled substances have been in place as early as 1918 [11], only recently has their implementation became ubiquitous throughout the country [12]. Because of lack of federal funding, PDMPs developed in a piecemeal, state-by-state fashion, with varying characteristics (e.g., some PDMPs report all scheduled medications, while others report only schedule II or III, and the time from filling a prescription to database entry varies widely) [13].

Currently, PDMPs are either available or being developed statewide in every state except Missouri [14]. PDMPs are extremely beneficial in the ED environment, given that ED practitioners often do not have established relationships with patients, and it would otherwise be impossible to determine the origin of prior prescriptions for controlled medications. Furthermore, PDMPs can help detect high-risk behavior when the aforementioned high-risk factors are not present. PDMPs have largely supplanted the use of individual "frequent flier" files that many hospitals used to maintain for high-risk patients, which were deemed to be unethical and possibly illegal [15].

The true advantage of PDMPs is that they are all-inclusive. Unlike other databases that sample only certain pharmacies or certain payers, PDMPs collect and report data on prescriptions regardless of where they were filled in a state. Furthermore, even prescriptions purchased with cash as opposed to insurance (possibly another high-risk characteristic) will be captured in the database. Finally, states now have web portals that prescribers can access in real-time to aid in prospective decision-making prior to writing a new prescription. Nearly all states report schedule II and III medications (mainly opioids) and most also include schedules IV and V (including benzodiazepines and stimulants). Some states also track nonscheduled medications with abuse potential, such as carisoprodol. PDMPs can be a helpful addition to the clinical assessment for medication-seeking patients. One study compared the provider clinical assessment of "drug-seeking" behavior of 544 patients who presented to the ED with back pain, dental pain, and headache to evidence of medication-seeking behavior in the PDMP (≥4 opioid prescriptions and ≥4 prescribers for controlled medication prescriptions in the prior 12 months) [16]. This study reported that providers' ability to detect medication-seeking behavior was rather poor, with a positive predictive value of only 41.2%. This study also reported that having multiple visits for the same complaint (OR 2.50), requesting medication by name (OR 1.91), having a "suspicious history" (OR 1.88), and having symptoms out of proportion to the examination results (OR 1.83) were all associated with medication-seeking behavior as demonstrated by the PDMP. Therefore, presence of these four factors should also raise suspicion of medication-seeking behavior.

Although they are powerful tools, PDMPs are not a panacea and it is important to realize their numerous limitations (Table 11.3). Perhaps the most important limitation is that PDMPs only capture prescriptions written for that individual. A very large study determined that only 21% of nonmedical users of opioids obtained them from by a legitimate prescription [17]. That is, 79% of nonmedical users of opioids used pills that would not have been detected by the PDMP, which were most often obtained from family or friends for free (53%). Another limitation worth noting is that there are no evidence-based guidelines by which to interpret PDMP profiles [18]. One practitioner's interpretation of a profile may vary from another's, and it is not clear which features are more strongly associated with outcomes of interest, like overdose [19]. In addition, methadone prescribed and dispensed through a methadone maintenance program is often not included. Prescriptions filled in other states may not be available. Finally, there is typically at least some delay from the time a prescription is filled until database entry.

Utilization and effectiveness of PDMPs has been described as mixed in the literature. For example, one study found that the PDMP result changed the decision to prescribe an opioid for 9.5% of patients, more commonly in favor of prescribing the opioid instead of not. Another study found that PDMP review changed the ED management in 41% of patients, with the majority receiving fewer or no opioid medications prescribed than originally planned [20]. On an impact level, data is also mixed with one large study determining that PDMPs have no effect on drug overdose mortality rates [21], but another showing that states with PDMPs had sustained reductions in opioid prescribing by physicians [22].

The summary of PDMPs is that they are exceptionally useful tools, although not perfect. Because clinician gestalt for detecting medication-seeking behaviors is poor, we strongly recommend utilizing a PDMP (if available) prior to prescribing any new controlled substance. By doing this consistently, internal bias can be minimized. A suspicious PDMP profile (including multiple opioid prescriptions, prescriptions from multiple providers) can be used as a powerful tool to help prompt

Table 11.3 Limitations of prescription drug-monitoring programs (PDMPs)

1. PDMPs only capture prescriptions that were written for that individual (i.e., do not report diverted medications or use of illicit drugs).
2. The timeliness of reporting of filled prescriptions varies among states.
3. Many states do not share information with bordering states.
4. PDMPs typically identify providers but not their specialty nor the system with which they are affiliated
5. There are no evidence-based guidelines by which to interpret PDMP profiles.
6. PDMPs are often not integrated into routine clinical workflow/electronic health records.
7. Methadone prescribed and dispensed through a methadone program may not be entered

assessment and possible treatment referrals for patients who have substance-use disorder. However, since medication diversion occurs, a reassuring PDMP profile cannot rule out medication-seeking behavior. In this respect, it's best to think of the PDMP as a tool that is *specific* but not *sensitive*.

Approach to the Patient with Medication-Seeking Behavior

When approaching a patient with medication-seeking behavior, it is important to realize that this is not a homogeneous patient population in terms of motivation: a differential diagnosis must be considered [23, 24]:

- *Addiction*: The patient may have physical and/or psychological dependency on the medication, marked by escalating use, tolerance, craving, withdrawal, recurrent use despite physical, social, or occupational harm. The attempt to obtain a prescription in the ED may be to prevent the uncomfortable, and very real, symptoms of opioid withdrawal.
- *Pseudo-addiction:* The patient may have undertreated pain that leads him/her to use alcohol, street drugs, or to seek medications from multiple providers in order to achieve relief of pain. These behaviors mimic addiction but subside when the pain is adequately treated.
- *Psychiatric illnesses:* Patients may have additional underlying psychiatric illnesses, such as depression, bipolar disorder, or anxiety that influence or drive the use of substances. Opioids, and other substances, can numb the intense emotions triggered by psychiatric illnesses, or even serve as (ill-advised) "treatments" for psychological suffering.
- *Criminal intent:* Although this is likely less common than the other categories, there are patients who are seeking medication simply for the purpose of diversion/profit.

Recalling the patient with shoulder pain described at the beginning of the chapter, several important features should now emerge. The patient is visiting from out of town, so there is no corroborating clinical information in an electronic medical record, no local primary care physician to contact and no adequate follow-up, all of which should be viewed as a high-risk features. He has >10/10 pain and pain out of proportion to the clinical examination. He also requests medication by name. These factors are all demonstrated in multiple studies to be associated with medication-seeking behavior. In this case, his PDMP profile might show no filled prescriptions, given that he is visiting from out of state.

What are the next steps with a patient for whom you are concerned?

1. *Set the stage*. Although these interactions are difficult, they are also a unique opportunity to intervene and potentially help a patient in need, as well as break a cycle of harmful behaviors. It is important to be calm, nonconfrontational, objective, and always have the patient's best interest in mind. Clinicians working in

the ED face a challenge in that they are often meeting their patients for the first time. For this reason, it is acceptable to say: "I can't follow you longitudinally and patients on controlled medications need close monitoring. I therefore don't feel comfortable writing a prescription for you from the emergency department." It is also important to remove the paternalistic dynamic to decrease defensiveness. Walk in and sit down with the patient. Remember that you are treating a patient who needs help, although they may define the help they need differently than the clinician.

2. *Be empathetic.* A lack of perceived empathy by patients can escalate behavior. Express an understanding that the patient has a painful condition and that you wish to help them in the safest way possible. Acknowledge their pain. Remember that being in pain and misusing opioids are not mutually exclusive categories. Realize that sometimes people abuse pain medications for control of other psychiatric symptoms, such as anxiety or insomnia, and sometimes to avoid the very uncomfortable symptoms of withdrawal. Make sure you are listening to the patient's concerns and exhibit that you take them seriously.
3. *Avoid judgment.* There is an enormous stigma associated with opioid use, and all substance use, to which patients are sensitive. Making the patient feel like "an addict" can be extraordinarily detrimental to the therapeutic relationship. Many people, including health-care providers, can view patients with substance-use disorders as making purposeful decisions to use or lacking the will power to resist use. Furthermore, when confronted with possible medication-seeking behavior, patients may feel that they are being accused of illegal activity. It is best instead to treat this behavior as if it resulted from a medical condition. Be firm, state the facts, but avoid passing judgment.
4. *Educate.* We are in a new era regarding opioids. For many years, there were concerns of "oligoanalgesia"—the undertreatment of pain in the ED [25, 26]. Now, it is hard to go a day without hearing about the bad effects of the opioid epidemic. The President, Surgeon General, state governors, mayors, and many other public figures are now frequently talking about the issue. Overdose deaths of public figures like Heath Ledger, Amy Winehouse, and Prince have also brought the dangers of opioids to the forefront of public discussion. Therefore, patients may now be less surprised if you use a statement such as "I'm really concerned about you. I don't want to prescribe any more of these medications for you, because they're unhealthy for you and I'm worried about how much you're using them" [27].

   Apart from the obvious risks of abuse and addiction, there is evidence that opioid use over time increases the perception of pain (opioid-induced hyperalgesia) and can lead to physical and psychological sequelae such as narcotic bowel syndrome [28]. Clinicians can inform patients that these medications carry risks and that one's practice is to avoid them when possible. Clinicians can also share evidence like a recent study that showed that among patients with acute, nontraumatic, nonradicular low back pain presenting to the ED, adding oxycodone or a muscle relaxer to naproxen alone did not improve functional outcomes or pain at 1-week follow-up [29]. Again, it is important to be objective and share this information with patients just as for any other medical condition.

5. *Share PDMP Data.* As stated above, a reassuring PDMP profile does not exclude medication-seeking behavior, but a concerning profile is a powerful tool. Although there is no clear definition about what a "concerning" profile looks like, any patient with multiple controlled substance prescriptions from multiple providers (≥4 in 1 year) should raise concern. It is recommended that a hard copy be printed and shared with the patient. Allowing the patient to see the actual printout does several important things: (a) it alerts patients that such a database does exist, and that practitioners in your ED access it, (b) it allows patients the opportunity to explain why they are using so many practitioners, as there may be a valid reason (e.g., seeing multiple residents in the same clinic), and (c) it can be incredibly powerful when patients see their concerning behavior printed out from a state database—just the ability to see that information may be motivation for the patient to realize that s/he has a problem and consider accepting treatment for it.
6. *Use Guidelines.* Guidelines about opioid prescribing have been created by a number of entities, including cities, states, the Centers for Disease Control and Prevention (CDC), and professional societies [30, 31]. These guidelines should be used in clinical practice, and can help practitioners justify their decision not to prescribe controlled substances. The presence of a directive from a larger body can lend credibility to the provider and allows them to use statements like "I'm not allowed to refill your lost prescription per this document." Although there are multiple versions, there are many aspects in common. By way of example, the ED prescribing guidelines from the Massachusetts Hospital Association are demonstrated in Table 11.4 [32].
7. *Help the Patient.* Even brief interventions in the ED with patients struggling with opioid-use disorders may create opportunities for treatment referral. Engage your social workers, hospital and community for a plan of action for patients with opioid misuse. Ensure adequate follow-up with a primary care physician or SUD specialist. Be prepared to provide referrals to community resources.
8. *Don't Take It Personally.* It would be wonderful if every patient responded positively to interventions, but inevitably many encounters with the medication-seeking patient will be more conflictual. When informed that their requests will not be met for the desired medication, patients may often become frustrated, attempt to bargain for fewer pills or a "weaker" opioid, or even become confrontational and argumentative. Having made a thoughtful decision not to prescribe, emergency clinicians should be firm and remain steadfast in this stance, while conveying compassion and offering whatever is possible in the form of nonopioid pain medication and other adjunctive treatment. Giving even a small prescription of opioids could be detrimental to the medication-seeking patient felt to be at risk for opioid abuse [33].

The patient in this chapter's vignette likely came to the ED specifically for an opioid prescription and when he found out that it was not possible, his adaptive method was anger and threats. It would be highly unlikely that such a patient actually would invoke a law suit for this reason. Furthermore, while EDs have the obligation to

Table 11.4 Massachusetts Hospital Association Emergency Department Opioid Prescribing Guidelines [32]

1. Hospitals, in conjunction with ED personnel, should develop a process to screen for substance misuse.
2. When possible, consult the PDMP before writing an opioid prescription.
3. Hospitals should develop a process to share the ED visit history of patients with other providers and hospitals that are treating the patients in the Emergency Department by using a health information exchange system.
4. Hospitals should develop a process to coordinate the care of patients who frequently visit EDs.
5. For acute exacerbations of chronic pain, the ED provider should notify the patient's primary opioid prescriber or PCP of the visit and the medication prescribed.
6. ED providers should not provide prescriptions for controlled substances that were lost, destroyed, or stolen (and no methadone unless confirmed and medical treatment precludes them going to their usual clinic)
7. Unless otherwise clinically indicated, ED providers should not prescribe long-acting or controlled-release opioids.
8. When opioid medications are prescribed, counsel:
to store the medications securely, not share them with others, and dispose of them properly when their pain has resolved
to avoid using the medications for nonmedical purposes
to avoid using opioids and concomitant sedating substances due to the risk of overdose.
9. Provide no more than a short course and minimal amount of opioid analgesics for serious acute pain, lasting no more than 5 days.

perform a medical-screening evaluation under the Emergency Medical Treatment and Active Labor Act (EMTALA) law [34], and there are standards which direct the need to measure patients' pain, there are no mandates to treat pain with opioids.

As a corollary, there will be patients who "fool" you and, despite your due diligence, will be abusers of medications that you prescribe. Skilled medication-seekers are often highly educated and highly motivated [4]. As we struggle to balance the very real issue of inadequate pain control with avoiding new addiction, it will be impossible to avoid mistakes, and emergency practitioners need to be comfortable walking this fine line.

Many physicians are worried about receiving poor satisfaction scores by refusing to give opioids to some patients. It is helpful to remind oneself that the duty is to the safety of the patient (not a satisfaction survey) and that the literature has shown that receiving opioid prescriptions for painful conditions is not associated with increased satisfaction scores [35, 36]. When weighing the decision between providing responsible and safe patient care versus potential scores on a satisfaction survey, always chose safety.

Conclusions

Patients with medication-seeking behavior can be a cause of stress and doubt for emergency providers but knowledge will help facilitate management of these patients. Recognition of the common characteristics of medication-seeking behavior is helpful, as is utilization of the state PDMP to identify the subset of patients who use multiple providers to obtain controlled substance prescriptions. Patients can be approached in a stepwise and uniform fashion in order to avoid bias, and the clinician's primary goal should be to "do no harm." Clinicians should be firm and objective in patient encounters and take an empathic, nonjudgmental stance. Guidelines can be helpful to standardize treatment among providers and demonstrate to the patient the constraints within which providers practice. Finally, clinicians should be prepared to counsel and help every patient—medication-seeking patients may be in dire need of treatment, and having their suffering acknowledged and responded to with appropriate treatment referrals may make a significant difference in their lives.

References

1. Hansen GR. The drug-seeking patient in the emergency room. Emerg Med Clin North Am. 2005;23(2):349–65.
2. McCaffery M, Grimm MA, Pasero C, Ferrell B, Uman GC. On the meaning of "drug seeking". Pain Manag Nurs. 2005;6(4):122–36.
3. Mosby medical dictionary. 8th ed. St. Louis: Mosby Elsevier; 2008.
4. Millard WB. Grounding frequent flyers, not abandoning them: drug seekers in the ED. Ann Emerg Med. 2007 Apr;49(4):481–6.
5. Solis M. Ethical, legal, and professional challenges posed by "controlled medication seekers" to healthcare providers – part 1. Am J Clin Med. 2010;7(1):25–9.
6. Corini E, Zacharoff KL. Definitions related to aberrant drug-related behavior: is there correct terminology? Available at: www.painedu.org/articles_timely.asp?ArticleNumber=58.
7. Solis M. Ethical, legal, and professional challenges posed by "controlled medication seekers" to healthcare providers – part 2. Am J Clin Med. 2010;7(2):86–92.
8. Vukmir RB. Drug seeking behavior. Am J Drug Alcohol Abuse. 2004 Aug;30(3):551–75.
9. Grover CA, Close RJ, Wiele ED, Villarreal K, Goldman LM. Quantifying drug-seeking behavior: a case control study. J Emerg Med. 2012;42(1):15–21.
10. Grover CA, Elder JW, Close RJ, Curry SM. How frequently are "classic" drug-seeking behaviors used by drug-seeking patients in the emergency department? West J Emerg Med. 2012;13(5):416–21.
11. PDMP Training and Technical Assistance Center. History of prescription drug monitoring programs. Available at: www.pdmpassist.org/pdf/PPTs/LE2012/1_Giglio_HistoryofPDMPs.pdf. Accessed 28 June 2016.
12. National Alliance for Model State Drug Laws: prescription drug monitoring programs. Available at: http://www.namsdl.org/prescription-monitoring-programs.cfm. Accessed 28 June 2016.
13. Manasco AT, Griggs C, Leeds R, Langlois BK, Breaud AH, Mitchell PM, Weiner SG. Characteristics of state prescription drug monitoring programs: a state-by-state survey. Pharmacoepidemiol Drug Saf. 2016;25(7):847–51.
14. Howell J. Big push for tort reform this legislative session. Mo Med. 2014;111(6):458–9.
15. Geiderman JM. Keeping lists and naming names: habitual patient files for suspected nontherapeutic drug-seeking patients. Ann Emerg Med. 2003;41(6):873–81.
16. Weiner SG, Griggs CA, Mitchell PM, Langlois BK, Friedman FD, Moore RL, Lin SC, Nelson KP, Feldman JA. Clinician impression versus prescription drug monitoring program criteria in the assessment of drug-seeking behavior in the emergency department. Ann Emerg Med. 2013;62(4):281–9.
17. Substance Abuse and Mental Health Services Administration. Results from the 2013 national survey on drug use and health. Available at: www.samhsa.gov/data/sites/default/files/NSDUHresultsPDFWHTML2013/Web/NSDUHresults2013.pdf. Accessed 28 June 2016.

18. Weiner SG, Griggs CA, Langlois BK, Mitchell PM, Nelson KP, Friedman FD, Feldman JA. Characteristics of emergency department "doctor shoppers". J Emerg Med. 2015;48(4):424–31.
19. Grover CA, Garmel GM. How do emergency physicians interpret prescription narcotic history when assessing patients presenting to the emergency department with pain? Perm J. 2012 Fall;16(4):32–6.
20. Baehren DF, Marco CA, Droz DE, Sinha S, Callan EM, Akpunonu P. A statewide prescription monitoring program affects emergency department prescribing behaviors. Ann Emerg Med. 2010;56(1):19–23.
21. Paulozzi LJ, Kilbourne EM, Desai HA. Prescription drug monitoring programs and death rates from drug overdose. Pain Med. 2011;12(5):747–54.
22. Bao Y, Pan Y, Taylor A, Radakrishnan S, Luo F, Pincus HA, Schackman BR. Prescription drug monitoring programs are associated with sustained reductions in opioid prescribing by physicians. Health Aff (Millwood). 2016;35(6):1045–51.
23. Passik SD, Kirsh KL. Assessing aberrant drug-taking behaviors in the patient with chronic pain. Curr Pain Headache Rep. 2004;8(4):289–94.
24. American Society of Addiction Medicine. Definitions related to the use of opioids for the treatment of pain: consensus statement of the American Academy of Pain Medicine, the American Pain Society, and the American Society of Addiction Medicine. Available at: www.asam.org/docs/default-source/public-policy-statements/1opioid-definitions-consensus-2-011.pdf?sfvrsn=0. Accessed 28 June 2016.
25. Fosnocht DE, Swanson ER, Barton ED. Changing attitudes about pain and pain control in emergency medicine. Emerg Med Clin North Am. 2005;23(2):297–306.
26. Rupp T, Delaney KA. Inadequate analgesia in emergency medicine. Ann Emerg Med. 2004;43(4):494–503.
27. Butterfield S. Dealing with drug-seeking behavior. ACP Hospitalist, 2014 Feb. Available at: www.acphospitalist.org/archives/2014/02/coverstory.htm. Accessed 28 June 2016.
28. Benyamin R, Trescot AM, Datta S, Buenaventura R, Adlaka R, Sehgal N, Glaser SE, Vallejo R. Opioid complications and side effects. Pain Physician. 2008;11(2 Suppl):S105–20.
29. Friedman BW, Dym AA, Davitt M, Holden L, Solorzano C, Esses D, Bijur PE, Gallagher EJ. Naproxen with cyclobenzaprine, oxycodone/acetaminophen, or placebo for treating acute low back pain: a randomized clinical trial. JAMA. 2015;314(15):1572–80.
30. Dowell D, Haegerich TM, Chou R. CDC guideline for prescribing opioids for chronic pain – United States, 2016. JAMA. 2016;315(15):1624–45.
31. Weiner SG, Perrone J, Nelson LS. Centering the pendulum: the evolution of emergency medicine opioid prescribing guidelines. Ann Emerg Med. 2013;62(3):241–3.
32. Massachusetts Hospital Association. MHA guidelines for emergency department opioid management. Available at: www.mhalink.org/Content/NavigationMenu/Newsroom/SubstanceAbuse/default.htm. Accessed 28 June 2016.
33. Parran T Jr. Prescription drug abuse. A question of balance. Med Clin North Am. 1997;81(4):967–78.
34. Hyman DA, Studdert DM. Emergency Medical Treatment and Labor Act: what every physician should know about the federal antidumping law. Chest. 2015;147(6):1691–6.
35. Zgierska A, Miller M, Rabago D. Patient satisfaction, prescription drug abuse, and potential unintended consequences. JAMA. 2012;307(13):1377–8.
36. Schwartz TM, Tai M, Babu KM, Merchant RC. Lack of association between Press Ganey emergency department patient satisfaction scores and emergency department administration of analgesic medications. Ann Emerg Med. 2014;64(5):469–81.

Chapter 12
Substance Use in Children and Adolescents

Peter Jackson, Michelle Chaney, and Laura M. Prager

Introduction

Drug and alcohol misuse is a major and potentially preventable threat to the health and well-being of adolescents. The peak onset of substance use is during adolescence. Furthermore, ongoing and significant substance use during adolescence can result in a higher likelihood of substance use disorders in adulthood [1]. Adolescents frequently present to the ED with a chief complaint related to substance use or with evidence of active substance use, in addition to other psychiatric or somatic symptoms. As an ED visit may represent an adolescent's first presentation with a clear substance-related issue, careful evaluation can provide a unique opportunity for providers to diagnose specific substance use disorders, to screen for ongoing substance use, to consider brief interventions if indicated, and to offer education and guidance to both the patient and his/her family about potential risks with ongoing use and available resources for treatment within the community.

P. Jackson (✉)
University of Vermont Medical Center, Burlington, VT, USA

Massachusetts General Hospital, Department of Psychiatry, Waltham, MA, USA
e-mail: peter.jackson@uvmhealth.org

M. Chaney
Resident in Child and Adolescent Psychiatry, Massachusetts General Hospital and McLean Hospital, Boston, MA, USA

Massachusetts General Hospital, Department of Psychiatry, Boston, MA, USA
e-mail: mchaney@partners.org

L. M. Prager
Harvard Medical School, Boston, MA, USA

Child Psychiatry Emergency Consult Service, Massachusetts General Hospital, Boston, MA, USA
e-mail: lmprager@partners.org

A. L. Donovan, S. A. Bird (eds.), *Substance Use and the Acute Psychiatric Patient*, Current Clinical Psychiatry, https://doi.org/10.1007/978-3-319-23961-3_12

Epidemiology

According to 2015 data from the Monitoring the Future (MTF) study, the annual prevalence of illicit drug use among 8th, 10th, and 12th grade students was 15%, 28%, and 38%, respectively. Among all three age groups, both alcohol use and cigarette use have trended downward over the past two decades and continue to do so. However, illicit drug use (including cannabis) has generally remained steady over that time period in all age groups (Fig. 12.1). The decades-long MTF study has also demonstrated that, in general, rates of substance use have been inversely proportional to adolescents' report of perceiving substances as harmful. According to the National Comorbidity Survey-Adolescent Supplement, approximately 11% of teens aged 13 to 18 meet the criteria for a substance use disorder, with a sharp increase in incidence after age 15 [2].

The use of specific substances often follows regional or even state-specific trends, and ED providers should be aware of such trends. See Appendix Table 1 at the end of this book for a comprehensive list of potential substances of abuse.

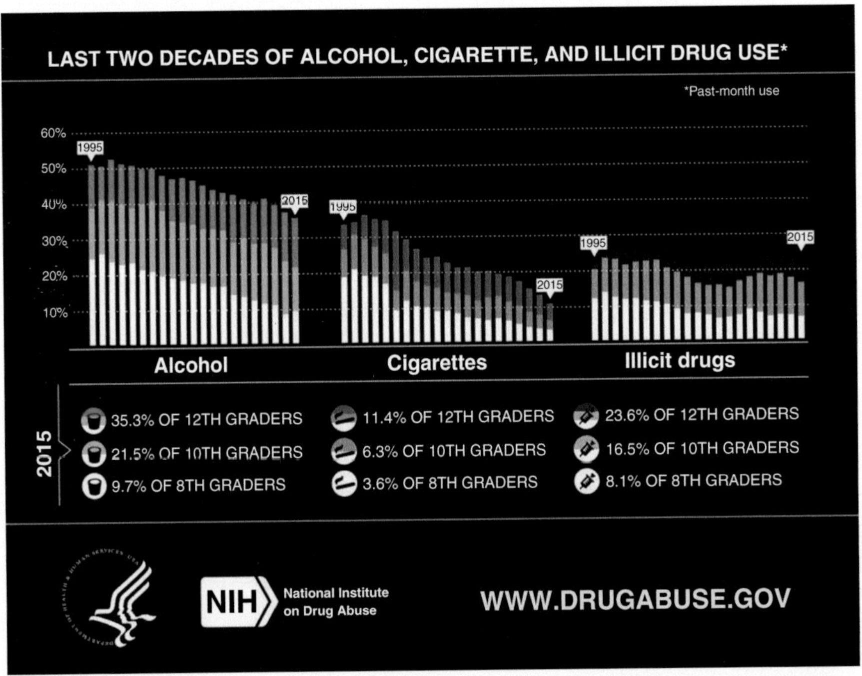

Fig. 12.1 Trends in adolescent alcohol, cigarette and illicit drug use over the past two decades. (Figure obtained from the National Institute on Drug Abuse, data from Monitoring the Future https://www.drugabuse.gov/related-topics/trends-statistics/infographics/monitoring-future-2015-survey-results)

Assessment

Adolescents who present to the ED are guaranteed a medical evaluation under Emergency Medical Treatment and Labor Act (EMTALA). Emergency medicine providers, ideally but not always with pediatric specialty training, perform a physical exam, review of systems, and mental status exam, including observation for common signs of intoxication or withdrawal. If the patient is presenting with an acute psychiatric crisis such as suicidality, psychosis, or behavioral dysregulation, the goal of the initial exam by an emergency medicine provider is increasingly defined as a determination of medical stability to ensure that preexisting or new-onset medical issues and acute intoxication are not causing the psychiatric symptoms [3]. Not all emergency medicine providers support obtaining standard laboratory tests or even urine toxicology screens. However, it can sometimes be very difficult to distinguish intoxication from, for example, psychosis or mania without objective evidence of the former. Overuse of amphetamines can mimic new-onset psychosis; an adolescent "crashing" after a cocaine binge can appear profoundly depressed. In many EDs, social workers, psychologists, psychiatric nurse practitioners, or psychiatrists conduct a subsequent evaluation (that may include screening laboratory studies) of the patient to characterize the relationship between the psychiatric symptoms and the presence/severity of new or chronic substance use disorders after the patient is deemed medically stable.

An evaluation of teens and young adults presenting with a chief complaint of a substance-related problem should include assessment for other mental health conditions, given very high comorbidity. The estimated prevalence of co-occurring mental illness (e.g., attention-deficit hyperactivity, mood, anxiety, and/or conduct disorders) in adolescents with a substance use disorder ranges from 60% to 75% [4, 5].

Finally, an emergency room assessment of adolescents should always include screening for other problems, such as active or prior legal issues, a history of violence, or risky sexual behaviors.

Confidentiality and Consent

Whenever possible, the interview with any adolescent in the ED, whether conducted by pediatric emergency medicine or by a psychiatrist or social worker, should include some time in which providers speak to the adolescent separately from their parents or primary caregivers. During this time, the limits of confidentiality should be explained clearly. Mental health clinicians routinely caution adolescents that they will break confidentiality if the teen verbalizes threat of intentional harm to self or others. In addition, providers must use their best clinical judgment about when to share information about an adolescent's otherwise risky and dangerous behavior with parents or guardians. Providers should consider the frequency and duration of substance use behaviors when deciding whether the adolescent's choices represent a threat to their own or others' safety. A good guideline to keep in mind is that a positive urine drug test does not indicate a pattern of drug use and a negative test does not preclude drug use [6]. However, toxicology screening can be illuminating, particularly if the teen has not disclosed the full extent (i.e., variety of drugs used) of his/her substance use or if he/she had not realized that a given substance was "laced" with other substances.

If an adolescent's substance use is a primary reason for the ED presentation, it is often reasonable to conclude that this represents a situation requiring a break in confidentiality. Red flags that might prompt a provider to break confidentiality include the following:

- Use in a high-risk situation, such as while driving
- Use when responsible for others, particularly a younger child
- A CRAFFT (a screening tool described later in chapter) score of 5 or higher in any adolescent, or of 2 or higher in anyone younger than 14
- Any intravenous drug use
- Prescription medication misuse
- More than a single use of heroin, cocaine, or methamphetamines
- Daily or near daily use of any substance
- Passing out or being brought in by friends due to a change in mental status
- History of physical altercation with injury or sexual assault

The laws governing confidentiality and consent in the treatment of adolescents vary from state to state in the United States, and listing them here is beyond the scope of this chapter. It is important that clinicians evaluating adolescents for mental health or substance use concerns be aware of both federal and state laws and regulations.

Nearly all states in the United States allow minors (individuals 18 years of age or younger in most states and 19 years of age or younger in a few states) to consent for treatment of substance use disorders. Many of these states permit, but do not require, parental notification for such treatment. Many parents are not aware that their minor adolescents are able to consent for substance use treatment on their own. In general, state laws tend to favor the rights of minor adolescents to obtain substance use treatment without parental consent, as well as the right to do so at an earlier age on average than for mental health treatment [7]. When in doubt, it is always prudent to check with the hospital's general counsel if there are questions regarding the legal rights of minors in a jurisdiction.

Drug Testing

Parents or guardians may at times request that drug testing be performed without the minor's knowledge. In this case, it is important for the clinician to meet with the parent/s to understand why they feel the testing is necessary, to inform parent/s about the limitations of drug testing and other methods of detecting substance use, and to discuss the potential harms of such a decision, including erosion of trust between an adolescent and parent or between an adolescent and the healthcare team [8]. Concerns raised by the parent should be discussed with the adolescent. The adolescent's assent, as well as permission to share results with the parent, should be obtained before testing.

The American Academy of Pediatrics (AAP) developed guidelines for drug testing adolescents in 1996 and again in 2014. Initially, it recommended that only in rare exceptions should drug testing be performed without the consent of an adolescent, including when the patient lacks decision-making capacity or when information gained from the history or examination is strongly suggestive of problematic substance use. The 2014 guidelines are even less flexible, stating that "drug testing of a competent adolescent without his or her consent is, at best, impractical and without his or her knowledge is unethical and illegal" [9]. Generally, providers should develop a plan, i.e., what will be the next steps, based on a positive or negative drug screen, before asking an adolescent to consent/assent to a urine or serum drug test.

Determining Severity of Substance Use

The American Academy of Pediatrics (AAP) has identified several stages of substance use in adolescents [10]. Emergency medicine providers should be aware of the patient's range of involvement and be familiar with appropriate interventions for each stage. Even a brief encounter with an informed, reassuring, yet definitive adult can be beneficial to a teen unsure of his or her choices.

Abstinence This refers to the period before an adolescent has ever tried drugs or imbibed more than a few sips of alcohol. If the teen denies use, the ED provider has an opportunity to applaud this behavior and reinforce the benefits of such a choice.

Experimentation The first few times a teen uses, he or she is often prompted by a desire to know how intoxication feels and to ally him or herself with peers who are already using substances. In this case, ED providers can promote patient strengths but discourage continuing activity by offering simple, clear medical advicc and educational counseling.

Limited Use Usually occurs with friends on weekends in relatively low-risk situations with few sequelae. ED providers should clarify which substances are being used and provide further education about risks inherent even in infrequent use.

Problematic Use This refers to use in a high-risk situations, such as when driving or babysitting. The use can be associated with problems such as legal charges, school suspension or fights, or unsafe sexual behavior. Substances may be used to relieve stress or to self-medicate mood or anxiety symptoms. ED providers should follow the same guidelines as noted in the approach to limited use but, in addition, offer close follow-up with a primary care provider and consider a referral to an outpatient appointment with a substance use specialist or even a partial hospital program (day treatment). At this stage, a provider should consider breaking confidentiality and sharing information about the adolescent's substance use with his or her parent or guardian.

Use Disorder The *Diagnostic and Statistical Manual of Mental Disorders*, Fifth Edition (DSM-5) identifies 11 criteria by which to gauge the severity of substance use. These include craving, using more or longer than intended, unsuccessful attempts to cut down or quit, excessive time spent obtaining substances, failure to fulfill academic, work or family responsibilities because of substance use, continued use despite recurring problems, stopping or reducing important personal activities because of use (e.g., quitting an athletic team), recurrent substance use in hazardous situations, continued use despite acknowledgment of physical or psychological problems associated with use, tolerance (diminished physical effect of the same dose or needing a higher dose to achieve desired effects), and withdrawal [11]. A substance use disorder is considered mild if two or three of the criteria are met within the same year, and a moderate substance use disorder is present when four to five criteria are met. Intervention goals for a mild or moderate substance use disorder, in addition to those mentioned above, should include brief motivational enhancement through exploration of ambivalence. Using a nonjudgmental tone, a provider should express a desire to understand why an adolescent is using substances. Sometimes it is helpful to ask what that adolescent enjoys about a substance before asking whether they have noticed any problems associated with use. After reviewing the adolescent's positive and negative feelings about their substance use, asking permission to provide feedback in the patient's own words demonstrates respect for the adolescent's autonomy. The clinician can then ask the adolescent if he/she is aware of any negative health impacts associated with a given substance and briefly discuss some of the risks. Adolescents with a substance use disorder should be referred for a comprehensive assessment and treatment to a substance use specialty clinic or, if that is not available, to an adolescent psychiatry clinic. Providers should strongly consider breaking confidentiality by informing a parent or guardian in these situations.

Severe Use Disorder Six or more of the above criteria indicate a severe substance use disorder. Emergency medicine providers should strongly consider breaking confidentiality and parental involvement is strongly encouraged. An adolescent with a severe substance use disorder should be referred for thorough assessment and intensive treatment in a dual diagnosis inpatient program, a residential program, or a partial hospitalization program.

Signs of Intoxication

As noted, ED physicians and other providers may be the first point of contact for a teen who is intoxicated. Appendix Table 2 at the end of this book includes a system-based list of possible signs and symptoms of acute substance ingestion/use.

Interventions in the ED

In addition to providing acute management of intoxication or withdrawal, ED providers have the opportunity to employ Screening, Brief Intervention, and Referral to Treatment (SBIRT) – a public health program designed by SAMHSA and endorsed by the American Academy of Pediatrics to identify individuals with problematic substance use and to try to change the trajectory of further use [12, 13]. SBIRT has three components – screening tools, brief intervention techniques, and referral to treatment – which are used to identify unhealthy substance use as soon as possible and increase the patient's awareness and insight about the risks of such use.

The most commonly used screening instrument for adolescents with suspected or known substance use is the CRAFFT (See Fig. 12.2). This tool has been validated for both outpatient clinic and ED use and has recently been updated for increased sensitivity in detecting substance use disorders in adolescents (CRAFFT 2.0) [14]. It is easily accessed, available in both clinician and self-administered forms, and can be freely used for clinical care. The individual letters stand for the words Car, Relax, Alone, Forget, Friends, and Trouble, which highlight the six topics covered in the assessment. Two or more yes answers suggest the need for further detailed assessment of substance use. There are additional, validated instruments, such as the Adolescent Drinking Inventory (ADI), that have been used by ED pediatricians to identify those teens whose alcohol-related presentations represent ongoing, problematic drinking [15]. The Screening to Brief Intervention (S2BI) includes a single screening question about frequency of past year use for seven different substance categories [16].

It is important to note that all of the abovementioned tools include not only screening questions but also recommendations for brief interventions to be done by the provider based on how the adolescent answers the screening questions. The most commonly recommended brief intervention for the ED setting is motivational interviewing (MI). There is some evidence to suggest that MI for adolescents who present to EDs with problematic alcohol use does reduce problematic use [17]. Although a recent review of the purported benefits of brief interventions with adolescents with problematic substance suggests that results are as yet inconclusive [18], the myriad risks of ongoing problematic substance use are so great that any attempt to mitigate the problem is worthwhile.

Family members are considered integral to management and treatment of adolescents who are using substances. Substance Abuse and Mental Health Services

The CRAFFT Screening Interview

Begin: "I'm going to ask you a few questions that I ask all my patients. Please be honest. I will keep your answers confidential."

Part A

During the PAST 12 MONTHS, did you:	**No**	**Yes**
1. Drink any <u>alcohol</u> (more than a few sips)? (Do not count sips of alcohol taken during family or religious events.)	☐	☐
2. Smoke any <u>marijuana or hashish</u>?	☐	☐
3. Use <u>anything else</u> to <u>get high</u>? ("anything else" includes illegal drugs, over the counter and prescription drugs, and things that you sniff or "huff")	☐	☐

For clinic use only: Did the patient answer "yes" to any questions in Part A?

No ☐ → **Ask CAR question only, then stop**

Yes ☐ → **Ask all 6 CRAFFT questions**

Part B	**No**	**Yes**
1. Have you ever ridden in a **<u>CAR</u>** driven by someone (including yourself) who was "high" or had been using alcohol or drugs?	☐	☐
2. Do you ever use alcohol or drugs to **<u>RELAX</u>**, feel better about yourself, or fit in?	☐	☐
3. Do you ever use alcohol or drugs while you are by yourself, or **<u>ALONE</u>**?	☐	☐
4. Do you ever **<u>FORGET</u>** things you did while using alcohol or drugs?	☐	☐
5. Do your **<u>FAMILY</u>** or **<u>FRIENDS</u>** ever tell you that you should cut down on your drinking or drug use?	☐	☐
6. Have you ever gotten into **<u>TROUBLE</u>** while you were useing alcohol or drugs?	☐	☐

CONFIDENTIALITY NOTICE:

The information recorded on this page may be protected by special federal confidentiality rules (42 CFR Part 2), which prohibit disclosure of this information unless authorized by specific written consent. A general authorization for release of medical information is NOT sufficient for this purpose.

Fig. 12.2 The CRAFFT Clinician Interview. (Reproduced with permission of Boston Children's Hospital)

Administration (SAMSHA) held a "national dialogue" in 2009 to learn what family members felt that they needed in order to help their adolescent. Top priorities included more educational resources for parents and increased access to treatment for youth [19]. It can be helpful to involve the family in the assessment of adolescents who present with substance use disorders. Cultural factors can play a role in parents' or other family members' understanding of the adolescent's patterns of use. In some families, the parents or caregivers may also have active substance use and may not be concerned about the adolescent's use. If the adolescent's substance use occurs within a home characterized by parental or guardian neglect, the family should be referred immediately to the state institution charged with the care and protection of children.

The final component of SBIRT is referral to treatment. Unfortunately, accessing outpatient and/or inpatient resources for adolescents with substance use disorders who present to EDs is challenging, even for motivated adolescents and their families. Available options differ from state to state, and access to a particular level of care is often dictated by third-party players. Possible options include outpatient programs that provide evaluation, psychopharmacologic management if indicated, group and individual treatment and family-based work, day treatment or partial hospitalization for those who can continue to live at home but need day-long care, and residential programs [20]. For substance use disorders uncomplicated by comorbid psychiatric illness, initial level of care is generally determined by severity of the use disorder, and treatment commonly proceeds in a step-down manner in which an adolescent receives more intensive treatment during early sobriety and gradually progresses to a lower level of care. While guidelines regarding placement criteria such as those proposed by the American Society of Addiction Medicine are becoming more commonly used, outcome studies of specific treatment matching guidelines are stronger for adult populations than for adolescents. Important factors to consider in deciding the most appropriate level of care include the presence and severity of comorbid psychiatric disorders, the immediate risk of medical problems from use or risk of withdrawal (suggesting the need for inpatient services), the short-term risk of relapse if returning to the home environment, the level of recovery support an adolescent has in their social circles, and the level of individual readiness for change. Red flags which should prompt an emergency room physician to consider an intensive level of care include the presence of suicidality or severe aggression; any IV drug use; using cocaine, heroin, or methamphetamine more than a single time; blackouts from alcohol use; a CRAFFT score of 5 or higher; and daily use of any substance. All levels of care are elective except when serious safety concerns are present necessitating involuntary commitment. Otherwise, participation depends on the willingness of the adolescent to accept the fact that he or she has a problem with substance use and to participate actively in a system of care. Should an adolescent patient present with a substance use disorder that the clinician considers life-threatening (such as anxiolytic or alcohol dependence that might result in a complicated withdrawal syndrome) and refuse treatment, the clinician should obtain consent from the patient's guardian to admit the patient to a pediatric inpatient medical unit for medical monitoring or to commit to an inpatient psychiatric unit where the staff feels comfortable monitoring for withdrawal syndromes. Regardless of whether the adolescent patient requires ongoing outpatient intervention or an inpatient stay, it can be helpful to alert the patient's pediatrician to the patient's ED visit prior to the patient's discharge, as it is possible that the patient will follow up with his/her pediatrician for ongoing drug monitoring once he/she has completed the acute phase of treatment.

Conclusion

Substance use in adolescents represents one of the primary risks to overall health and well-being in this population. Regular drug and alcohol use at a young age is a risk factor for developing a more severe and prolonged course of substance use later in life. The ED may represent the first and, at times only, contact a substance-misusing adolescent will have with healthcare providers. In addition to being the location for provision of acute care, this setting represents an opportunity for secondary or tertiary prevention in young patients presenting with substance-induced or substance-related symptoms. An understanding and appreciation of age-specific factors, such as rules surrounding confidentiality and consent, unique developmental differences, trends in use, and appropriate screening tools, will increase the efficacy of emergency evaluation and treatment of substance-using adolescents, a population particularly vulnerable to the adverse physical, psychosocial, and mental effects of drugs and alcohol.

References

1. Merikangas K, McClair V. Epidemiology of substance use disorders. Hum Genet. 2012;131(6):779.
2. Merikangas K, He J, Burstein M, Swanson S, Avenevoli S. Lifetime prevalence of mental disorders in US adolescents: results from the National Comorbidity Study–Adolescent Supplement (NCS-A). J Am Acad Child Adolesc Psychiatry. 2010;49(10).
3. Chun T, Mace S, Katz E. Evaluation and management of children and adolescent with acute mental health or behavioral problems. Part I: common clinical challenges of patient with mental health and or behavioral emergencies. Pediatrics. 2016;138(3).
4. Turner W, Muck R, Muck R, Stephens R, Sukumar B. Co-occurring disorder in the adolescent mental health and substance abuse treatment systems. J Psychoactive Drugs. 2004;36(4):455–62.
5. Hoffman N, Bride B, MacMaster S, Abrantes A, Estroff T. Identifying co-occurring disorders in adolescent population. J Addict Dis. 2004;23(4):41–53.
6. Weddle M, Kokotailo P. Confidentiality and consent in adolescent substance abuse: an update. Virtual Mentor. 2005;7(3).
7. Kerwin M, Kirby K, Speziali D, Duggan M, Mellitz C, Versek B, et al. What can parents do? A review of state laws regarding decision making for adolescent drug abuse and mental health treatment. J Child Adolesc Subst Abuse. 2015;24(3):166–76.
8. Weddle M, Kokotailo P. Adolescent substance abuse. Confidentiality and consent. Pediatr Clin N Am. 2002;49(2):301–15.
9. Levy S, Siqueira L, Ammerman S, Gonzalez P, Ryan S, Smith V. Testing for drugs of abuse in children and adolescents. Pediatrics. 2014;133(6):e1798–807.
10. Knight J, Roberts T, Gabrielli J, Van Hook S. Adolescent alcohol and substance use and abuse [Internet]. Performing Preventive Services: A Bright Futures Handbook. Retrieved 29 Dec 2016, from https://brightfutures.aap.org/Bright%20Futures%20Documents/Screening.pdf.
11. American Psychiatric Association. Diagnostic and statistical manual of mental disorders. 5th ed. Arlington: American Psychiatric Publishing; 2013.
12. Mitchell S, Gryczynski J, O'Grady K, Schwartz R. SBIRT for adolescent drug and alcohol use: current status and future directions. J Subst Abuse Treat. 2013;44(5):463–72.

13. SAMHSA-HRSA Center for Integrated Health Solutions. SBIRT screening, brief interventions, and referral to treatment. eSolutions newsletter. Retrieved 29 Dec 2016, from http://www.integration.samhsa.gov/clinical-practice/sbirt.
14. The Center for Adolescent Substance Abuse Research. The CRAFFT screening tool. Retrieved 29 Dec 2016, from http://www.childrenshospital.org/ceasar/crafft
15. Sindelair-Manning H, Lewander W, Chun T, Barnett N, Spirito A. Emergency department detection of adolescents with a history of alcohol abuse and alcohol problems. Pediatr Emerg Care. 2008;24(7):457–61.
16. Levy S, Weiss R, Sherritt L, Ziemnik B, Spalding A, Van Hook S, et al. An electronic screen for triaging adolescent substance use by risk levels. JAMA Pediatr. 2014;168(9):822–8.
17. Spirito A, Monti P, Barnett N, Colby S, Sindelar H, Rohsenow D, et al. A randomized clinical trial of a brief motivational intervention for alcohol-positive adolescents treated in the emergency department. J Pediatr. 2004;145(3):396–402.
18. Newton A, Dong K, Mabood N, Ata N, Ali S, Gokiert R, et al. Brief emergency department interventions for youth who use alcohol and other drugs: a systematic review. Pediatr Emerg Care. 2013;29(5):673–84.
19. Substance Abuse and Mental Health Services Administration (SAMSHA) 2009. Families of youth with substance use addiction: a national dialogue. US Department of Health and Human Services. Retrieved 29 Dec 2016, from http://www.drugfree.org/news-service/families-of-youth-with-substance-use-addiction-a-national-dialogue/
20. NIDA. Principles of adolescent substance use disorder treatment: a research-based guide. 2014. Retrieved December 29, 2016, from https://www.drugabuse.gov/publications/principles-adolescent-substance-use-disorder-treatment-research-based-guide.

Chapter 13
Emergency Management of Substance Use in Pregnant Patients

Allison S. Baker and Charlotte S. Hogan

Introduction

Intoxication from alcohol and other illicit substances is a frequent reason for emergency department visits. Clinicians who encounter patients with substance use disorders in the ED have a privileged opportunity to intervene with evidence-based treatments and a chance to help patients move toward the highest level of health possible.

This is a particularly compelling clinical scenario when the patient is pregnant and using substances. While pregnancy was once thought to be a period of decreased risk for psychiatric illness, it is now understood that mental illness and substance use disorders continue, and sometimes worsen, during a woman's pregnancy. It is critical that screening for substance use disorders occurs during every emergency department visit, particularly for pregnant women and women of reproductive potential.

In the field of addiction medicine, it is firmly established that a clinician's nonjudgmental attitude powerfully and positively influences the efficacy of their intervention [1]. Despite this, many clinicians may struggle with maintaining a nonjudgmental attitude, especially in the clinical encounter with a pregnant woman using substances. This issue is worthy of emphasis because, in the authors' experience, pregnant women using substances often feel particularly shameful and guilty about their substance use, and as a result of that shame may be inclined to avoid treatment, including prenatal care [2]. Clinicians should do their best to establish a clinician-patient relationship without discrimination or stigmatization. All important information about the risks of substance use and the benefits of treatment should be communicated in a nonjudgmental, respectful, non-stigmatizing, and empathic manner [3].

A. S. Baker · C. S. Hogan (✉)
Perinatal Psychiatry, MGH Center for Women's Mental Health, Boston, MA, USA

Massachusetts General Hospital, Department of Psychiatry, Boston, MA, USA
e-mail: chogan9@partners.org

A. L. Donovan, S. A. Bird (eds.), *Substance Use and the Acute Psychiatric Patient*, Current Clinical Psychiatry, https://doi.org/10.1007/978-3-319-23961-3_13

The use of alcohol, illicit substances and psychoactive drugs is common in pregnancy and can lead to multiple health and social problems for both the mother and her baby [4]. In this chapter, we will review the risks associated with the following substances: alcohol, benzodiazepines, cannabis, opioids, stimulants (including cocaine and amphetamine), and nicotine. We will specifically review the risks to the mother and the developing fetus, as well as the potential risks and benefits of emergency department interventions used to treat these substance use disorders. Attention will be given to relevant legal and ethical issues and the goals of the emergency department encounter will be identified.

Alcohol

Chronic alcohol use during pregnancy (as defined by the ingestion of 2 or more drinks/day) can lead to both adverse obstetrical outcomes and negative effects on fetal development [5]. In terms of obstetric risk, alcohol use is associated with a threefold increase in preterm deliveries, as well as increased rates of other serious complications including spontaneous abortion, low-birth-weight infants, placental abruption, amnionitis, and overall perinatal mortality [3].

Maternal alcohol use during pregnancy is also associated with an increased risk of fetal alcohol syndrome (FAS): a pattern of neurologic, behavioral, and cognitive deficits that can interfere with growth, learning, and socialization. FAS has three major components: a characteristic pattern of facial abnormalities (small eye openings, indistinct or flat philtrum, thin upper lip), growth deficiencies, and central nervous system abnormalities that include structural, neurological, and functional deficits [6].

Alcohol use on a regular basis can put a pregnant woman at risk for a withdrawal syndrome that can be severe and even life-threatening, which often requires emergency care. Given the potential risks associated with alcohol withdrawal, the lack of significant harm that has been demonstrated from short-term benzodiazepine use in pregnancy, and the evidence supporting the use of benzodiazepines in the management of alcohol withdrawal in the general population, the World Health Organization (WHO) recommends that hospitalization for medically monitored detoxification be considered in the withdrawal management of pregnant women with alcohol dependence [6]. The WHO also recommends that alcohol withdrawal management be facilitated by the use of an alcohol-withdrawal scale such as the CIWA-Ar, and include administration of folate, multivitamin, and thiamine. While not specifically stated by the WHO, it is generally considered good clinical practice to consult OB while the patient is admitted for medically monitored detoxification.

Benzodiazepines

Studies concerning the teratogenicity of benzodiazepines have produced conflicting results. Recent studies, however, have not provided substantive evidence that in-utero exposure to benzodiazepines causes an increase in any specific malformation or pattern of malformations [7]. Early studies that reported an association with adverse outcomes were criticized because of recall bias and possible exposure to multiple drugs [8]. Infants of mothers taking chronic doses of benzodiazepines near term are at risk for developing withdrawal symptoms postnatally [9]. For this reason, women should be counseled to discontinue use well before delivery. If abstinence is not possible, the lowest possible dose should be used, and one of the shorter-acting benzodiazepines should be considered, such as lorazepam [10].

Many women who are taking benzodiazepines may have psychiatric illnesses, epilepsy, or be dependent on other drugs or alcohol. Maternal illness or illicit drug use is likely to create an environment that is not conducive to optimal infant development, both prenatally and in the postpartum period. Each of these conditions is a risk factor during pregnancy and, therefore, it is difficult to discern negative clinical effects due specifically to benzodiazepines, especially in relation to subsequent neurobehavioral dysfunction.

If a pregnant woman presents to the ED intoxicated with benzodiazepines, abrupt cessation of use can lead to withdrawal, which can be severe and result in seizures or delirium. As such, long-acting benzodiazepines such as clonazepam should be used to manage benzodiazepine withdrawal. In addition, psychosocial interventions should be offered throughout the period of benzodiazepine withdrawal, and inpatient care should be strongly considered in the withdrawal management of pregnant women with benzodiazepine dependence.

An important additional component of emergency care for alcohol and benzodiazepine use disorders in pregnancy is referral to further treatment. This can begin in the ED setting with a consultation referral to social work services, who can then assist in establishing adequate psychiatric, substance use and general medical follow-up. Subsequent to assessment and stabilization in the ED, continued care would ideally include integrated obstetric, psychiatric, substance use treatment, and case management assistance. Patients may benefit from an intensive outpatient treatment program or a residential program, such as the Day Hospital at Women and Infant's Hospital in Providence, RI (http://www.womenandinfants.org/services/behavioral-health/day-hospital.cfm).

Cannabis

Marijuana use – both medical and recreational – is on the rise in reproductive-aged women [11]. This is no surprise given that many states have legalized or are now moving forward with legalization of medical marijuana. It is estimated that roughly half of female marijuana users continue to use during pregnancy [12]. While marijuana is often considered to be a relatively benign substance and is viewed by some as being safer than traditional medications for the treatment of depression and anxiety, data show that the developing fetus may be particularly vulnerable to its effects.

The use of cannabis during pregnancy has been associated with a spectrum of risks to the developing fetus. These include increased risk of intrauterine growth restriction, low birth weight, increased risk of stillbirth, and cognitive delays and deficits, including poor executive functioning [13]. Infants prenatally exposed to cannabis had decreased birth weight and were more likely to need placement in the neonatal intensive care unit or intensive care unit compared to infants whose mothers did not use cannabis during pregnancy.

Women who use cannabis have been shown to have an increased risk of anemia during pregnancy. One study has demonstrated a risk for precipitous labor [14]. In terms of breastfeeding, there are insufficient data to evaluate the effects of marijuana use on infants during lactation and breastfeeding, and in the absence of such data, marijuana use is discouraged [13].

While there are well-documented risks stemming from maternal exposure to cannabis, nonetheless there appears to be a growing number of people who view marijuana as a more effective or safer option than traditional pharmacologic interventions for the treatment of a variety of conditions, including nausea and vomiting, depression, anxiety, and insomnia. At this point, there is no data to support the use of marijuana for the management of these symptoms. The American Academy of Obstetrics and Gynecology recommends that pregnant women or women contemplating pregnancy should be counseled to discontinue use of marijuana for medicinal purposes in favor of an alternative therapy for which there is better data regarding reproductive safety [13].

Opioids

Opioid use disorders are a rising nationwide trend, and pregnant women are included in the significant impact of this problem. The prevalence of opioid use disorders during pregnancy has increased by 127% from 1998 to 2011 [15]. Opioid use carries significant risk during pregnancy, including increased risk of obstetrical maternal mortality [16]. Opioid use during pregnancy has also been associated with significant increases in fetal risk. During maternal opioid intoxication, respiratory suppression can cause fetal hypoxemia, which can lead to intrauterine growth restriction, placental insufficiency, low birth weight, and other complications [16]. During maternal opiate withdrawal, increased autonomic arousal may cause uterine contraction, potentially resulting in miscarriage or premature labor [17]. A major adverse neonatal outcome is neonatal abstinence syndrome (NAS), which is a neonatal drug withdrawal syndrome that often requires neonatal intensive care and is associated with significant medical complications [17]. For all these reasons, it is essential to facilitate treatment for pregnant women with opioid use disorders presenting in the emergency department with the goal of minimizing potential risks to both mother and fetus.

In the emergency department, if a woman presents with opioid intoxication, she should receive close monitoring and attentive supportive care. To avoid precipitating acute withdrawal, the use of naloxone should be reserved for cases of life-threatening maternal overdose [18]. A thorough psychiatric and addiction evaluation should take place as soon as she is able to participate, in order to identify any acute safety concerns, comorbid psychiatric illness, and other substance use disorders. In addition to urine toxicology screening, medical work-up should include liver function tests and electrocardiogram (to assist in determining best treatment, as given below). With informed consent, it is prudent to consider screening for hepatitis B and C, HIV, and other conditions for which the patient may be at risk due to her opioid use disorder; however if the patient's expected emergency department stay is shorter than the time it would take for these tests to return, it may be appropriate to defer these tests to a treatment setting in which more reliable follow-up of test results can occur.

Given significant risk of maternal and fetal complications if left untreated, opioid withdrawal should be addressed diligently; the standard of care is initiation of maintenance therapy (and prevention of withdrawal) with substitution agents, either buprenorphine or methadone. If a patient is beginning to show signs of withdrawal during her ED stay, one of these medications should be initiated during that visit, with the ultimate plan for inpatient admission. Otherwise, initiation of substitution therapy could be deferred to the inpatient treatment setting, where acute withdrawal can be most safely managed. Maintenance therapy is preferred to medical detoxification off opioids completely because it may improve maternal and infant outcomes, and because it decreases risk of relapse [19]. Both methadone and buprenorphine have been demonstrated as effective treatment strategies in preventing prenatal opioid withdrawal and in maintenance of abstinence [20]. Specific studies are limited, but there are no major congenital malformations associated with either when used during pregnancy, although there is still a risk of NAS [21].

Both methadone and buprenorphine are compatible with breastfeeding as the amount of either drug transferred into the breast milk is low [22], and breastfeeding is generally recommended for stable mothers on methadone or buprenorphine maintenance therapy (who are not concurrently using illicit substances) because doing so may decrease the severity of NAS [23].

Methadone has been the drug of choice for treating opioid use disorders during pregnancy for decades. Methadone can prolong the QT interval, so it is appropriate to obtain an EKG before administration. In the acute setting, for a pregnant patient in opioid withdrawal, an initial single dose of methadone 10–20 mg could be started, with subsequent doses of methadone 5–10 mg given every 4–6 hours as needed until signs and symptoms of withdrawal are suppressed. If opioid withdrawal begins in the ED, then this process should be started while the patient is there, in order to avoid fetal distress or adverse pregnancy outcomes. Treatment can then be continued after she is admitted for ongoing medical care in the inpatient setting.

A growing collection of data supports buprenorphine as an equally good option for maintenance therapy during pregnancy, and this may be used to treat acute withdrawal if it is the chosen option for ongoing treatment. Again, treatment should be started in the ED setting if the patient is already in withdrawal at that time, with continued dose titration during an inpatient medical admission. Compared to methadone, it has been associated with less severe NAS and has fewer drug-drug interactions [21]. Baseline liver function tests should be obtained prior to initiation of buprenorphine due to concerns about potential buprenorphine-induced hepatotoxicity. A combined formulation of buprenorphine with naloxone (i.e., Suboxone) is *not* recommended during pregnancy because of the risks of precipitating withdrawal with naloxone if it is used improperly [19]. Buprenorphine, as a partial opioid receptor agonist, can precipitate withdrawal symptoms if administered too soon after a full opioid receptor agonist. Therefore, buprenorphine should not be administered unless a patient is showing signs of at least moderate withdrawal, and should be given no less than 24 hours after last use of a short-acting opioid (such as heroin).

The decision of which agent to use in the treatment of opioid withdrawal and for potential initiation of maintenance therapy should be made with the patient's participation, factoring in what has worked for the patient previously, patient preference, access to care (availability of methadone clinic versus access to buprenorphine prescriber), and medical comorbidities.

An important additional component of emergency care is referral to further treatment. Most experts recommend inpatient admission for medical management of withdrawal and for initiation of substitution therapy acutely [24]. Subsequently, continued care would ideally include integrated obstetric, psychiatric, substance use treatment, and case management assistance. Patients may benefit from a subsequent intensive outpatient treatment program or a residential program. Referrals should be made to a clinic for ongoing treatment with methadone or buprenorphine. In many areas, there are programs specifically designed to care for pregnant women with opioid use disorders, and it is often possible to bypass usually long waitlists for care.

Stimulants (Cocaine and Methamphetamine)

Cocaine use during pregnancy is associated with adverse maternal and fetal outcomes, including increased risk for premature rupture of membranes, placental abruption, preterm birth, low birth weight, small for gestational age infants, decreased fetal head circumference, and adverse effects on childhood cognitive/social development [18]. Methamphetamine use during pregnancy is associated with adverse effects similar to those of cocaine, including low birth weight, preterm birth, intrauterine fetal death, gestational hypertension, preeclampsia, and abnormal childhood neurocognitive development [18, 25]. Given these significant risks, if a pregnant woman with a stimulant use disorder presents to the ED, in addition to medical and obstetrical assessments, effort should be made to engage her in motivational interviewing to promote sobriety and to connect her to addiction treatment. If a pregnant woman presents to the ED intoxicated on stimulants, treatment with benzodiazepines and/or antipsychotic medications (from either the typical or atypical antipsychotic class) for the management of acute agitation, anxiety, or psychosis may be appropriate and necessary interventions, and in this scenario, the benefit of acute treatment would likely outweigh risks of fetal exposure to these medications. In the case of acute agitation of a pregnant woman, all efforts should be made to avoid physical restraints. If restraints are required, in the second half of pregnancy, a woman should not be restrained in supine position given potential for obstruction of venous return to the heart by the gravid uterus [26]; left lateral or Fowler's position would be preferred. There is no pharmacologic intervention necessary for stimulant withdrawal; however, the possibility of depressed mood may prompt screening for safety issues during this period [27].

Nicotine

Smoking during pregnancy has been associated with a number of negative outcomes, including spontaneous abortion, impaired fetal growth, placenta previa, placental abruption, and preterm delivery [28]. Recommendations on the use of nicotine replacement therapy during pregnancy are not yet clear; data on the efficacy of nicotine replacement therapy in aiding smoking cessation are not consistent [29]. Nicotine replacement therapy exposes the mother to continuous low doses of nicotine thus avoiding acute nicotine spikes, which may be safer to the fetus, given that concentrations of nicotine are higher in the placenta, amniotic fluid, and fetal serum than in maternal serum [28]. While nicotine replacement therapy may carry some risks itself during pregnancy, in general, nicotine replacement is considered less harmful to the fetus than smoking [30]. The American College of Obstetrics and Gynecologists (ACOG) published recommendations in 2010 advising that nicotine replacement should only be used with clear resolve of the patient to quit smoking, and with discussion of the known risks of continued smoking, as well as the possible risks of nicotine replacement therapy [28]. Acutely in the ED, a decision regarding the use of nicotine replacement therapy should also take into account the potential for nicotine withdrawal to impair the patient's ability to participate in important care of comorbid conditions, often making it an appropriate intervention (Table 13.1).

Table 13.1 Review of risks and management

Substance	Maternal risk	Fetal risk	Intoxication management	Withdrawal management	Disposition
Alcohol/ benzodiazepines	Increased rates of spontaneous abortion, low-birth-weight infants, placental abruption, increased perinatal mortality, amnionitis, and preterm deliveries	Fetal alcohol syndrome (FAS): craniofacial dysmorphism, impaired prenatal & postnatal growth, central nervous system abnormalities, cardiac defects. Congenital malformations, genitourinary defects, and learning disabilities	Supportive care	Long-acting benzodiazepines	Inpatient detox, followed by outpatient or residential addiction treatment
Cannabis	Modest increase in preterm birth	Low birth weights, smaller lengths and head circumferences. Abnormal neurocognitive development	n/a	Mood/safety monitoring, monitor nausea/ vomiting	Referral to outpatient treatment (motivational interviewing, address psychiatric comorbidities)
Opioids	Obstetrical maternal mortality, miscarriage, premature labor	Intrauterine growth restriction, placental insufficiency, neonatal abstinence syndrome	Supportive care, monitoring. Naloxone only in life threatening overdose.	Methadone or suboxone	Inpatient detox, followed by outpatient or residential addictions treatment
Stimulants	Premature rupture of membranes, placental abruption, preterm birth, gestational hypertension, preeclampsia	Small for gestational age, decreased head circumference, abnormal neurocognitive development	Benzodiazepines, Antipsychotics if agitated/anxious	Mood/safety monitoring	Referral to outpatient or residential addictions treatment
Nicotine	Spontaneous abortion, placenta previa, placental abruption, preterm delivery	Impaired fetal growth	n/a	+/− Nicotine patch	Referral to outpatient treatment (CBT, motivational interviewing, bupropion)

Conclusion

Substance use disorders during pregnancy are common – in 2012, a large survey indicated that in the USA approximately 6% of pregnant women used illicit drugs, 8.5% drank alcohol, and 16% smoked cigarettes [31]. In addition to the risks discussed above, women with substance use disorders during pregnancy are more likely to receive inadequate prenatal care, have poor nutrition, experience poverty and domestic violence, and have comorbid psychiatric illness [32] – all of which should be screened for during the emergency department visit in addition to treatment of acute medical conditions related to substance use.

An encounter in the emergency department offers enormous potential for identifying at-risk pregnant women struggling with substance use disorders, and engaging them in treatment. Given that many of these patients experience shame and guilt about their use, and with the awareness that some will avoid medical or addiction treatment as a result, the ED provider has an opportunity to offer a nonjudgmental introduction to treatment. Some women will also avoid care due to concerns about legal ramifications, not without reason. It is important as a provider to have a familiarity with relevant state laws regarding substance use during pregnancy – some states have declared substance use during pregnancy to be child abuse under civil child welfare statutes, and a few states consider substance use as grounds for civil commitment of pregnant women; some states also require providers to report suspected prenatal drug use [33]. While these laws may be intended to protect the fetus and possibly compel maternal treatment, they often pose yet another challenge for the provider in developing rapport and trust with the patient at a time when the treatment relationship is perhaps needed most.

Overall, goals in the emergency department treatment of a pregnant patient with a substance use disorder include safely managing acute intoxication/withdrawal; engaging the patient with a nonjudgmental empathic approach; screening for comorbid medical, psychiatric, and social problems; and connecting the patient to ongoing addiction care.

References

1. Center for Substance Abuse Treatment. Substance abuse treatment for persons with co-occurring disorders. Treatment Improvement Protocol (TIP) Series 42. DHHS Publication No. (SMA) 05-3922. Rockville: Substance Abuse and Mental Health Services Administration; 2005.
2. Wilson J, Thorp Jr. J. Glob libr women's med, (ISSN: 1756-2228) 2008. https://doi.org/10.3843/GLOWM.10115.
3. Whitlock EP, Polen MR, Green CA, Orleans T, Klein J, U. S. Preventive Services Task Force. Behavioral counseling interventions in primary care to reduce risky/harmful alcohol use by adults: a summary of the evidence for the U.S. Preventive Services Task Force. Ann Intern Med. 2004;140(7):557–68.

4. Stinson FS, Grant BF, Dawson DA, Ruan WJ, Huang B, Saha T. Comorbidity between DSM-IV alcohol and specific drug use disorders in the United States: results from the National Epidemiologic Survey on Alcohol and Related Conditions. Drug Alcohol Depend. 2005;80(1):105–16. https://doi.org/10.1016/j.drugalcdep.2005.03.009.
5. World Health Organization (WHO). Guidelines for the identification and management of substance use and substance use disorders in pregnancy. Geneva: World Health Organization (WHO); 2014.
6. Bertrand J, Floyd RL, Weber MK, O'Connor M, Riley P, Johnson KA, Cohen DE, National Task Force on FAS/FAE. Fetal alcohol syndrome: guidelines for referral and diagnosis. Atlanta: Centers for Disease Control and Prevention; 2004.
7. Bellantuono C, Tofani S, Di sciascio G, Santone G. Benzodiazepine exposure in pregnancy and risk of major malformations: a critical overview. Gen Hosp Psychiatry. 2013;35(1):3–8.
8. Chisolm MS, Payne JL. Management of psychotropic drugs during pregnancy. BMJ. 2016;532:h5918.
9. National Guideline Clearinghouse (NGC). Guideline summary: Guidelines for the identification and management of substance use and substance use disorders in pregnancy. In: National Guideline Clearinghouse (NGC) [Web site]. Rockville: Agency for Healthcare Research and Quality (AHRQ); 2014 Jan 01. Available: https://www.guideline.gov.
10. McElhatton PR. The effects of benzodiazepine use during pregnancy and lactation. Reprod Toxicol. 1994;8(6):461–75.
11. National Institute on Drug Abuse. Trends & Statistics. Retrieved from https://www.drugabuse.gov/related-topics/trends-statistics on 28 Aug 2016.
12. Passey ME, Sanson-Fisher RW, D'Este CA, Stirling JM. Tobacco, alcohol and cannabis use during pregnancy: clustering of risks. Drug Alcohol Depend. 2014;134:44–50.
13. Marijuana use during pregnancy and lactation. Committee Opinion No. 637. American College of Obstetricians and Gynecologists. Obstet Gynecol. 2015;126:234–8.
14. van Gelder MM, Reefhuis J, Caton AR, Werler MM, Druschel CM, Roeleveld N, National Birth Defects Prevention Study. Characteristics of pregnant illicit drug users and associations between cannabis use and perinatal outcome in a population-based study. Drug Alcohol Depend. 2010;109:243–7.
15. Maeda A, Bateman BT, Clancy CR, Creanga AA, Leffert LR. Opioid abuse and dependence during pregnancy: temporal trends and obstetrical outcomes. Anesthesiology. 2014;121(6):1158–65.
16. Wilder CM, Winhusen T. Pharmacologic management of opioid use disorder in pregnant women. CNS Drugs. 2015;29(8):625–36.
17. Forray A, Foster D. Substance use in the perinatal period. Curr Psychiatry Rep. 2015;17:91.
18. The American College of Obstetricians and Gynecologists (ACOG): Committee Opinion. Opioid Abuse, Dependence, and Addiction in Pregnancy. 2014. Number 524.
19. Mozurkewich EL, Rayburn WF. Buprenorphine and methadone for opioid addiction during pregnancy. Obstet Gynecol Clin N Am. 2014;41(2):241–53.
20. Noormohammadi A, Forinash A, Yancey A, Crannage E, Campbell K, Shyken J. Buprenorphine versus methadone for opioid dependence in pregnancy. Ann Pharmacother. 2016;50(8):666–72.
21. Zedler BK, Mann AL, Kim MM, Amick HR, Joyce AR, Murrelle EL, et al. Buprenorphine compared with methadone to treat pregnant women with opioid use disorder: a systematic review and meta-analysis of safety in the mother, fetus, and child. Addiction. 2016;111:2115. https://doi.org/10.1111/add.13462. [Epub ahead of print].
22. D'Apolito K. Breastfeeding and substance abuse. Clin Obstet Gynecol. 2013;56(1):202–11.
23. Bagley SM, Wachman EM, Holland E, Brogly SB. Review of the assessment and management of neonatal abstinence syndrome. Addict Sci Clin Pract. 2014;9(1):19.
24. Young JL, Martin PR. Treatment of opioid dependence in the setting of pregnancy. Psychiatr Clin N Am. 2012;35(2):441–60.

25. Kwiatkowski MA, Roos A, Stein DJ, Thomas KG, Donald K. Effects of prenatal methamphetamine exposure: a review of cognitive and neuroimaging studies. Metab Brain Dis. 2014;29(2):245–54.
26. Ladavac AS, Dubin WR, Ning A, Stuckeman PA. Emergency management of agitation in pregnancy. Gen Hosp Psychiatry. 2007;29(1):39–41.
27. Rayburn WF, Bogenschutz MP. Pharmacotherapy for pregnant women with addictions. Am J Obstet Gynecol. 2004;191(6):1885–97.
28. The American College of Obstetricians and Gynecologists (ACOG): Committee Opinion. Smoking Cessation During Pregnancy. 2010. Number 471.
29. Coleman T, Chamberlain C, Davey MA, Cooper SE, Leonardi-Bee J. Pharmacological interventions for promoting smoking cessation during pregnancy. Cochrane Database Syst Rev. 2015;(12):CD010078.
30. Berard A, Zhao JP, Sheehy O. Success of smoking cessation interventions during pregnancy. Am J Obstet Gynecol 2016. pii: S0002-9378(16)30432-X. https://doi.org/10.1016/j.ajog.2016.06.059. [Epub ahead of print].
31. Forray A. Substance use during pregnancy. F1000Res. 2016;5:F1000 Faculty Rev-887.
32. Gopman S. Prenatal and postpartum care of women with substance use disorders. Obstet Gynecol Clin N Am. 2014;41(2):213–28.
33. McLafferty LP, Becker M, Dresner N, Meltzer-Brody S, Gopalan P, Glance J, et al. Guidelines for the management of pregnant women with substance use disorders. Psychosomatics. 2016;57(2):115–30.

Appendices

A. L. Donovan, S. A. Bird (eds.), *Substance Use and the Acute Psychiatric Patient*, Current Clinical Psychiatry, https://doi.org/10.1007/978-3-319-23961-3

Appendix Table 1 Additional information on drugs commonly used

Substance	Street names	Neurobiological effects	Signs and symptoms of intoxication	Withdrawal symptoms	Comments
Alcohol		Central CNS depressant via potentiation of GABA effect at $GABA_A$ receptors	Euphoria and disinhibition at low levels, sedation, ataxia, and slurred speech at higher levels	Tremor, anxiety, insomnia, transient hallucinations; severe forms include seizure, autonomic instability, delirium	Rates of use are additionally elevated among college enrollees. Advise about risk of even single episodes of binge drinking
Tobacco	Bidis, hookahs, snuff, chew	CNS stimulant via activation of nicotinic receptors	Elevated blood pressure, respiratory rate and heart rate	Irritability, insomnia, inattention, increased appetite	As cigarette smoking has steadily declined, e-cigarette use among adolescents is on the rise. Important to ask about chewing tobacco and not just smoking
Marijuana	Weed, hash, joint, bud, dope, reefer, grass, hemp	Main active ingredient, THC, binds to cannabinoid receptors throughout the brain (CB1 > CB2)	Enhanced sensory perception and euphoria followed by drowsiness, increased appetite, slowed reaction time, and impaired coordination; hallucinations, anxiety, panic, and psychosis at higher doses	Irritability, insomnia, decreased appetite, anxiety	Possible loss of IQ points with early, repeated use Most commonly used illicit drug by teens, nearly 50% of 12th graders have used it Used in concentrated forms (hash or honey oil, wax or “budder,” “shatter” which can deliver much higher amounts of THC per use
Prescription stimulants	Speed, uppers, MPH, the smart drug, black beauties	Central CNS stimulants	Alertness, increased energy, increased BP and pulse, hyperthermia	Depression, tiredness, sleep problems	Most commonly misused drug is Adderall Often associated with other SUDs, academic decline

Prescription opioids	Many names depending on drug	Opioid agonists at the mu-opioid receptor	Euphoria, drowsiness, diminished reflexes, respiratory depression	Body aches, restlessness, diarrhea, chills	Most commonly used are Vicodin and OxyContin. Risk for progression to heroin use Advise family members to dispose of old/unused prescriptions
Inhalants (aerosols, paint thinner, gasoline, permanent markers, glue, nitrous oxide)	Whippets, poppers, snappers, laughing gas	Generally, CNS depressants Nitrates lead to vasodilation	Euphoria, giddiness, somnolence, confusion, disinhibition, slurred speech, dizziness	Nausea, loss of appetite, mood swings, sweating, tics	More commonly used by younger adolescents Facial rash or eye irritation
Synthetic cannabinoids	K2, spice, incense, black mamba, fire, skunk, yucatan, fake weed	Bind to cannabinoid receptors, often more strongly than THC	Tachycardia, agitation, confusion, anxiety, paranoia, increased BP	Headache, depression, anxiety, irritability	Persistent withdrawal symptoms not uncommon in chronic users Chemical composition of many products is unknown and they can produce unpredictable health effects
Cough medicine (dextromethorphan or DXM, codeine)	Triple C, robo, robotripping	Opioid-like actions	Euphoria, dissociation, slurred speech, increased BP and pulse	Unknown	Consider effects of other ingredients as well, i.e., antihistamines
Prescription tranquilizers/sedative hypnotics	Candy, downers, tranks	Prominent GABA effects	Drowsiness, sedation, amnesia, impaired coordination and reaction time, confusion, respiratory depression	Headache, tension, anxiety, restlessness, numbness in hands and feet, hallucinations, seizures, delirium	Withdrawal can be dangerous, detox/taper requires medical supervision Some in this category, i.e., Rohypnol (flunitrazepam), are used as date rape drugs Increased concern for overdose when used with alcohol

(continued)

Appendix Table 1 (continued)

Substance	Street names	Neurobiological effects	Signs and symptoms of intoxication	Withdrawal symptoms	Comments
MDMA (Ecstasy)	Molly, Adam, Eve, lover's speed, peace, uppers, "E"	Mixed serotonin and norepinephrine/dopamine effects, additional increase in serotonin release compared to amphetamines	Enhanced sensory perception, disinhibition, increased BP and pulse, bruxism, confusion, hyperthermia, dehydration	Fatigue, loss of appetite, depression, poor concentration	Molly often contains more methamphetamine constituent Other adulterants frequently found in tablets include cocaine, caffeine, ephedrine
Hallucinogens Classic: LSD, psilocybin, peyote, DMT, ayahuasca Dissociative drugs: PCP, ketamine, DXM, salvia	Acid, angel dust, vitamin K, shrooms	Prominent serotonergic properties, particularly in the prefrontal cortex Dissociative drugs disrupt glutamate activity at NMDA receptors	Varied effects depending on drug used; visual, auditory, and tactile hallucinations; nightmares; increased energy; tachycardia; psychosis	Varied effects depending on drug used, commonly includes headache, sweating	Long-term effects can include persistent psychosis or perceptual disturbances
Heroin	Dope, junk, skunk, white horse, china white, brown sugar	Direct mu-opioid receptor agonist	Euphoria, constricted pupils, alternating wakefulness and drowsiness, clouded thinking, itching, slowed respiratory rate and heart rate	Restlessness, body aches, diarrhea, vomiting, chills, restless legs, insomnia	Often preceded by prescription opioid use Overdose antidote is naloxone Buprenorphine and naltrexone are approved treatments for older adolescents
Cocaine	Coke, crack, rock, blow, bump, snow, flake, charlie	Blockade of the dopamine transporter, preventing reuptake of dopamine into the presynaptic neuron	Increased energy, euphoria, enlarged pupils, hypertension, hyperthermia, headache, aggression, paranoia, psychosis	Fatigue, insomnia, restlessness, depression, increased appetite, vivid nightmares	Risk of stroke, myocardial infarction or bowel infarction due to vasoconstriction

Adapted from Table 23.5, Goldstein, *The Mass General Hospital for Children Adolescent Medicine Handbook*, pp. 259–81, December 2016, with permission
CNS central nervous system, *GABA* gamma-aminobutyric acid, *THC* tetrahydrocannabinol, *CB* cannabinoid, *BP* blood pressure, *NMDA* N-methyl-D-aspartate

Appendix Table 2 Symptoms and signs of substance abuse

System	Symptom/sign	Substance
Vital signs	Hypertension	Cocaine, amphetamine, anabolic steroids, LSD, phencyclidine, Ecstasy, ketamine, bath salts
	Hypotension	Opiates, barbiturates
	Tachycardia	Marijuana, cocaine, LSD, amphetamine, Ecstasy, ketamine, bath salts
	Hyperthermia	Cocaine, amphetamine, LSD, Ecstasy
	Hypothermia	Heroin
Skin	Track marks, abscesses	Intravenous drugs
	Acne, stretch marks	Anabolic steroids
	Itchiness	Opiates
Eyes/nose	Injected conjunctivae	Marijuana
	Dilated pupils	Marijuana, cocaine, amphetamine, LSD, ketamine
	Constricted pupils	Heroin/opiates
	Nystagmus	Benzodiazepines, barbiturates
	Lacrimation	LSD
	Nasal irritation, mucosal erosion	Cocaine, glue sniffing
Heart	Arrhythmia	Heroin, cocaine, amphetamines Inhalants, PCP
GI	Constipation	Opiates
	Increased appetite	Marijuana
Neurologic	Hyperreflexia and hyporeflexia	Marijuana, cocaine, amphetamines, bath salts
	Ataxia	Amphetamines, alcohol, psilocybin, ketamine, inhalants
	Seizure	Cocaine, PCP
Mental status	Decreased libido	Anabolic steroids
	Rapid speech	Amphetamines, cocaine, bath salts
	Slurred speech	Alcohol, benzodiazepines, inhalants
	Drowsiness	Marijuana, benzodiazepines
	Hallucinations	LSD, psilocybin, amphetamines, ketamine, inhalants, synthetic marijuana
	Agitation	PCP, amphetamines *Salvia divinorum* Amphetamines
	Trance-like state	Ketamine, PCP
	Paranoia	PCP, LSD
	Rage Flashbacks	Anabolic steroids, cocaine, psilocybin, ketamine

Adapted from Table 23.4, Goldstein, *The Mass General Hospital for Children Adolescent Medicine Handbook*, pp. 259–81, December 2016, with permission

Index

A. L. Donovan, S. A. Bird (eds.), *Substance Use and the Acute Psychiatric Patient*, Current Clinical Psychiatry, https://doi.org/10.1007/978-3-319-23961-3

Printed in the United States
By Bookmasters